MW01101893

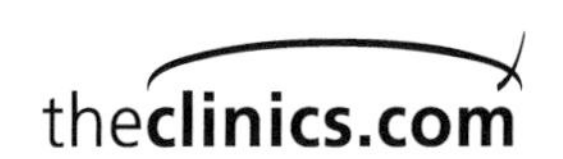

INFECTIOUS DISEASE CLINICS OF NORTH AMERICA

Infections of the Head and Neck

GUEST EDITOR
Anthony W. Chow, MD

June 2007 • Volume 21 • Number 2

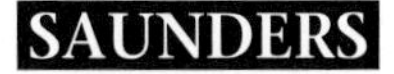

An Imprint of Elsevier, Inc.
PHILADELPHIA LONDON TORONTO MONTREAL SYDNEY TOKYO

W.B. SAUNDERS COMPANY
A Division of Elsevier Inc.

Elsevier, Inc., 1600 John F. Kennedy Blvd., Suite 1800, Philadelphia, PA 19103-2899.

http://www.theclinics.com

INFECTIOUS DISEASE CLINICS OF NORTH AMERICA
June 2007
Editor: Karen Sorensen

Volume 21, Number 2
ISSN 0891–5520
ISBN-10: 1-4160-4327-6
ISBN-13: 978-1-4160-4327-0

Infectious Disease Clinics of North America (ISSN 0891–5520) is published in March, June, September, and December (For Post Office use only: volume 20 issue 4 of 4) by Elsevier Inc., 360 Park Avenue South, New York, NY 10010-1710. Business and Editorial Offices: 1600 John F. Kennedy Blvd., Suite 1800, Philadelphia, PA 19103-2899. Customer Service Office: 6277 Sea Harbor Drive, Orlando, FL 32887-4800. Periodicals postage paid at New York, NY and additional mailing offices. Subscription prices are $184.00 per year for US individuals, $308.00 per year for US institutions, $92.00 per year for US students, $216.00 per year for Canadian individuals, $373.00 per year for Canadian institutions, $243.00 per year for international individuals, $373.00 per year for international institutions, and $119.00 per year for Canadian and foreign students. To receive student rate, orders must be accompained by name of affiliated institution, date of term, and the *signature* of program/residency coordinator on institution letterhead. Orders will be billed at individual rate until proof of status is received. Foreign air speed delivery is included in all *Clinics* subscription prices. All prices are subject to change without notice. **POSTMASTER**: Send address changes to *Infectious Disease Clinics of North America*, Elsevier Periodicals Customer Service, 6277 Sea Harbor Drive, Orlando, FL 32887-4800. **Customer Service: 1-800-654-2452 (US). From outside of the US, call 1-407-345-4000. E-mail: elspcs@elsevier.com**.

Infectious Disease Clinics of North America is also published in Spanish by Editorial Inter-Médica, Junin 917, 1er A 1113, Buenos Aires, Argentina.

Reprints. For copies of 100 or more, of articles in this publication, please contact the Commercial Reprints Department, Elsevier Inc., 360 Park Avenue South, New York, New York 10010-1710. Tel. (212) 633-3813, Fax: (212) 462-1935, email: reprints@elsevier.com.

Infectious Disease Clinics of North America is covered in *Index Medicus, Current Contents/Clinical Medicine, Science Citation Alert, SCISEARCH,* and *Research Alert.*

Printed in the United States of America.

GUEST EDITOR

ANTHONY W. CHOW, MD, FRCPC, FACP, Professor Emeritus, Division of Infectious Diseases, Department of Medicine, University of British Columbia, Vancouver Hospital Health Sciences Centre, Vancouver, British Columbia, Canada

CONTRIBUTORS

MARIA L. ALCAIDE, MD, Division of Infectious Diseases, Department of Medicine, University of Miami Miller School of Medicine; Medical Service, Infectious Diseases Section (111-1), Miami Veterans Affairs Healthcare System, Miami, Florida

NAWAF AL-DAJANI, MD, Fellow, Division of Infectious and Immunological Diseases, Department of Pediatrics, BC Children's Hospital, University of British Columbia, Vancouver, British Columbia, Canada

ALAN L. BISNO, MD, Professor of Medicine Emeritus, Division of Infectious Diseases, Department of Medicine, University of Miami Miller School of Medicine; Medical Service (111), Miami Veterans Affairs Healthcare System, Miami, Florida

ITZHAK BROOK, MD, MSc, Professor of Pediatrics and Medicine, Department of Pediatrics and Medicine, Georgetown University School of Medicine, Washington, DC

ANTHONY W. CHOW, MD, FRCPC, FACP, Professor Emeritus, Division of Infectious Diseases, Department of Medicine, University of British Columbia, Vancouver Hospital Health Sciences Centre, Vancouver, British Columbia, Canada

JOEL B. EPSTEIN, DMD, MSD, FRCD(C), Professor and Head, Department of Oral Medicine and Diagnostic Sciences, College of Dentistry; and Director, Oral Cancer Biology, Detection and Treatment, Chicago Cancer Center, University of Illinois at Chicago, Chicago, Illinois

MANRAJ K.S. HERAN, MD, FRCPC, Clinical Assistant Professor, Division of Neuroradiology, Vancouver General Hospital, Vancouver, British Columbia, Canada

LINDA HOANG, MSc, MD, DTM&H, FRCPC, Clinical Assistant Professor, Department of Pathology and Laboratory Medicine, University of British Columbia; and Head, Bacteriology and Mycology Program, British Columbia Centre for Disease Control Laboratory Services, Provincial Health Services Authority, Vancouver, British Columbia, Canada

MARK W. HULL, MD, FRCPC, Fellow, Division of Infectious Diseases, Department of Medicine, University of British Columbia, Vancouver, British Columbia, Canada

MICHAEL C. HURLEY, MRCPI, FRCR, FFR(RCSI), Fellow, Division of Neuroradiology, Vancouver General Hospital, Vancouver, British Columbia, Canada

KEVIN B. LAUPLAND, MD, MSc, FRCPC, Associate Professor, Department of Medicine; and Department of Critical Care Medicine; and Department of Pathology and Laboratory Medicine; and Department of Community Health Sciences, University of Calgary, Calgary, Alberta, Canada

WALTER LOESCHE, DMD, PhD, Marcus Ward Emeritus Professor of Dentistry, Department of Biological and Material Sciences, School of Dentistry; and Emeritus Professor of Microbiology and Immunology, Department of Microbiology and Immunology, School of Medicine, University of Michigan, Ann Arbor, Michigan

JOHN H. POWERS, MD, FACP, FIDSA, Senior Medical Scientist, Scientific Applications International Corporation in support of the Collaborative Clinical Research Branch, National Institute of Allergy and Infectious Diseases, National Institutes of Health; Assistant Clinical Professor of Medicine, George Washington University School of Medicine, Washington, DC; University of Maryland School of Medicine, Baltimore, Maryland

STEVEN C. REYNOLDS, MD, FRCPC, Specialist in Infectious Diseases; and Fellow, Division of Critical Care Medicine, Department of Medicine, University of British Columbia, Vancouver Hospital, Vancouver, British Columbia, Canada

DIANE L. ROSCOE, MD, FRCPC, Clinical Professor, Department of Pathology and Laboratory Medicine, University of British Columbia; and Head, Division of Medical Microbiology and Infection Control; and Regional Microbiology Lead, Vancouver General Hospital and Vancouver Coastal Health, Vancouver, British Columbia, Canada

ABDU A. SHARKAWY, BMSc, MD, FRCPC, Assistant Professor of Medicine, Department of Medicine, Division of Infectious Diseases, University of Toronto and Toronto Western Hospital, Toronto, Ontario, Canada

ELLEN R. WALD, MD, Alfred Dorrance Daniels Professor on Diseases of Children; and Chair, Department of Pediatrics, University of Wisconsin School of Medicine and Public Health, Madison, Wisconsin

SUSAN H. WOOTTON, MD, Clinical Instructor, Division of Infectious and Immunological Diseases, Department of Pediatrics, BC Children's Hospital, University of British Columbia, Vancouver, British Columbia, Canada

CONTENTS

FORTHCOMING ISSUES

September 2007

Infection in High-Risk Populations
Nancy Khardori, MD, and
Romesh Kardori, MD, *Guest Editors*

December 2007

Fever of Unknown Origin
Burke A. Cunha, MD, *Guest Editor*

March 2008

Infectious Disease Emergencies
David A. Talan, MD, *Guest Editor*

RECENT ISSUES

March 2007

HIV/AIDS
Kenneth H. Mayer, MD,
Guest Editor

December 2006

Infections and Rheumatic Diseases
Luis R. Espinoza, MD, *Guest Editor*

September 2006

Fungal Infections
Thomas F. Patterson, MD, *Guest Editor*

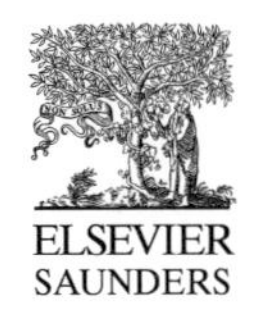

INFECTIOUS DISEASE CLINICS OF NORTH AMERICA

Infect Dis Clin N Am 21 (2007) xi–xiii

Preface

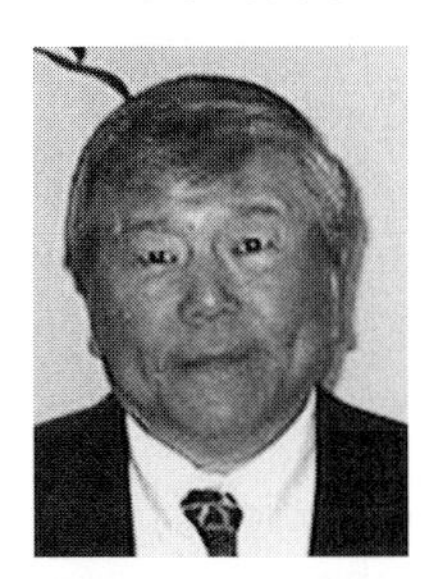

Anthony W. Chow, MD, FRCPC, FACP
Guest Editor

It was with relish and appreciation that I gratefully accepted the invitation to be Guest Editor of the current issue of *Infectious Disease Clinics of North America* devoted to infections of the head and neck. After all, to be invited back a second time almost 2 decades later, after serving in a similar capacity for an earlier issue published in March 1988 (“Infectious Syndromes of the Head and Neck”), speaks to the importance of the subject matter and offers a rare opportunity to marvel at the incredible advances in medicine and technology in this interim. On the other hand, it also was reassuring that the basic tenets of careful clinical observation, deductive reasoning, and adherence to the scientific method have remained the cornerstone to the diagnosis and treatment of infections of the head and neck. This issue serves to highlight the multispecialty nature of these infections which are seen by family physicians, internists, pediatricians, emergency physicians, dentists, oral surgeons, ophthalmologists, radiologists, and otorhinolaryngologists alike.

Similar to the previous issue, this issue is organized into two sections to present both the basic and clinical information necessary for providing patients the best possible care. The section “General Considerations”, emphasizes the tightly regulated ecologic niches of the indigenous microflora and the highly efficient innate immune system in the head and neck region and highlights the importance of anaerobic bacteria in head and neck infections by Hull and myself. The role of the clinical microbiology laboratory in the

0891-5520/07/$ - see front matter
doi:10.1016/j.idc.2007.05.001

microbiologic investigation of head and neck infections is reviewed, with particular emphasis on recent developments of rapid molecular techniques and the need to distinguish between normal flora and true pathogens by Brook. An important technological advance has been the refinement of imaging techniques by multidetector CT and MRI, which have revolutionized the ability to visualize fascial borders of soft tissues as well as vascular integrity and parameningeal foci in complex head and neck infections (Hurley and Heran). A selection of radiographic images is offered to illustrate their value in identifying vital structures in head and neck infections, such as the airway, cervical vessels, orbits, paranasal sinuses, deep fascial spaces, intracranial structures, and the spinal canal. Finally, the principles of antimicrobial management for head and neck infections based on suspected source, likely pathogens, predicted susceptibility or resistance patterns, and pharmacokinetic and pharmacodynamic considerations are discussed by Roscoe and Hoang. Although the emerging resistance among respiratory pathogens and oral gram-negative anaerobes is emphasized, the use of empiric coverage for resistant pathogens should be dictated by relative risks based on the severing of infection, nature of comorbid disease, and prior exposure to antimicrobial agents rather than merely on the recovery of resistant micro-organisms in mixed culture. In the section "Specific Syndromes," a variety of head and neck infections are considered, including periorbital and orbital infections (Wald), acute otitis media (Powers), acute and chronic bacterial sinusitis (Brook), pharyngitis and epiglottitis (Alcaide and Bisno), dental caries and periodontitis as two contrasting infectious diseases (Loesche), mucositis in the cancer patient and immunosuppressed host (Epstein), cervical lymphadenitis, suppurative parotitis, thyroiditis, and infected cysts (Al-Dajani and Wootton), cervicofacial actinomycosis and mandibular osteomyelitis (Sharkawy), life-threatening peripharyngeal and deep fascial space infections (Reynolds and myself), and vascular and parameningeal infections of the head and neck (Laupland). The article "Diagnosis and Treatment of Acute Otitis Media: Evaluating the Evidence" is particularly poignant in pointing out the paucity of quality evidence supporting the clinical diagnosis and decisions regarding the initiation, choice, and duration of antimicrobial therapy. This paucity of evidence-based data persists even though a diagnosis of acute otitis media is the most common reason for prescribing an antimicrobial agent to children and it is one of the most common reasons overall for anyone in the United States to receive an antimicrobial agent. It is likely the same assessment applies to the diagnosis and treatment of acute bacterial sinusitis, emphasizing the critical need for further research to help clinicians make more informed decisions.

I am deeply indebted to so many close colleagues and former trainees who contributed to this issue. I thank Dr. Robert Moellering, Jr., Consulting Editor of the *Infectious Disease Clinics of North America*, for his prodding and encouragement to take on this task, and Karen Sorensen of Elsevier Saunders for her expert assistance and indulgence. We hope this update will continue to serve as a useful resource for the clinician caring for patients and for the investigator to stimulate further research, which clearly is needed in this important area.

Anthony W. Chow, MD, FRCPC, FACP
Division of Infectious Diseases
Department of Medicine
University of British Columbia
Vancouver Hospital Health Sciences Centre
2733 Heather Street, Vancouver
British Columbia, Canada V5Z 3J5

E-mail address: tonychow@interchange.ubc.ca

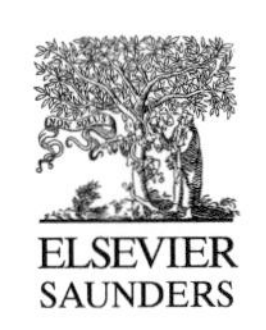

ELSEVIER
SAUNDERS

Infect Dis Clin N Am 21 (2007) 265–282

INFECTIOUS
DISEASE CLINICS
OF NORTH AMERICA

Indigenous Microflora and Innate Immunity of the Head and Neck

Mark W. Hull, MD, FRCPC[a], Anthony W. Chow, MD, FRCPC, FACP[b,*]

[a]*Division of Infectious Diseases, Department of Medicine, University of British Columbia, Vancouver, BC, Canada*

[b]*Division of Infectious Diseases, Department of Medicine, University of British Columbia, Vancouver Hospital Health Sciences Centre, 2733 Heather Street, Vancouver, BC, Canada V5Z 3J5*

The indigenous microflora

From the earliest days of the study of microbiology, the mouth has been identified as a habitat for large numbers of micro-organisms. The seventeenth-century microscopist, Anton van Leeuwenhoek, provided initial descriptions of the differing bacteria found within the oral cavity. Since then, studies of the human bacterial flora in health and disease have progressed rapidly, keeping pace with technological advances in scientific investigation. The introduction of anaerobic culture techniques has greatly aided the characterization of the normal oral flora. The availability of molecular and bioinformatic tools, such as real-time and quantitative polymerase chain reaction, has greatly facilitated the study of previously uncultivable species and has clarified their taxonomic relationships [1]. Study of the normal oral flora has generated, among others, the seminal hypothesis of Miller [2] on the causation of dental caries. Miller, a student of Koch, linked the intake of refined carbohydrates and the production of organic acids by oral bacteria to demineralization of the tooth surface, ultimately leading to the formation of dental caries. More recent studies of various oral bacteria and the host inflammatory responses to their infections have allowed the generation of hypotheses linking dental disease with various systemic conditions including coronary heart disease and cerebrovascular accidents [3].

* Corresponding author.
E-mail address: tonychow@interchange.ubc.ca (A.W. Chow).

doi:10.1016/j.idc.2007.03.015

id.theclinics.com

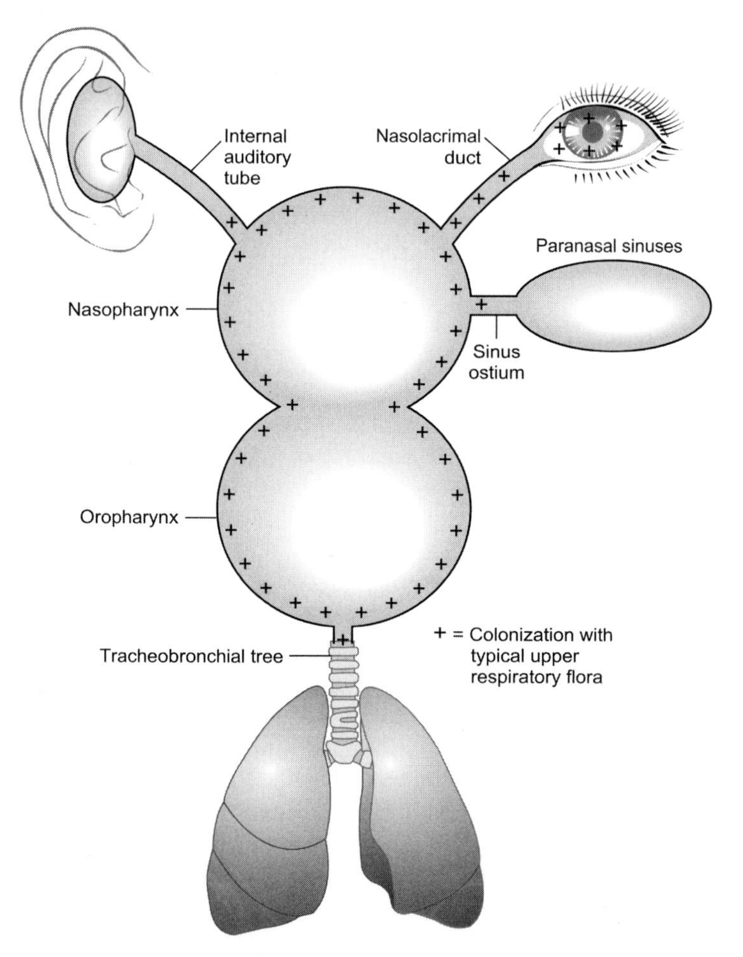

Fig. 1. The anatomic relationship and distribution of the indigenous microflora of the head and neck. (*Adapted from* Todd JK. Bacteriology and clinical relevance of nasopharyngeal and oropharyngeal cultures. Pediatr Infect Dis 1984;3(2):160; with permission.)

The oral cavity, upper respiratory tract, and certain regions of the ears and eyes have an indigenous microflora. Because of the close anatomic relationship of these structures, the resident flora of these regions shares many common pathogens (Fig. 1). Within a given microenvironment, however, certain microbes that constitute the normal flora are associated with distinct anatomic sites (Table 1). Thus, the normal flora exists within complex ecosystems at different sites and interacts closely with different bacterial species and with the host epithelial layers [4]. This indigenous microflora is known to change over time, and host age, underlying disease, and chemotherapeutic agents affect its composition [5–8].

Components of the normal flora exist as commensals in a symbiotic relationship with the host and prevent colonization and subsequent disease by

Table 1
Micro-organisms found at various sites of the head and neck in the healthy human host

Predominant genus or family	Mouth (saliva, tooth surface)[a]	Oropharynx[a]	Nose, nasopharynx[a]	External ear[a]	Conjunctiva[a]
Facultative					
Gram-positive cocci					
Streptococci (viridans group)	4[a]	4	3	1	-
Streptococcus mutans	4	3	-	-	-
Streptococcus sanguis	4	4	-	-	-
Streptococcus mitior	4	4	-	-	-
Streptococcus salivarius	4	4	-	-	-
Streptococcus pneumoniae	-	2	2	±	±
Streptococcus pyogenes	-	1	1	-	±
Streptococcus faecalis	1	-	-	±	-
Staphylococcus aureus	-	-	2	±	2
Staphylococcus epidermidis	4	3	4	4	4
Gram-positive bacilli					
Corynebacterium	2	4	4	3	4
Gram-negative cocci					
Moraxella	1	2	3	-	1
Neisseria spp	2	3	1	1	±
Neisseria meningitidis	-	-	1	-	-
Gram-negative bacilli					
Eikenella	1	-	-	-	-
Enterobacteriaceae	1	±	±	1	±
Haemophilus influenzae	-	2	2	-	1
Haemophilus parainfluenzae	-	3	3	-	2
Anaerobic					
Gram-positive cocci					
Peptostreptococcus	4	4	-	1	-
Gram-positive bacilli					
Actinomyces	4	-	-	-	-
Lactobacillus	4	-	-	-	-
Propionibacterium	-	-	-	1	3
Gram-negative cocci					
Veillonella	4	-	-	-	-
Gram-negative bacilli					
Fusobacterium	3	4	-	-	-
Bacteroides, Porphyromonas, Prevotella	4	4	-	-	-
Other					
Miscellaneous bacteria					
Pseudomonas	-	-	-	1	-
Acinetobacter	1	1	-	-	-
Spirochetes					
Treponema	3	-	-	-	-
Fungi					
Candida	2	1	±	±	±

[a] Approximate prevalence of organisms at site indicated: ±, rare; 1, 0%–10%; 2, 11%–30%; 3, 30%–60%; 4, 0%–60%.

Data from Roscoe DL, Chow AW. Normal flora and mucosal immunity of the head and neck. Infect Dis Clin North Am 1988;2(1):6–7.

more pathogenic species. *Neisseria meningitidis*, for example, can be recovered from cultures of the oropharynx of healthy individuals but is contained at levels too low to cause disease [9]. Although the mechanisms for regulation and control of potential pathogens by the normal flora are poorly understood, the protective role of the normal flora is clearly established. It is somewhat paradoxical, therefore, that some constituents of the normal flora are low-virulence organisms that also can cause disease when local mucosal defenses are impaired.

To understand the microbial etiology of head and neck infections, familiarity with the normal flora of the pertinent structures is required. Knowledge of the baseline flora will help determine the likely causative agent of an infection and guide antimicrobial therapy. In addition, appreciation of the role of the normal flora in regulating host defense against more pathogenic species may temper a clinical inclination to introduce broad-spectrum antibiotics unnecessarily, thus altering this beneficial balance with potentially serious consequences.

Acquisition of the normal flora

Establishment of a normal flora occurs in a sequential manner. The first exposure of the mucosal surfaces of a sterile neonate is to the maternal genital microflora during its passage through the birth canal. Select species are able to colonize a specific site through bacterial–tissue interactions. Ecosystems mature as other species are encountered and interbacterial aggregation and signaling occur within the mucosal biofilm. A variety of conditions affect successful colonization of the mucosal surface in the oral cavity, including factors such as epithelial cell turnover, salivary flow, and dentition. Conditions within the microenvironment, such as the supply of nutrients, oxygen tension, and pH, also are important factors that influence the predilection of different bacterial species for certain intraoral locales.

Initial binding of bacteria to mucosal surfaces is facilitated by nonspecific factors such as van der Waals forces between the microbial coat and a tooth surface [10]. These weak physicochemical interactions facilitate reversible adherence. More specific interactions between surface molecules on the bacterial surface (adhesins) and host receptor proteins result in more irreversible binding. Oral streptococcal species produce several adhesins, notably antigen I/II, which have multiple receptor binding sites [11] for host receptor proteins containing sialic acid moieties, such as salivary proteins [12]. Other host molecules, such as fibronectin, also are associated with bacterial adhesion. Fibronectin is a glycoprotein found in the extracellular matrix and tissue fluids of vertebrates. Many gram-positive bacteria, including several staphylococcal and streptococcal species, produce an array of surface molecules collectively known as "microbial surface components recognizing adhesive matrix molecules" (MSCRAMM), which target fibronectin and other molecules for binding to host cells [13]. In the absence of fibronectin, adherence of gram-positive cocci is diminished, while that of gram-negative bacilli may be enhanced [14]. Colonization by certain bacterial species within the oral cavity may be aided by the presence of other bacteria that alter the local environment sufficiently to permit growth or allow colonization simply by providing a means of attachment at that site through coaggregation. Many bacterial species possess fimbriae that serve to allow coadhesion to other micro-organisms. Oral flora (eg, *Prevotella* species) is able to coaggregate by fimbriae with *Actinomyces* species or oral streptococci [15]. In this manner interbacterial interactions allow increased species diversity within certain microenvironments within the oral cavity. Attachment of bacteria to host surfaces and other bacterial species promotes cell division and production of extracellular polymers, leading to the formation of biofilms and dental plaques on the tooth surface. The plaque biofilm has channels within its architecture, and bacteria are organized in a way that allows interbacterial contact and metabolic interactions, including synergistic degradation of more complex nutrients within the oral cavity [16,17].

In addition to interbacterial interactions, other factors may affect colonization of specific bacterial species at certain locales within the oral cavity. These factors include physical retention resulting from bacteria becoming entrapped within dental fissures or gingival crevices. The mechanical effects of the constant flow of salivary fluids over surfaces play a role in decreasing bacterial colony density. Host dietary intake also may contribute to the balance of oral bacterial species. Diets high in refined sugars may promote the growth of *Streptococcus mutans*, whereas foods containing lectins may promote enhanced adherence by other streptococcal species such as *Streptococcus sanguinis*. These lectins serve to bind mucosal cells and act as receptors for these bacteria.

Composition of the oral flora

An estimated 300 to 500 bacterial species coexist within the oral cavity, of which approximately 50% are currently uncultivable [1,5]. Streptococcal species, diphtheroids, and Veillonellae make up 80% of the cultivable flora of the oral cavity. Quantitative studies indicate that obligate anaerobes constitute a large and important part of the residential oral flora. Overall, *Streptococcus*, *Peptostreptococcus*, *Veillonella*, *Lactobacillus*, *Corynebacterium*, and *Actinomyces* species account for more than 80% of the total cultivable oral flora. Facultative gram-negative bacilli are uncommon in healthy adults but may be more prominent in seriously ill, hospitalized, and elderly patients. Unique ecologic niches are observed (Table 2).

Gram-positive cocci

The predominant components of oral flora are streptococcal species, most commonly members of the alpha-hemolytic viridans group. Currently, 26 different species of viridans streptococci are recognized [18]. They are

Table 2
Predominant cultivable bacteria from various sites of the oral cavity

Type	Predominant Genus or Family	Total Viable Count (Mean %)			
		Gingival Crevice	Dental Plaque	Tongue	Saliva
Facultative					
Gram-positive cocci	Streptococcus	28.8	28.2	44.8	46.2
	S mutans group	(0–30)	(0–50)	(0–1)	(0–1)
	S sanguinis	(10–20)	(40–60)	(10–20)	(10–30)
	S mitis	(10–30)	(20–40)	(10–30)	(30–50)
	S salivarius	(0–1)	(0–1)	(40–60)	(40–60)
Gram-positive bacilli	Lactobacillus	15.3	23.8	13.0	11.8
Gram-negative cocci	Moraxella	0.4	0.4	3.4	1.2
Gram-negative bacilli	Enterobacteriaceae	1.2	ND	3.2	2.3
Anaerobic					
Gram-positive cocci	Peptostreptococcus	7.4	12.6	4.2	13.0
Gram-positive bacilli	Actinomyces, Eubacterium, Leptotrichia	20.2	18.4	8.2	4.8
Gram-negative cocci	Veillonella	10.7	6.4	16.0	15.9
Gram-negative bacilli		16.1	10.4	8.2	4.8
	Fusobacterium	1.9	4.1	0.7	0.3
	Bacteroides, Porphyromonas, Prevotella	4.7	ND	0.2	ND

Abbreviation: ND, not detected.

Data from Chow AW. Infections of the oral cavity, neck and head. In: Mandell GL, Bennett JE, Dolin R, editors. Principles and practice of infectious diseases. 6th edition. Philadelphia: Elsevier Churchill Livingstone; 2005. p. 787.

divided into five major groups on the basis of phenotypic and molecular properties, including *S mutans*, *Streptococcus salivarius*, *Streptococcus anginosus*, *S sanguinis* (formerly *S sanguis*), and *Streptococcus mitis* groups. Other gram-positive cocci include anaerobic Peptostreptococcus species. Within the mutans group, the two most common species isolated from the human oral cavity are *S mutans* and *Streptococcus sobrinus*. *S mutans*, and *S sobrinus* to a lesser extent, are associated with caries formation [17]. The salivarius group has three main species in the human oral microflora—*S salivarius*, *Streptococcus vestibularis*, and *Streptococcus infantarius*. *S mitis* and *S oralis* are the major components within the mitis group; *S sanguinis*, *Streptococcus parasanguinis*, and *Streptococcus gordonii* are the main constituents of the sanguinis group. The anginosus group consists of three species—*S anginosus*, *S milleri*, and *Streptococcus intermedius*. This group differs from other viridans streptococci in that these isolates may exhibit beta-hemolysis and frequently are associated with suppurative infections of the head and neck, with a propensity for hematogenous spread into pleural spaces, liver, and the brain [19–21]. In comparison, the other viridans streptococci are not commonly associated with pyogenic infections but are more commonly associated with infective endocarditis

[22] and bacteremia in the setting of fever and neutropenia following chemotherapy for hematologic malignancies [23].

Gram-positive bacilli

A variety of gram-positive rods can be isolated from the human oral cavity. Lactobacilli are found soon after birth but drop in number as the neonate ages. Pleomorphic or filamentous gram-positive rods, the so-called "diphtheroids," are common inhabitants of the oral cavity but do not seem to play an important role in oral disease [5]. Other branching filamentous rods found within the oral cavity belong to the *Actinomyces* species, including *Actinomyces israelii, Actinomyces viscosus, Actinomyces naeslundii,* and *Actinomyces odontolyticus*. These facultative anaerobes are associated with a variety of human diseases, including dental root caries, cervicofacial actinomycosis, mandibular osteomyelitis, and actinomycosis involving the chest, abdomen, and the female genital tract [17,24,25].

Gram-negative cocci

Anaerobic gram-negative cocci also are found as part of the normal oral flora. *Veillonella* species such as *Veillonella parvula, Veillonella dispar*, and *Veillonella atypica* are found on the soft tissues of the mouth such as the tongue surface and in the saliva and may constitute up to 5% of the dental plaque biomass [26]. *Veillonella* species isolated from subgingival dental plaques demonstrate the ability to coaggregate with streptococcal species, a property vital to the formation of diverse biofilms, whereas those from the tongue and saliva have limited coaggregation properties [27]. Veillonellae are unable to ferment sugars directly and instead rely on fermentation products, such as lactic acid, produced by streptococci. This close relationship with streptococcal species may play a contributory role in the pathogenesis of dental caries [28].

Gram-negative bacilli

Among the most numerous and varied components of the oral flora are the gram-negative rods. Anaerobic gram-negative rods constitute approximately 16% of the normal flora in the gingival crevice (see Table 2). Commonly identified species include the black-pigmented rods previously classified within the *Bacteroides* genus but now renamed as *Prevotella* or *Porphyromonas* species [29]. Bile-sensitive saccharolytic *Bacteroides* species now are classified within the genus *Prevotella*; bile-sensitive asaccharolytic species are classified within the genus *Porphyromonas*. Apart from being the dominant microflora in the healthy gingival crevice, some seem to play a unique role in certain disease states. For example, *Prevotella intermedia* and *Porphyromonas gingivalis* are among the predominant species found in advanced periodontal disease. Species such as *Bacteroides forsythus* are also identified [30]. Numerous other gram-negative anaerobic or facultative rods within the oral cavity can contribute to different disease states. These include *Actinobacillus actinomycetemcomitans*, *Fusobacterium* species, and *Eikenella corrodens*. *Actinobacillus* has been identified as an intraoral pathogen that contributes to localized juvenile periodontitis; *Fusobacterium* species such as *Fusobacterium nucleatum* may play an important role in acute dental abscesses [31–33]. *Fusobacterium* species also are associated with suppurative infections and thrombosis of the internal jugular vein (Lemierre syndrome); systemic dissemination by *E corrodens* and *A actinomycetemcomitans* are associated with the formation of cardiac valve vegetations and infective endocarditis [34,35].

Spirochetes

Spirochetes belonging to the genus *Treponema* are found within the normal anaerobic flora of the oral cavity. A variety of morphotypes has been observed, but many remain uncultivable and are identifiable only by molecular techniques [36]. The most common species in the human oral flora include *Treponema denticola*, *Treponema orale*, and *Treponema vincentii*. The anaerobic nature of the treponemes favors their isolation from subgingival tissues and within periodontal pockets. In disease states, treponemes, particularly *T denticola*, have been associated with periodontal destruction, whereas others are linked to acute necrotizing ulcerative gingivitis [37–39].

Distribution of the normal flora within the oral cavity

Tongue and saliva

Viridans streptococci, particularly *S salivarius*, and *Veillonella* species predominate on the dorsum of the tongue and the buccal mucosa. The saliva, another major reservoir of the oral microflora, is estimated to contain 6×10^9 micro-organisms/mL [40].

Tooth surface and gingival crevice

In the gingival crevice of healthy adults, the total microscopic counts averaged 2.7×10^{11} micro-organisms/g wet weight [41]. Whereas cultivable facultative or aerobic bacteria averaged 2.2×10^{10} micro-organisms/g wet weight, anaerobic bacteria were isolated at approximately 1.8×10^{11} micro-organisms/g, an eightfold difference [42,43]. In the gingival crevice, which provides a more anaerobic microenvironment, predominant isolates include *Fusobacterium*, *Prevotella*, and *Porphyromonas* species as well as oral anaerobic spirochetes. Plaque-associated bacteria below the gingival margin also comprise mainly anaerobic gram-negative rods and spirochetes. The clean surface of a tooth is coated in a layer of bacteria-free salivary protein polymers known as the "acquired pellicle." Oral microflora sequentially colonize this pellicle in the formation of a dental plaque. Streptococcal species such as *S mutans* predominate on the tooth surface, although *Actinomyces*, *Eubacterium*, and *Peptostreptococcus* species and black-pigmented anaerobic gram-negative rods are also isolated. Attachment of *S mutans* to tooth surfaces is enhanced in the presence of dietary sucrose, which leads to the production of extracellular dextrans by the bacteria.

The oropharynx

Viridans streptococci, including species within the *S salivarius*, *S mutans*, and *S anginosus* groups, constitute the most prevalent components of the normal oropharyngeal flora [40]. Gram-negative diplococci, including *N meningitidis*, are found in 5% to 10% of healthy asymptomatic individuals [44,45]. Facultative gram-negative bacilli are isolated rarely from healthy individuals. An increased rate of colonization is noted in chronically ill or hospitalized patients and in the elderly. This transition from colonization with gram-positive organisms to gram-negative bacteria contributes to the development of ventilator-associated pneumonias in mechanically ventilated patients [46].

Alterations related to age and underlying disease

The oral microflora constantly evolves with age and with the underlying conditions of the host. The oral cavity is sterile at birth but rapidly becomes colonized following exposure to the maternal birth canal. Organisms, including anaerobic species such as lactobacilli and *Veillonella* species, are detectable within a few hours [47]. Streptococcal species, predominantly *S mitis* and *S salivarius,* become established within 2 days of birth and predominate during the first year of life, accounting for 70% of the total flora [48,49]. New niches are created with the eruption of teeth, and other streptococcal species, including *S mutans* and *S sanguinis,* then are able to colonize dental surfaces. In one study, the acquisition of *S mutans* occurred at a median of 26 months [50]. Sampling of the tongue and tooth surfaces in children aged 6 to 36 months yielded a wide diversity of the microflora by DNA hybridization techniques, including *S sobrinus*, *S mutans*, *P gingivalis*, and *A actinomycetemcomitans* [51]. The flora remains relatively constant throughout early childhood and puberty, and *S salivarius*, *S oralis*, and *S mitis* remain prominent [6]. With the eruption of secondary teeth, conditions favoring the growth of anaerobic and spirochete populations are created. As teeth are lost during aging, spirochetes and lactobacilli are reduced markedly, as are populations of *S mutans* and *S sanguinis*. After lost teeth are replaced with dentures, the flora returns to predentition levels [52].

Important differences in bacterial compositions have been noted for dental caries, gingivitis, and different forms of periodontal disease when compared with cultures from healthy tissues (Fig. 2). On the plaque-free

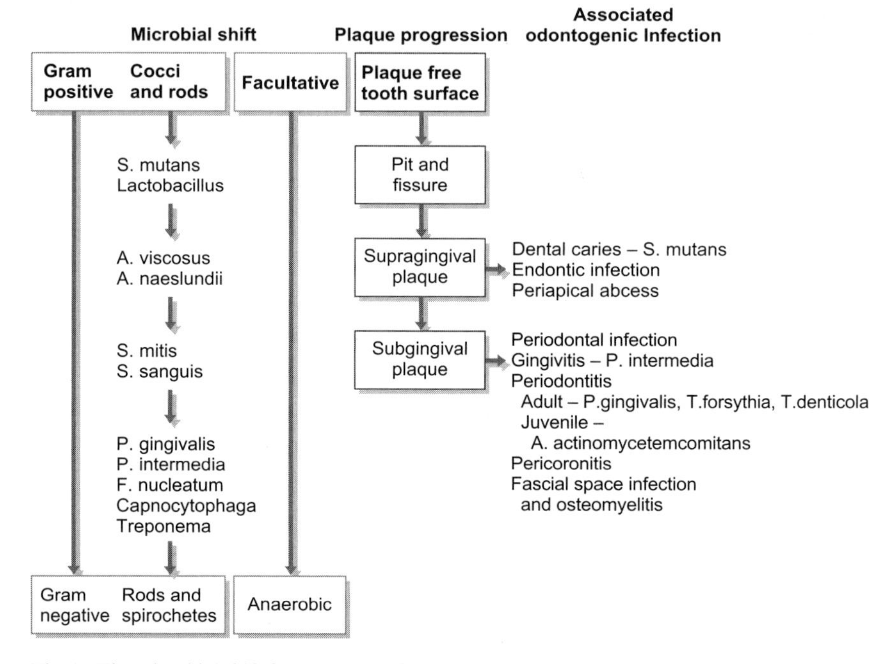

Fig. 2. The microbial shift from a plaque-free tooth surface to colonization of the supragingival plaque and progression to a subgingival plaque and various associated odontogenic infections. (*From* Chow AW. Infections of the oral cavity, neck and head. In: Mandell GL, Bennett JE, Dolin R, editors. Principles and practice of infectious diseases. 6th edition. Philadelphia: Elsevier Churchill Livingstone; 2005. p. 788; with permission.)

tooth surface, gram-positive facultative bacteria predominate. As pits and fissures appear, the supragingival plaque develops, and the predominant flora switches to *Streptococcus mutans* and *Actinomyces* species. This predominance gradually progresses to the subgingival plaque in which anaerobic gram-negative bacilli and spirochetes predominate, leading to periodontal disease and loss of dentition. Micro-organisms residing within the supragingival plaque are characterized by their ability to adhere to the tooth surface and by their saccharolytic activity. Micro-organisms in the subgingival plaque frequently are asaccharolytic and need not be adherent. The microbiology of odontogenic infections generally reflects this acquisition of a unique microflora during the development and progression of the supragingival and subgingival dental plaques.

Normal flora at other sites

The nares and nasopharynx

The normal flora colonizing the nasopharynx reflects that of the surrounding contiguous structures. Viridans streptococci again predominate. Species identified with infections within the middle ear have also been found in the nasopharynx of healthy children. These organisms include *S pneumoniae*, *H influenzae*, and *Moraxella catarrhalis*. Children younger than 2 years of age harbor these organisms more commonly than those aged 11 to 15 years [53], and they also may be more common in children who are prone to episodes of otitis media [54]. Carriage of *S pneumoniae* is reduced by the introduction of effective pediatric vaccination [55]. Bacteria common within the anterior nares include diphtheroids, coagulase-negative staphylococci, and *Staphylococcus aureus*. The recent U.S. National Health and Nutrition Examination Survey, conducted during 2001 and 2002, identified a nasal carriage rate for *S aureus* in 32.4% of the general population, with methicillin-resistant *S aureus* being isolated in 0.8% [56].

The paranasal sinuses in healthy individuals generally are considered to be sterile. Because there is a close anatomic link between these spaces and other body sites that normally are heavily populated by an endogenous flora, microbial access to these passageways is easily attained (see Fig. 1). This population usually is transient, however, because the organisms are cleared quickly by local defense mechanisms.

The external ear and eye

The inner and middle ear also are considered sterile environments in the healthy state. Examination of the normal flora inhabiting the external ear canal reveals micro-organisms predominantly associated with the skin flora. *Corynebacterium* species, coagulase-negative staphylococci, and *S aureus* are the main isolates in healthy children and adults [57,58]. *Pseudomonas aeruginosa* is found also, particularly in individuals who have diabetes mellitus. Bacterial strains associated with otitis externa are found to bind more tightly to the epithelial cells of the outer ear canal [59].

The conjunctiva, lacrimal apparatus, and eyelids harbor normal flora. Bacteria at these sites resemble the flora of the surrounding skin or within the upper respiratory tract. Most common isolates include *Staphylococcus* species and diphtheroids, with gram-negative cocci or bacilli isolated only occasionally.

Mucosal immunity

It is a tribute to the local defenses in the healthy host that infections within the oral cavity are not more common. Despite ongoing exposure to commensal bacteria and potential pathogens, microbial invasion into healthy tissues is infrequent. The mucosal surface serves as the first line of defense by acting as a mechanical barrier. The continuous cell shedding and turnover of the mucosal epithelium and the constant flow of saliva containing a myriad of antimicrobial peptides serve to prevent bacterial colonization or infection. Additionally, various salivary constituents may inhibit microbial attachment to the oral epithelium, either by competition for cellular receptor sites or clumping of micro-organisms. These defense mechanisms are multifaceted in nature with both nonspecific and specific components that constitute the innate and the acquired immunity of the head and neck.

Mechanical barriers

The mucosa acts as a physical barrier to microbial invasion. It consists of a layer of interconnected epithelial cells resting on a basal membrane. Junctions between these epithelial cells are tightly regulated for the passage of molecules into the underlying connective tissues, lymphatics, or regional microcirculation. Interspersed with the epithelial cells are mucin-producing goblet cells that line the surface of the nasal cavity and the oropharynx. These cells produce a thick layer of mucin glycoproteins that coat the surrounding epithelia, forming a protective glycocalyx. This layer may trap and block bacteria from adhering to the underlying epithelial cells [60]. In addition, bacteria seeking to colonize mucosal surfaces must develop a strategy to deal with the constant turnover of the epithelial cell layer.

The normal commensal microflora contributes to mucosal defense by preventing colonization and invasion by more pathogenic species through bacterial interference ("colonization resistance"). Displacement of the normal resident microflora can lead to the influx of other more pathogenic species, as seen when antibiotic use leads to overgrowth of oral *Candida* species, ultimately leading to opharyngeal candidiasis. The yeast is able to fill the vacant ecologic niche. The normal flora reoccupies these sites when the antibiotic selection pressure is removed [5,61]. The mechanisms of bacterial interference include competition for binding sites, availability of nutrients, and alterations of the microenvironment such as local pH or redox potential. Bacterial interference occurs in the nasopharynx and in locales such as the anterior nares where coagulase-negative staphylococci or diphtheroids may prevent growth of *S aureus* [62], and non-pathogenic *Neisseria* species may inhibit colonization and invasion by *N meningitidis* [45].

Salivary antimicrobial peptides and chemical inhibitors

Saliva acts as an antimicrobial agent in addition to its role in digestion, taste, and phonation [63]. The saliva consists of secretions from the major and minor salivary glands and also sloughed cells, food and bacterial particulates, and secreted chemical inhibitors, immunoglobulins, and antimicrobial peptides. Mechanically, saliva serves to coat the teeth and contribute to the protective pellicle. In addition, it flushes the oral cavity, clearing away bacteria and their by-products as well as food debris that may aid bacterial growth and colonization. Disruptions in salivary flow rates have been associated with caries formation, and individuals who have impaired salivary flow experience a high incidence of dental caries

[64]. The buffering capacity of saliva contributes to the maintenance of salivary pH. Alterations in pH also are associated with the development of dental caries [63].

Numerous chemical inhibitors of bacterial growth are found within the saliva. These inhibitors include lysozyme, lactoferrin, defensins, and the peroxidase system. Lysozyme is ubiquitous within human body secretions and is able to lyse bacteria by catalyzing breakdown of the bacterial cell wall in a manner akin to the action of penicillin. Lysozyme also is active against gram-negative bacteria in the presence of complement and antibody, which disrupts the lipopolysaccharide coat in the cell wall [40]. Lactoferrin serves to sequester iron from the environment, thus inhibiting bacterial growth, particularly facultative and aerobic species that are dependent on iron for metabolism. In addition, lactoferrin can inhibit growth of *S mutans* in an iron-independent manner [63]. Lactoferrin has a hidden domain that is exposed after undergoing proteolysis, resulting in antimicrobial activity against various microbes, including *A actinomycetemcomitans* [65,66]. Other antimicrobial peptides include histamines and the β-defensins that are produced in the ductal cells of salivary glands and have broad antibacterial and antifungal properties [67]. Human beta-defensin (hBD)-1 is expressed constitutively in epithelial tissues, whereas hBD-2 and hBD-3 are expressed in response to bacterial stimuli or inflammation. Recent studies have found that commensal and pathogenic bacteria use different signaling pathways in hBD-2 induction and suggest that epithelial cells from different body sites may use common signaling mechanisms to distinguish commensal and pathogenic bacteria [68]. Salivary lactoperoxidase and myeloperoxidase are generated by polymorphonuclear leukocytes within the gingival crevices and have potent bactericidal properties. Lactoperoxidase generates a hypothiocyanate molecule that is toxic to bacteria [69].

Cellular and humoral innate and acquired immunity

The epithelial cells of the oral cavity and salivary glands have an innate system for recognizing pathogenic microbes by the activation of toll-like receptors (TLRs). TLRs are transmembrane proteins, of which 10 members currently are known to exist in humans. TLRs function as pathogen-recognition receptors that interact with conserved domains on micro-organisms (so-called "pathogen-associated molecular patterns," PAMPS) [70,71]. These PAMPS include protein motifs (TLR4, -5), lipids or lipoproteins (TLR1, -2), and nucleic acid sequences (TLR9) [72]. Activation of TLRs leads to a cascade of signaling pathways, ultimately leading to the nuclear translocation of nuclear factor kappa B and the transcription and increased production of various proinflammatory (eg, interleukin [IL]-1α, IL-6, IL-12, tumor necrosis factor-α, and others) or anti-inflammatory cytokines (eg, IL-10, transforming growth factor-β, and others) and chemokines (eg, regulated on activation, normal T expressed and secreted (RANTES), macrophage inflammatory protein-1, IL-8, and others) that are critical for nonspecific defense in the head and neck region [73,74].

The mucous membranes have a full complement of immunocompetent cells, including lymphocytes, macrophages, dendritic cells, natural killer cells, and eosinophils, located in the lamina propria beneath the epithelial layer. Mucosa-associated lymphoreticular tissue (MALT) is common throughout the nasopharynx, bronchi, and gut. Aggregate sites within the oropharynx include the tonsils and adenoids. Together with the diffuse collections of lymphoid cells comprising MALT, dendritic cells are able to process foreign antigens for presentation to and activation of T cells and T-cell–dependent B-cell activation. Antigen-stimulated B cells travel to sites within the mucosal lymphoreticular tissue and expand and differentiate in a clonal fashion to become immunoglobulin-secreting plasma cells. The primary immunoglobulin secreted at these sites within salivary and other exocrine glands is IgA; however, some IgM- and IgG-secreting plasma cells are present also [75]. The concentrations of IgA, IgG, and IgM isotypes in whole saliva are 200 mg, 2 mg, and 1 mg/1000 mL of saliva, respectively [76]. The primary route for IgG to enter saliva is through the gingival crevice [77]. Secretory IgA (sIgA) exists as a dimeric molecule, with two IgA antibodies joined by a bridge known as the "secretory component." The secretory component stabilizes the sIgA against proteolytic enzymes that commonly are found within the saliva. The secretory component is synthesized by epithelial cells and added to IgA molecules as they move through the mucosal surface. The major role of sIgA is inhibition of bacterial adherence [78]. Salivary sIgA antibodies directed against common mucosal bacteria, such as *S mitis* and *S salivarius,* appear within the first weeks of life, and responses to *S mutans* antigens are highest between 30 and 65 years of age [79]. Although this response plays a role in preventing tooth decay, the presence of sIgA does not seem to be vital, because IgA-deficient individuals are not at higher risk of dental caries [78]. Within the lacrimal gland, plasma cells also secrete IgA, which is detected in tears and is active against both *Streptococcus* species and *Haemophilus influenzae* [80].

In addition to humoral and cellular immunity, various phagocytic cells in the oral mucosa also seem to be important. Phagocytic cells such as leukocytes and macrophages are abundant in the lamina propria and presumably contribute to the removal of foreign matter that has breached the epithelial barrier.

References

[1] Harper-Owen R, Dymock D, Booth V, et al. Detection of unculturable bacteria in periodontal health and disease by PCR. J Clin Microbiol 1999;37(5):1469–73.
[2] Miller WD. Microorganisms of the human mouth. Philadelphia: SS White; 1890.
[3] Li X, Kolltveit KM, Tronstad L, et al. Systemic diseases caused by oral infection. Clin Microbiol Rev 2000;13(4):547–58.

[4] Tlaskalova-Hogenova H, Stepankova R, Hudcovic T, et al. Commensal bacteria (normal microflora), mucosal immunity and chronic inflammatory and autoimmune diseases. Immunol Lett 2004;93(2–3):97–108.
[5] Schuster GS. Oral flora and pathogenic organisms. Infect Dis Clin North Am 1999;13(4): 757–74, v.
[6] Lucas VS, Beighton D, Roberts GJ. Composition of the oral streptococcal flora in healthy children. J Dent 2000;28(1):45–50.
[7] Dreizen S, McCredie KB, Bodey GP, et al. Microbial mucocutaneous infections in acute adult leukemia. Results of an 18-year inpatient study. Postgrad Med 1986;79(8):107–18.
[8] Mirowski GW, Bettencourt JD, Hood AF. Oral infections in the immunocompromised host. Semin Cutan Med Surg 1997;16(4):249–56.
[9] Todd JK. Bacteriology and clinical relevance of nasopharyngeal and oropharyngeal cultures. Pediatr Infect Dis 1984;3(2):159–63.
[10] Busscher HJ, van der Mei HC. Physico-chemical interactions in initial microbial adhesion and relevance for biofilm formation. Adv Dent Res 1997;11(1):24–32.
[11] Kolenbrander PE, London J. Adhere today, here tomorrow: oral bacterial adherence. J Bacteriol 1993;175(11):3247–52.
[12] Jenkinson HF, Demuth DR. Structure, function and immunogenicity of streptococcal antigen I/II polypeptides. Mol Microbiol 1997;23(2):183–90.
[13] Joh D, Wann ER, Kreikemeyer B, et al. Role of fibronectin-binding MSCRAMMs in bacterial adherence and entry into mammalian cells. Matrix Biol 1999;18(3):211–23.
[14] Abraham SN, Beachey EH, Simpson WA. Adherence of streptococcus pyogenes, Escherichia coli, and Pseudomonas aeruginosa to fibronectin-coated and uncoated epithelial cells. Infect Immun 1983;41(3):1261–8.
[15] Hamada S, Amano A, Kimura S, et al. The importance of fimbriae in the virulence and ecology of some oral bacteria. Oral Microbiol Immunol 1998;13(3):129–38.
[16] Wood SR, Kirkham J, Marsh PD, et al. Architecture of intact natural human plaque biofilms studied by confocal laser scanning microscopy. J Dent Res 2000;79(1):21–7.
[17] Marsh PD. Microbiologic aspects of dental plaque and dental caries. Dent Clin North Am 1999;43(4):599–614, v–vi.
[18] Facklam R. What happened to the streptococci: overview of taxonomic and nomenclature changes. Clin Microbiol Rev 2002;15(4):613–30.
[19] Schuman NJ, Turner JE. The clinical significance of beta hemolytic streptococci of the milleri group in oral abscesses. J Clin Pediatr Dent 1999;23(2):137–42.
[20] Corredoira J, Casariego E, Moreno C, et al. Prospective study of Streptococcus milleri hepatic abscess. Eur J Clin Microbiol Infect Dis 1998;17(8):556–60.
[21] Shinzato T, Saito A. The Streptococcus milleri group as a cause of pulmonary infections. Clin Infect Dis 1995;21(Suppl 3):S238–43.
[22] Mylonakis E, Calderwood SB. Infective endocarditis in adults. N Engl J Med 2001;345(18): 1318–30.
[23] Ahmed R, Hassall T, Morland B, et al. Viridans streptococcus bacteremia in children on chemotherapy for cancer: an underestimated problem. Pediatr Hematol Oncol 2003;20(6):439–44.
[24] Miller M, Haddad AJ. Cervicofacial actinomycosis. Oral Surg Oral Med Oral Pathol Oral Radiol Endod 1998;85(5):496–508.
[25] Yildiz O, Doganay M. Actinomycoses and Nocardia pulmonary infections. Curr Opin Pulm Med 2006;12(3):228–34.
[26] Mager DL, Ximenez-Fyvie LA, Haffajee AD, et al. Distribution of selected bacterial species on intraoral surfaces. J Clin Periodontol 2003;30(7):644–54.
[27] Hughes CV, Kolenbrander PE, Andersen RN, et al. Coaggregation properties of human oral Veillonella spp.: relationship to colonization site and oral ecology. Appl Environ Microbiol 1988;54(8):1957–63.
[28] Delwiche EA, Pestka JJ, Tortorello ML. The Veillonellae: gram-negative cocci with a unique physiology. Annu Rev Microbiol 1985;39:175–93.

[29] Jousimies-Somer H, Summanen P. Recent taxonomic changes and terminology update of clinically significant anaerobic gram-negative bacteria (excluding spirochetes). Clin Infect Dis 2002;35(Suppl 1):S17–21.
[30] Loesche WJ, Grossman NS. Periodontal disease as a specific, albeit chronic, infection: diagnosis and treatment. Clin Microbiol Rev 2001;14(4):727–52, table of contents.
[31] Mandell RL, Socransky SS. A selective medium for Actinobacillus actinomycetemcomitans and the incidence of the organism in juvenile periodontitis. J Periodontol 1981;52(10):593–8.
[32] Zambon JJ, Umemoto T, De Nardin E, et al. Actinobacillus actinomycetemcomitans in the pathogenesis of human periodontal disease. Adv Dent Res 1988;2(2):269–74.
[33] Dahlen G. Microbiology and treatment of dental abscesses and periodontal-endodontic lesions. Periodontol 2000 2002;(28):206–39.
[34] Golpe R, Marin B, Alonso M. Lemierre's syndrome (necrobacillosis). Postgrad Med J 1999; 75(881):141–4.
[35] Brouqui P, Raoult D. Endocarditis due to rare and fastidious bacteria. Clin Microbiol Rev 2001;14(1):177–207.
[36] Moter A, Hoenig C, Choi BK, et al. Molecular epidemiology of oral treponemes associated with periodontal disease. J Clin Microbiol 1998;36(5):1399–403.
[37] Simonson LG, Goodman CH, Bial JJ, et al. Quantitative relationship of Treponema denticola to severity of periodontal disease. Infect Immun 1988;56(4):726–8.
[38] Riviere GR, DeRouen TA, Kay SL, et al. Association of oral spirochetes from sites of periodontal health with development of periodontitis. J Periodontol 1997;68(12):1210–4.
[39] Loesche WJ, Syed SA, Laughon BE, et al. The bacteriology of acute necrotizing ulcerative gingivitis. J Periodontol 1982;53(4):223–30.
[40] Roscoe DL, Chow AW. Normal flora and mucosal immunity of the head and neck. Infect Dis Clin North Am 1988;2(1):1–19.
[41] Chow AW. Infections of the oral cavity, neck and head. In: Mandell GL, Bennett JE, Dolin R,, editors. Principles and practice of infectious diseases. 6th edition. Philadelphia: Elsevier Churchill Livingstone; 2005. p. 787–802.
[42] Gordon DF, Stutman M, Loesche WJ. Improved isolation of anaerobic bacteria from the gingival crevice area of man. Appl Microbiol 1971;21(6):1046–50.
[43] Chow AW, Roser SM, Brady FA. Orofacial odontogenic infections. Ann Intern Med 1978; 88(3):392–402.
[44] Greenfield S, Sheehe PR, Feldman HA. Meningococcal carriage in a population of "normal" families. J Infect Dis 1971;123(1):67–73.
[45] Caugant DA, Hoiby EA, Magnus P, et al. Asymptomatic carriage of Neisseria meningitidis in a randomly sampled population. J Clin Microbiol 1994;32(2):323–30.
[46] O'Neal PV, Brown N, Munro C. Physiologic factors contributing to a transition in oral immunity among mechanically ventilated adults. Biol Res Nurs 2002;3(3):132–9.
[47] Carlsson J, Gothefors L. Transmission of Lactobacillus jensenii and Lactobacillus acidophilus from mother to child at time of delivery. J Clin Microbiol 1975;1(2):124–8.
[48] McCarthy C, Snyder ML, Parker RB. The indigenous oral flora of man. I. The newborn to the 1-year-old infant. Arch Oral Biol 1965;10:61–70.
[49] Smith DJ, Anderson JM, King WF, et al. Oral streptococcal colonization of infants. Oral Microbiol Immunol 1993;8(1):1–4.
[50] Caufield PW, Cutter GR, Dasanayake AP. Initial acquisition of mutans streptococci by infants: evidence for a discrete window of infectivity. J Dent Res 1993;72(1):37–45.
[51] Tanner AC, Milgrom PM, Kent R Jr, et al. The microbiota of young children from tooth and tongue samples. J Dent Res 2002;81(1):53–7.
[52] Theilade E, Budtz-Jorgensen E, Theilade J. Predominant cultivable microflora of plaque on removable dentures in patients with healthy oral mucosa. Arch Oral Biol 1983;28(8): 675–80.
[53] Stenfors LE, Raisanen S. Occurrence of middle ear pathogens in the nasopharynx of young individuals. A quantitative study in four age groups. Acta Otolaryngol 1990;109(1–2):142–8.

[54] Bernstein JM, Faden HF, Dryja DM, et al. Micro-ecology of the nasopharyngeal bacterial flora in otitis-prone and non-otitis-prone children. Acta Otolaryngol 1993;113(1): 88–92.
[55] Dagan R, Melamed R, Muallem M, et al. Reduction of nasopharyngeal carriage of pneumococci during the second year of life by a heptavalent conjugate pneumococcal vaccine. J Infect Dis 1996;174(6):1271–8.
[56] Kuehnert MJ, Kruszon-Moran D, Hill HA, et al. Prevalence of Staphylococcus aureus nasal colonization in the United States, 2001-2002. J Infect Dis 2006;193(2):172–9.
[57] Stenfors LE, Raisanen S. Quantity of aerobic bacteria in the bony portion of the external auditory canal of children. Int J Pediatr Otorhinolaryngol 2002;66(2):167–73.
[58] Dibb WL. The normal microbial flora of the outer ear canal in healthy Norwegian individuals. NIPH Ann 1990;13(1):11–6.
[59] Sundstrom J, Agrup C, Kronvall G, et al. Pseudomonas aeruginosa adherence to external auditory canal epithelium. Arch Otolaryngol Head Neck Surg 1997;123(12):1287–92.
[60] Lamont JT. Mucus: the front line of intestinal mucosal defense. Ann N Y Acad Sci 1992;664: 190–201.
[61] Knight L, Fletcher J. Growth of Candida albicans in saliva: stimulation by glucose associated with antibiotics, corticosteroids, and diabetes mellitus. J Infect Dis 1971;123(4):371–7.
[62] Uehara Y, Nakama H, Agematsu K, et al. Bacterial interference among nasal inhabitants: eradication of Staphylococcus aureus from nasal cavities by artificial implantation of Corynebacterium sp. J Hosp Infect 2000;44(2):127–33.
[63] Hicks J, Garcia-Godoy F, Flaitz C. Biological factors in dental caries: role of saliva and dental plaque in the dynamic process of demineralization and remineralization (part 1). J Clin Pediatr Dent 2003;28(1):47–52.
[64] Papas AS, Joshi A, MacDonald SL, et al. Caries prevalence in xerostomic individuals. J Can Dent Assoc 1993;59(2):171–4, 177–9.
[65] Bellamy W, Takase M, Yamauchi K, et al. Identification of the bactericidal domain of lactoferrin. Biochim Biophys Acta 1992;1121(1–2):130–6.
[66] Groenink J, Walgreen-Weterings E, Nazmi K, et al. Salivary lactoferrin and low-Mr mucin MG2 in Actinobacillus actinomycetemcomitans-associated periodontitis. J Clin Periodontol 1999;26(5):269–75.
[67] Amerongen AV, Veerman EC. Saliva—the defender of the oral cavity. Oral Dis 2002;8(1): 12–22.
[68] Chung WO, Dale BA. Innate immune response of oral and foreskin keratinocytes: utilization of different signaling pathways by various bacterial species. Infect Immun 2004; 72(1):352–8.
[69] Lenander-Lumikari M, Loimaranta V. Saliva and dental caries. Adv Dent Res 2000;14:40–7.
[70] Medzhitov R, Janeway C Jr. Innate immune recognition: mechanisms and pathways. Immunol Rev 2000;173:89–97.
[71] Akira S, Hemmi H. Recognition of pathogen-associated molecular patterns by TLR family. Immunol Lett 2003;85(2):85–95.
[72] Beutler B, Hoebe K, Du X, et al. How we detect microbes and respond to them: the Toll-like receptors and their transducers. J Leukoc Biol 2003;74(4):479–85.
[73] Kopp E, Medzhitov R. Recognition of microbial infection by Toll-like receptors. Curr Opin Immunol 2003;15(4):396–401.
[74] Takeda K, Kaisho T, Akira S. Toll-like receptors. Annu Rev Immunol 2003;21:335–76.
[75] Russell MW, Mestecky J. Induction of the mucosal immune response. Rev Infect Dis 1988; 10(Suppl 2):S440–6.
[76] Slavkin HC. Changing patterns of disease and mucosal immunity. J Am Dent Assoc 1999; 130(5):735–8.
[77] Tenovuo J, Grahn E, Lehtonen OP, et al. Antimicrobial factors in saliva: ontogeny and relation to oral health. J Dent Res 1987;66(2):475–9.

[78] Tenovuo J. Antimicrobial function of human saliva—how important is it for oral health? Acta Odontol Scand 1998;56(5):250–6.
[79] Smith DJ, King WF, Taubman MA. Salivary IgA antibody to oral streptococcal antigens in predentate infants. Oral Microbiol Immunol 1990;5(2):57–62.
[80] McClellan KA. Mucosal defense of the outer eye. Surv Ophthalmol 1997;42(3):233–46.

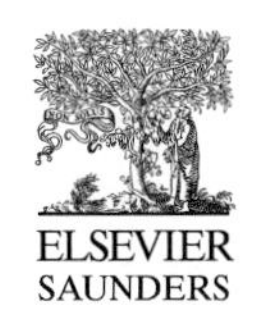

ELSEVIER
SAUNDERS

INFECTIOUS DISEASE CLINICS OF NORTH AMERICA

Infect Dis Clin N Am 21 (2007) 283–304

Microbiologic Investigations for Head and Neck Infections

Diane L. Roscoe, MD, FRCPC[a,b,*], Linda Hoang, MSc, MD, DTM&H, FRCPC[a,c]

[a]*Department of Pathology and Laboratory Medicine, University of British Columbia, Vancouver, BC, Canada*

[b]*Division of Medical Microbiology and Infection Control, Vancouver General Hospital and Vancouver Coastal Health, Room 1112A JPPN Microbiology, 855 W. 12th Avenue, Vancouver, BC, Canada V5Z 1M9*

[c]*Bacteriology and Mycology Program, British Columbia Centre for Disease Control Laboratory Services, Provincial Health Services Authority, 655 W. 12th Avenue, Vancouver, BC, Canada V5Z 4R4*

Determination of the specific cause of head and neck infections is challenging for several reasons. There is a diverse population of normal resident flora containing both organisms with low virulence and those commonly considered true pathogens, all or none of which may be the true cause of these infections. In addition, appropriate collection of specimens from the infected site without contamination by normal flora often is difficult and sometimes is not possible. Communication with the laboratory of patient information regarding relevant risk factors or atypical clinical presentations, or when unusual pathogens are suspected, is key to adequate analysis of specimens. Similarly, laboratories should advise clinicians of the sensitivity and specificity of the routine tests available in their facility and should recommend special testing when indicated. These aspects of the microbiologic investigation of head and neck infections are reviewed here.

Normal flora or true pathogen?

Two main anatomic areas are heavily colonized with normal flora that may contribute to the development of head and neck infections: the oral

* Corresponding author. Division of Medical Microbiology and Infection Control and Regional Microbiology Lead, Vancouver General Hospital and Vancouver Coastal Health, Room 1112A JPPN Microbiology, 855 W. 12th Avenue, Vancouver, BC, Canada V5Z 1M9.

E-mail address: diane.roscoe@vch.ca (D.L. Roscoe).

doi:10.1016/j.idc.2007.03.012

cavity/upper respiratory tract and the skin. The flora at these two sites is similar qualitatively but may differ quantitatively. Organisms generally considered as commensals include coagulase-negative staphylococci, nonhemolytic and viridans streptococci, *Corynebacterium* spp, micrococci, saprophytic *Neisseria* spp, *Haemophilus* spp, and a wide range of anaerobes including Propionibacterium, Lactobacillus, Peptostreptococcus, and Veillonella. Other organisms commonly found at these sites but often thought of as pathogens include *Staphylococcus aureus*, *Streptococcus pneumoniae*, beta-hemolytic streptococci, *Neisseria meningitidis*, *Haemophilus influenzae* (serotype B, other serotypes, and non-typeable strains), *H parainfluenza*, *Moraxella catarrhalis*, and *Eikenella*, *Fusobacterium*, *Bacteroides*, *Prevotella*, *Porphyromonas,* and *Actinomyces* spp [1,2]. Spirochetes also are present in the oral cavity [3]. Gram-negative facultative organisms such as *Escherichia coli* and environmental organisms such as *Pseudomonas* spp are not generally part of the normal flora at these sites in healthy individuals. Fungi other than *Candida* spp and parasites are not components of the normal flora in the head and neck region. Viruses also are not part of the normal flora; however, some, such as the herpes viruses, can remain latent and become reactivated. Thus, recovery of these agents such as cytomegalovirus (CMV), herpes simplex virus (HSV), and varicella zoster virus (VZV), must be interpreted in the clinical context.

The diversity of anatomic structures and their microenvironment adds complexity, because both the type and number of the resident normal flora may vary at each site. In addition, the normal flora may change depending on age, general health, hygiene, antibiotics, smoking, hospitalization, and other conditions [2,4]. For example, an antecedent viral respiratory tract infection is known to increase colonization by *S aureus* and gram-negative bacilli [5]. In the presence of predisposing factors, such as immunosuppression, local tissue trauma, or dental disease, this complex flora consisting mostly of low-virulence organisms leads to local infections that often are polymicrobial. Unfortunately, even with organisms considered true pathogens, there is no fool-proof way to distinguish in the laboratory whether the organism detected is just a commensal or is the true offending agent. This difficulty underscores the importance of proper specimen collection and the need to correlate laboratory data with clinical information. In particular, relevant host factors should be kept in mind when interpreting microbiologic data and considering empiric antimicrobial therapy.

Specimen collection

The proper collection of specimens is a critical step in the accurate determination of the organism responsible for various infections of the head and neck [6]. The first challenge is to consider the likely differential diagnosis so that the best specimen (blood, serum, swab, aspirate, or tissue biopsy) is collected. Further challenges are (1) gaining access to the anatomically complex infection site, (2) avoiding contamination by overgrowth of normal flora that may affect interpretation of the culture results, and (3) maintaining viability of fastidious organisms within the specimen during transport.

Specimen collection should occur before administration of any anti-infective agents, if possible. If serologic testing is required, blood should be collected before intravenous immunoglobulin therapy. Timing of serologic tests in relation to the onset of symptoms is important because it may affect the ability to detect acute (presence of IgM) versus previous infection (presence of IgG alone).

Specimens should be collected in sufficient quantity, particularly if both direct examination and appropriate culture methods or special tests are required. Tissues or fluids from the site of infection are preferred, and the desired tests should be prioritized. The collection of specimens for fungal work-up requires a larger volume for inoculation to enhance the recovery of pathogenic fungi. Specimens should be labeled with at least the patient's name, the patient identification number, source of specimen, date and hour of collection, ordering physician's name, and any special requests.

Tissue biopsies are the preferred specimens and can be submitted in leak-proof sterile containers. Aspirates of pus or fluid specimens also can be submitted in a sterile container if the expected transport time to the microbiology laboratory is less than 2 hours. If a delay in transport to the laboratory is anticipated, the aspirate should be injected into aerobic and anaerobic transport tubes. Syringes should not be used for transport of specimen, both for safety and for specimen integrity. Collection of specimens with swabs should be avoided, particularly when a fastidious organism is suspected or if aspirates or biopsies are obtainable. If swabs are used, it is best to submit two separate specimens, one for direct examination and the second for culture. Cotton swabs, which may contain fatty acids that can inhibit the survival of certain fastidious organisms, should be avoided. Dacron or Rayon polyester-tipped swabs may be used if submitted in the appropriate transport media, such as Amies or Stuart's medium. Care should be taken to avoid drying out of the swab. Commercially available viral transport medium stabilizes viruses, inhibit overgrowth by bacteria and fungi, and should be used for swab specimens. Viral transport medium also is appropriate for viral antigen detection and nucleic acid tests [7]. For specimens from sterile sites such as vitreous fluid, transport in a sterile container is preferred, and viral transport medium is not required.

Specimens should be transported to the microbiology laboratory as soon as possible. Swabs may remain stable in transport medium for up to 48 hours. For viral testing, swabs and tissues should be submitted in viral transport medium if a delay in transport of more than 2 hours is anticipated. The specimens should be kept at 4°C if transport time is longer than 1 hour and frozen at −60°C and transported in dry ice if additional delay is expected. Many viruses are susceptible to freeze–thaw cycles, which can drastically compromise their viability. Specimens for fungal work-up also should be transported to the laboratory as soon as possible. Because their viability is easily affected by cold and heat, transport at room temperature is recommended. The exception is when the specimen is likely to be contaminated with bacterial flora, when 4°C conditions are required to inhibit bacterial overgrowth during transport. These temperature and time requirements apply to culture techniques, antigen detection methods, and nucleic acid testing.

Laboratory investigations

A variety of routine and special laboratory tests are available for the microbiologic investigation of head and neck infections. The most common causative agents in various head and neck infections and the laboratory methods recommended for their investigation are summarized in Table 1.

Examination of direct smears

The Gram stain is perhaps the only truly rapid and comprehensive test in diagnostic microbiology. Developed more than a century ago, it remains the first step in the microbiologic evaluation of most clinical specimens. A properly prepared Gram stain allows the detection of the number and general type of bacteria and also of the presence and nature of the inflammatory response. This information is particularly important for assessing whether the specimen sampled is from an infected site or whether the organisms present are more representative of the commensal flora. Also, the Gram stain is more likely to provide information about the most predominant organisms at the infected site, whereas cultures favor more rapidly growing bacteria that may mask other, more fastidious organisms that may be the true pathogens. When assessing the inflammatory response, the presence of many polymorphonuclear white blood cells suggests a bacterial cause, whereas the predominance of mononuclear white blood cells suggests viral or other agents that cause more chronic infections. Visualizing organisms within neutrophils (eg, the lancet-shaped gram-positive diplococci typical of *S pneumoniae*) suggests a causal relation with the patient's infection. Unfortunately, the Gram stain lacks specificity, and only rarely is the Gram stain appearance sufficient for a definitive identification; additional testing is usually necessary.

Direct examination for some microorganisms requires special stains that must be explicitly requested. *Mycobacteria* spp have a very lipid-rich cell wall that results in intense staining that cannot be removed by an acid decolorizing agent, hence the name "acid-fast bacilli." Examples of acid-fast stains include the auramine or auramine-rhodamine stain, Kinyoun stain, and Ziehl-Neelsen stain. The auramine stain is based on nonspecific binding

Table 1
Common laboratory procedures for the microbiologic diagnosis of head and neck infections

Infection	Common causative agents	Direct smear	Antigen detection	Serology	Histopathology	Molecular techniques	Culture
Ocular infections							
Conjunctivitis	Bacterial, viral	X	X				X
Blepharitis and dacryoadenitis	Bacterial, fungal, viral	X	DFA		X		X
Keratitis	Bacterial, viral, parasitic, fungal	X	DFA		X	X	X
Orbital and periorbital (preseptal) cellulitis	Mixed aerobes and anaerobes	X					X
Endophthalmitis	Bacterial, fungal	X			X	X	X
Chorioretinitis	Bacterial, fungal, viral, parasitic			X		X	X
Otitis externa and media	Bacterial, fungal	X					X
Sinusitis							
Acute	Bacterial	X					X
Chronic	Bacterial, fungal	X			X		X
Oropharyngeal infections							
Tonsillopharyngitis	Bacterial, viral	X	X			X	X
Epiglottitis	Bacterial, viral						X
Peritonsillar abscess	Bacterial	X					X
Mucositis and stomatitis	Bacterial, fungal, viral	X	X			X	X
Mandibular osteomyelitis and actinomycosis	Bacterial	X	X				X
Deep fascial space infections	Bacterial	X			X		X
Cervical lymphadenitis	Bacterial, fungal, viral, parasitic	X	X	X	X	X	X

Abbreviations: DFA, direct fluorescent immunoassay; X, procedure available.

of fluorochromes to mycolic acids present in the mycobacterial cell wall and is more sensitive and rapid than the other stains. *Nocardia* spp may be detected by Gram stain as long, slender, gram-positive branching bacilli but are partially acid-fast and can be identified more definitively using a modified acid-fast stain similar to that used for mycobacteria but with a less harsh decolorizing agent. Fungi may be seen on Gram stain but often are overlooked and are best visualized in specimens using a wet-mount made with calcofluor white. The latter is a nonspecific fluorochrome that binds to cellulose and chitin, allowing detection of fungal elements using a fluorescent microscope [8]. Calcofluor white is often combined with potassium hydroxide that helps breakdown the background cellular material, allowing better visualization of hyphae and yeasts. Potassium hydroxide can be used alone to prepare wet mounts for the detection of fungi if calcofluor white is not available but is less sensitive because of difficulty in visualizing fungal elements. Viruses can only be seen directly by electron microscopy. Parasites are detected primarily by examination of smears after concentration and staining, and specific requests should be submitted.

Direct detection of microbial antigens

A variety of commercial products is available to detect antigens of microorganisms directly in specimens or from organisms growing in culture. These assays fall under the large umbrella of immunoassays, because most use antibodies or antigens to detect complementary antigen or antibody in clinical specimens or from culture growth. Examples of these methods include precipitation reactions, latex agglutination, flocculation, direct and indirect fluorescent immunoassays, enzyme-linked immunoassays, and optical immunoassays. These methods have evolved extensively since first introduced, with improvements in ease of performance, sensitivity, specificity, cost effectiveness, and the adaptation to automation. These tests have several advantages including (1) detection of organisms before culture results are available, (2) detection of uncultivable or fastidious pathogens, (3) detection of organisms that might be unsafe to handle in the laboratory, and (4) detection of microbial products such as toxins. The pathogen-specific nature of these assays also is one of their disadvantages, however, because it limits each test to a single pathogen, and the tests often are valid for a limited range of specimen types. Some organisms that can be detected using these tests include *Chlamydia trachomatis*, *Legionella pneumophila*, *Neisseria gonorrhoeae*, group A streptococci, *Cryptococcus neoformans*, and a variety of viruses including influenza A and B, parainfluenza virus 1, 2, and 3, adenovirus, respiratory syncytial virus, HSV, and VZV. An antigen-detection method is available for the presence of *S pneumoniae,* group B streptococcus, *N meningitidis*, and *H influenzae* type B in sterile body fluids. Most *H influenzae* involved in head and neck infections are non-typeable, however, and these methods reportedly are no more sensitive than an accurately performed and interpreted Gram stain, making them not very useful clinically [9]. The early diagnosis of invasive aspergillosis by the detection of circulating Aspergillus cell wall antigens (galactomannan and beta-D-glucan) has been evaluated primarily in patients who had hematologic malignancies. The combination of galactomannan enzyme-linked immunoassays with polymerase chain reaction (PCR) seems to improve sensitivity and specificity for the detection of Aspergillus in bronchoalveolar lavage specimens, but its application in head and neck infections remains to be determined [10–13].

Microbial antigen detection can also be used for the rapid identification of organisms grown in culture. Common applications include the identification of beta-hemolytic streptococci as Lancefield groups A, B, C, and G, *N gonorrhoeae*, *L pneumophila*, and many viral agents.

Serology

The detection of antibodies against specific pathogens is one of the cornerstones of diagnosis of infectious diseases. The presence and type of antibodies in acute and convalescent sera can be helpful to determine the specific cause, particularly in the diagnosis of viral and parasitic infections. The diagnosis of infections such as measles, mumps, rubella, Epstein-Barr virus, CMV, and toxoplasmosis relies heavily on serologic testing. The presence of IgM suggests a recent infection, whereas IgG alone suggests that the infection may have been acquired some time in the past. In some cases the need to have both acute and convalescent serology to determine a change in titer limits the usefulness of serologic testing to a retrospective diagnosis.

Histopathologic examination

In conjunction with cultures, examination of tissue samples obtained by biopsies and stained with hematoxylin and eosin (H&E) offers the opportunity to detect microorganisms, assess their invasiveness, and evaluate the host response (eg, acute versus chronic or granulomatous inflammation). Tissue Gram stains are not very helpful for bacterial infections, but histopathologic examination can be most valuable when fungi, parasites, and other unusual organisms are suspected. Special stains are performed according to preliminary evaluation of the H&E sections. Some fungi have characteristic histopathologic morphology when evaluated by special stains such as Gomori methenamine silver, periodic acid-Schiff, and mucicarmine. Tissue acid-fast stains may detect *Mycobacterium* spp. H&E is particularly valuable to confirm Acanthamoeba infections of the cornea.

Molecular techniques

Molecular techniques have revolutionized the field of diagnostic microbiology and have become increasingly available, particularly in tertiary and quaternary centers. In most situations, molecular tests supplement but do not replace the more routine testing methods. The major advantages of genome-based tests include a reduced turn-around time for reporting, increased sensitivity for specimens in which low organism counts limit the detection by culture, and the ability to identify noncultivable organisms or detect potential pathogens when the patient has been treated with anti-infective agents [14]. Molecular methods, however, require special technical expertise and infrastructure and substantially increase the costs and complexity to the diagnostic microbiology laboratory.

Molecular techniques generally comprise of three procedural concepts: probe-based hybridization, DNA amplification, and nucleic acid detection assays. Probe-based assays rely on the detection of nucleic acid sequences that are complementary to that of the probe. These sequences are specific for a genus or species. Hybridization can be applied directly to clinical specimens, organisms isolated from culture, or nucleic acids extracted from clinical specimens, cultures, or amplified nucleic acids. The advantages and disadvantages of these tests depend on the specimen type, turn-around time, sensitivity, specificity, and costs [15]. Commercial hybridization assays (eg, AccuProbe, Gen-Probe, San Diego, CA, USA) are available for bacteria, mycobacteria, and fungi. Because of their relatively low sensitivity, probe-based assays have been limited to rapid identification of amplified nucleic acid products or cultures of mycobacteria and dimorphic fungi.

PCR is the most widely used and versatile procedure for nucleic acid amplification. With the existence of other amplification methods such as transcription-mediated amplification and strand displacement amplification, molecular testing should be referred to more appropriately as "nucleic acid amplification testing" (NAT or NAAT). There are numerous NAT assays for the detection of various bacteria, viruses, and parasites directly from clinical specimens, but these tests tend to be organism specific. For example, PCR tests with primers specifically targeting influenza A virus or *Bordetella pertussis* genomes are available and can be used routinely to detect these organisms from nasopharyngeal washes [16,17]. Detection of specific virulence genes is also available, such as PCR for shiga-like toxins from fecal samples in patients who have bloody diarrhea. The unique advantages and disadvantages of each amplification procedure are beyond the scope of this article. Depending on the assay used, the sensitivity, specificity, cost, and speed may vary. Sequence-based analysis is particularly useful for organisms that are poorly cultivable or for accurate species identification when traditional phenotypic methods have failed. In particular, analysis of *16S* rRNA gene sequences has greatly expanded the phylogenic identification of bacteria. The *16S* rRNA gene is universal and is highly conserved in bacteria but has sufficient variability in certain regions to allow genus- or species-specific identification. The gene sequences are compared with a large, publicly available reference databank to determine identical or closest-related organisms. Such assays have been particularly useful for the enumeration and characterization of the noncultivable indigenous microflora in the gingival crevice and dental surfaces in health and disease [18]. Currently, *16S* rRNA gene sequencing is used primarily by reference microbiology laboratories for the accurate identification of bacteria in pure cultures [19]. The use of molecular diagnostic tools for fungal infections is in the early stages of development.

After amplification, a detection method is required to evaluate the presence of specific gene sequences. Products can be detected by visualization on an agarose gel with or without prior restriction enzyme digestion, by enzyme immunoassay, by hybridization assays or direct DNA sequencing, and even by real-time PCR (the immediate detection of amplified product while the PCR reaction is underway).

The increased sensitivity of NAT assays is counterbalanced by the presence of intrinsic DNA or RNA enzyme inhibitors and by low copy numbers of target organisms in clinical specimens. Before a test is made available, it must undergo stringent evaluation and validation. One of the major challenges is defining the criterion to establish sensitivity and specificity of the test. For example, how does one know that a positive result indicates presence of the targeted pathogen in the clinical specimen rather than a nonspecific reaction or contamination by commensals? Similarly, how does one know that a negative result indicates true absence of the targeted gene in the sample tested and not a result of mutations in the genome of the organism?

Currently, very few molecular techniques have been evaluated for the rapid diagnosis of head and neck infections (see Table 1). It is best to consult the microbiology laboratory for their role and availability in the clinical setting.

Culture

Culture remains the mainstay of microbiologic investigation for head and neck infections. In general, the organisms of interest are not particularly fastidious, and with improvements in the isolation and identification of clinically important anaerobic organisms, culture is perhaps the most sensitive and readily available laboratory method to detect potential pathogens. The main drawback is difficulty in determining the specificity and significance of the culture results, because it often is impossible to ascertain which of the many organisms isolated are the most important for therapeutic decisions. Blood cultures are perhaps the best way to determine the most likely causative agent during an invasive infection and always should be obtained for seriously ill patients.

Specimens should be plated promptly, and a Gram stain should be prepared and interpreted in conjunction with the culture results. The routine battery of media for bacterial culture includes a nutrient agar plate with 5% sheep blood and a chocolate agar plate for more fastidious organisms such as *Haemophilus* spp. Anaerobic culture media and incubation should be included for tissue aspirates and biopsy specimens. Specimens from the mouth always grow anaerobes and are not cultured routinely for such. The morphology of oral organisms can be very characteristic based on Gram stain examination and may be a more reliable indicator for the presence of anaerobes. Specimens should be incubated at 35°C to 37°C and examined daily for up to 7 days. Most bacterial pathogens grow within 48 to 72 hours, but more fastidious organisms, such as *Haemophilus aphrophilus*, *Actinomyces* spp, and *Nocardia* spp, may take longer. Cultures for mycobacteria must be requested specifically so that the appropriate media are inoculated, and cultures are incubated for up to 8 weeks. Recent advances in automated culture technology using liquid media have greatly improved recovery and decreased the time to detection by several weeks [20]. Cultures for Chlamydia and Chlamydophila require special facilities and are rarely performed in the clinical microbiology laboratory except in research centers.

Rapidly growing yeasts and fungi, such as Aspergillus and Mucor, also grow in the routine battery of media set up for bacterial culture. If other fungi are suspected, however, a special fungal culture should be requested to ensure plating in special media to inhibit bacterial overgrowth and prolonged incubation for the more slowly growing organisms. Unfortunately, culturing to identify the etiology of invasive fungal disease has poor sensitivity, and the offending agent often is not recovered. *Aspergillus*, Zygomycetes, and *Fusarium* spp are common fungi that might be involved in these infections.

Viral cultures should be set up in appropriate cell lines and checked weekly for several weeks. Potential growth is identified by observing typical cytopathic effects, by comparing growth patterns in different cell lines, and by fluorescent antibody staining against the suspected agent. With the availability of direct antigen detection and molecular tests, viral cultures are performed less frequently than previously but still have a role in epidemiologic investigations for strain typing and for antiviral susceptibility testing.

With the exception of Acanthamoeba in suspected corneal infections, cultures are seldom performed for parasitic infections. Culture for Acanthoemeba requires co-inoculation of media previously seeded with a lawn of *E coli* or *Enterobacter aerogenes*. Cultures are observed under low-power (10×) microscopy and can be positive in as early as 2 to 3 days [21].

Antimicrobial susceptibility testing

The emergence of antibiotic resistance among many upper respiratory and oral organisms has made the performance of antimicrobial susceptibility testing an important priority. Among the common pathogens in head and neck infections, concern is greatest for methicillin-resistant *S aureus* (MRSA), penicillin-resistant *S pneumoniae*, macrolide-resistant group A streptococci, and beta-lactam resistant *H influenzae*. Molecular tools for the detection of resistance genes (eg, mecA in MRSA) have become more readily available. There also are excellent guidelines from the Clinical and Laboratory Standards Institute (CLSI, formerly NCCLS) for routine susceptibility testing of most bacteria, including strict anaerobes and fastidious organisms involved in head and neck infections [22–25]. These guidelines also address the detection of resistance in relevant pathogens.

Disk diffusion remains a common method for antibiotic susceptibility testing, and categorical results (S, susceptible; I, intermediate; or R, resistant) are reported. Microbroth dilution techniques provide more accurate assessment by determine the minimum inhibitory concentration (MIC), and results usually are translated according to accepted breakpoints and reported as susceptibility categories (S, I, or R). MIC information for certain antibiotics (eg, penicillin susceptibility of *S pyogenes* or *S pneumoniae*) may be useful for some deep-seated head and neck infections and can be requested from the clinical laboratory, if required.

Commercially available susceptibility testing systems are used widely in diagnostic microbiology laboratories. These systems generally use microbroth techniques and can either provide serial dilution MIC or breakpoint MIC results. Another widely used system is the Etest (AB Biodisk, Solna, Sweden), which allows MIC determination of antibiotics using antibiotic-impregnated strips and a predetermined antibiotic gradient. This technology is readily available in most clinical laboratories and has been validated for a wide range of microorganisms compared with reference methods, including anaerobes and fastidious microbes [26,27].

Susceptibility testing for strict anaerobes is not performed routinely in many laboratories and usually is restricted to isolates recovered from blood cultures, normally sterile body fluids, or for serious infections. As with other organisms, antibiotic resistance has been increasingly recognized for oral anaerobes against penicillin, cefoxitin, and clindamycin, and periodic surveillance testing is warranted to provide information on local susceptibility patterns within specific health care centers [28].

Antifungal susceptibility testing has lagged because of technical difficulties and uncertainty in the interpretation of results. As these methods become better standardized, critical information on the correlation between laboratory results and clinical outcome becomes better understood. Guidelines for the performance of antifungal susceptibility testing by both broth dilution and disk diffusion, primarily for *Candida* spp, are also available from the CLSI [29,30]. Antifungal susceptibility testing of molds is under development also but is much more difficult to standardize because of the dimorphic growth characteristics of these organisms.

Considerations in specific head and neck infections

A wide variety of etiologic agents may be encountered in various head and neck infections. The more common pathogens and their laboratory diagnosis are summarized in Table 1 and are discussed briefly here.

Ocular infections

Conjunctivitis

Conjunctivitis is caused most commonly by bacterial and viral pathogens. Bacterial causes include *S aureus*, *S pneumoniae*, *H influenzae*, *M catarrhalis*, *N gonorrhoeae*, *N meningitides*, *C trachomatis*, and less commonly by enteric gram-negative rods including *E coli*, Proteus, and Klebsiella. Viral causes include adenovirus (serotypes 8, 11, and 19 can cause epidemic keratoconjunctivitis), herpes viruses (HSV and VZV), and Coxsackie and enteroviruses. A moist swab should be passed over the conjunctiva, avoiding the eyelids and lashes that may harbor resident skin flora, and the specimen should be placed in bacterial and/or viral transport medium for appropriate examination. The confirmation of chlamydial conjunctivitis is difficult, because commercial NAT systems for Chlamydia are approved for testing genital specimens only. Currently, direct fluorescent immunoassay is one option to confirm this infection [31]. Another alternative is the examination of conjunctival scrapings stained with Giemsa and examined for the presence of intracytoplasmic inclusions, but this method is less sensitive.

Blepharitis and dacryocystitis

Common organisms implicated in blepharitis and dacryocystitis, including Staphylococci, Streptococci, *Haemophilus* spp, enteric gram-negative bacilli, and anaerobic organisms, normally are present also in the nasal passages and/or contiguous skin, [32]. *Actinomyces israeli* is the most commonly identified pathogen in dacryocystitis, but many other pathogens including *Candida* spp, Aspergillus, HSV, and VZV have been implicated also. Purulent material should be sent for direct examination and appropriate culture.

Keratitis

Corneal ulcers can be caused by bacterial, viral, parasitic, and fungal pathogens. The major bacterial causes are *Staphylococcus* spp, *S pneumoniae*, beta-hemolytic streptococci, *Bacillus* spp, particularly *B cereus*, Haemophilus, Moraxella, Pseudomonas, and gram-negative enteric bacilli. *Mycobacterium* spp and *Nocardia* spp are increasingly recognized in postsurgical and post-trauma patients. Contact lens wearers are at risk for fungal infections, particularly *Fusarium* spp, as well as Pseudomonas and Acanthamoeba infections. Corneal scrapings should be collected with a sterile platinum spatula. Direct examination may not be very helpful for bacterial and fungal identification, but direct antigen detection may be valuable for the rapid diagnosis of viral causes, particularly herpesviruses and adenoviruses. Molecular tests by PCR are available also for these agents. The detection of Acanthamoeba requires special culture procedures, as described previously. Alternately, a corneal biopsy for histopathologic examination may detect the presence of parasites.

Preseptal (periorbital) and orbital cellulitis

Preseptal cellulitis generally arises from a local bacterial infection, such as conjunctivitis or impetigo, whereas orbital cellulitis may result as an extension of infection from the adjacent sinuses. The causative organism may vary according to predisposing conditions. When associated with spread from sinus infections, *S pneumoniae*, *H influenzae* (usually nontypeable), *S aureus*, and *M catarrhalis* are the most common organisms. Fungal causes such as aspergillosis and mucormycosis are encountered occasionally, and histopathologic examination along with cultures may be helpful. Blood cultures should be collected but seldom are positive.

Endophthalmitis

Endophthalmitis most commonly occurs following penetrating ocular trauma, intraocular surgery, and sometimes after hematogenous seeding. It may be caused by a range of pathogens, most commonly Staphylococcus, Streptococcus, Propionibacterium, *Candida albicans*, and occasionally enteric gram-negative bacteria. Superficial swabs are not useful for microbiologic diagnosis, and vitreous or aqueous aspirates are required for appropriate culture. Vitreous biopsies may also be obtained. Negative cultures do not rule out an infectious cause, because the sensitivity of cultures is poor. Culture of vitreous washings after filtration may increase the yield, and blood cultures always should be obtained. Molecular diagnostic tools are being investigated [33].

Chorioretinitis

Chorioretinitis syndromes pose a diagnostic challenge for many of the reasons cited previously. A wide range of organisms can cause chorioretinitis, and the clinical presentation is not always diagnostic. Appropriate specimens for investigation are difficult to collect without compromising vision. Tissue examination usually is not possible until late in the disease, and other available techniques are not sensitive enough for early diagnosis. The most common causes include VZV, HSV 1 and 2, and, less commonly, CMV, *Toxoplasma gondii*, *Treponema pallidum*, *Candida* spp, *Mycobacterium tuberculosis*, and Toxocara. HIV-infected patients may have disease caused by other fungi (eg, Histoplasma, Coccidioides, Pneumocystis), bacteria (eg, *Mycobacterium avium-intracellulare*) or viruses (eg, *Mulloscum contagiosum*). To date, the diagnosis of chorioretinitis primarily is made clinically, and the suspected cause is confirmed by serologic tests, if available. Newer molecular assays on aqueous or vitreous fluid for specific viruses, the most common cause of this syndrome, offer some promise [34].

Otitis externa and interna

Otitis externa

The normal flora of the skin extends into the external ear canal; hence, *S aureus* is a common cause of external otitis. Prior colonization with other organisms may follow certain activities, such as swimming ("swimmer's ear"), and gram-negative rods, particularly *Pseudomonas* spp, *E coli*, and *Proteus* spp may be isolated. Fungi such as *Aspergillus niger* and *C albicans* may be causative agents. A more serious form is malignant otitis externa, an invasive infection most often caused by *Pseudomonas aeruginosa*. The most common predisposing factor is diabetes mellitus [35]. This infection may begin in the external canal but aggressively invades the soft tissues, including cartilage and temporal bone, and may lead to petrous osteomyelitis. Cultures of purulent drainage from the external canal or biopsy specimens reveal the offending pathogen.

Otitis media

Determination of the exact cause of otitis media requires aspiration of the middle ear effusion by tympanocentesis. The primary pathogens in this setting usually are aerobic and facultative bacteria and occasionally may involve anaerobes. In younger children, the most common organisms are *S pneumoniae*, *M catarrhalis*, and nontypeable *H influenzae*. In older children and adults, the most common pathogens are *S pneumoniae*, group A streptococcus, *S aureus*, and, less commonly, *H influenzae*. Chronic otitis media may be caused more commonly by gram-negative bacteria and by *S aureus*. Routine aerobic and anaerobic cultures determine the bacterial cause in most cases. Viral cultures usually are not performed, even though an antecedent viral upper respiratory tract infection is the most likely predisposing factor leading to a secondary bacterial infection of the middle ear.

Acute and chronic sinusitis

The microbiologic diagnosis of acute sinusitis can be achieved reliably only by sinus puncture or endoscopic procedures. Collection through the nasal cavity results in contamination by the resident flora including *S aureus*. Appropriate specimens should be collected from sinus washings, aspirates, scrapings, or tissue biopsies.

Acute sinusitis

Predominant organisms in acute maxillary and ethmoid sinusitis usually are *S pneumoniae* and non-typeable *H influenzae* [36,37]. One study found the incidence of acute rhinosinusitis caused by MRSA to be 2.7%, with nasal surgery and prior antibiotic use as the major risk factors [38]. Increasing prevalence rates of penicillin- and macrolide-resistant *S pneumoniae* are noted [39]. Predominant anaerobic bacteria include *Prevotella*, *Porphyromonas*, *Fusobacterium*, and *Peptostreptococcus* spp, primarily in cases of maxillary sinusitis secondary to odontogenic infections. Very few studies have examined for atypical bacteria such as *Chlamydophila pneumoniae* and *Mycoplasma pneumoniae*; however, PCR tests for these organisms have been evaluated for respiratory specimens [40]. Viral cultures usually are not performed, even though a viral upper respiratory tract infection is the most common antecedent event of a purulent bacterial sinusitis.

Unlike community-acquired sinusitis, which frequently results from a viral respiratory infection, nosocomial sinusitis most commonly occur after nasopharyngeal intubation in mechanically ventilated patients. Infections are often polymicrobial and include gram-negative bacilli such as *P aeruginosa*, *Serratia marcescens*, *Klebsiella pneumoniae*, *Enterobacter* spp, and *Proteus mirabilis* [41,42].

Chronic sinusitis

The predominant pathogens in chronic sinusitis usually are anaerobes and *S aureus*, as well as fungi [43]. The fungi include *Aspergillus* spp, *Pseudoallescheria* (*P boydii*), and Zygomycetes (eg, *Mucor* spp, *Rhizopus* spp, and *Cunninghamella* spp). Identification of fungal elements on direct examination is highly suggestive of their pathogenic role, but histopathologic confirmation from tissue biopsy of the sinus cavity is required.

Oropharyngeal infections

Tonsillopharyngitis

Acute tonsillopharyngitis is caused most commonly by viruses or atypical bacterial agents including *M pneumoniae* and *C pneumoniae*, usually as part of an upper respiratory tract infection. Common viral causes include rhinovirus, coronavirus, adenovirus, influenza and parainfluenza viruses, Coxsackie virus, HSV, EBV, and CMV. Primary HIV infection also is associated with acute pharyngitis and viremia. Investigation for the specific viral cause of acute tonsillopharyngitis usually is not performed except when HIV or infectious mononucleosis is suspected. Approximately 30% of the cases of acute tonsillopharyngitis are caused by bacteria, most commonly group A streptococci [44]. Because it is not possible to distinguish bacterial from viral causes by clinical presentation alone, laboratory studies should be performed to exclude the possibility of group A streptococcus to avoid unnecessary antibiotic therapy. Other beta-hemolytic streptococci, such as groups C and G, also have been reported to cause acute pharyngitis but rarely are associated with postinfectious complications. *Arcanobacterium hemolyticum* has been reported to cause a scarlet fever-like syndrome that occurs primarily in late adolescents and young adults [45,46]. Other less common causes of acute pharyngitis include *N gonorrhoeae*, *Corynebacterium diphtheriae*, *Corynebacterium ulcerans*, *Yersinia enterocolitica*, *T pallidum*, and *Francisella tularensis*. If these agents are suspected, this suspicion should be communicated to the clinical microbiology laboratory because special media and techniques are required for their detection.

Swab specimens should be obtained by rubbing the tonsils and the posterior pharynx. These specimens can be submitted either for routine throat culture or rapid antigen detection methods. The diagnosis of group A streptococcal pharyngitis has been one of the widest applications of rapid detection technology. A variety of commercial kits are available. Because the specificity of these tests is high, usually 95% or greater, a positive rapid test can be considered equivalent to a positive throat culture, and culture confirmation is unnecessary. Because the sensitivity of these tests only ranges from 70% to 90%, a negative test should be confirmed by routine throat culture [47–49]. False-negative cultures are uncommon when performed properly by trained technologists using appropriate culture methods. Culture is also necessary for the detection of other beta-hemolytic streptococci such as group C or G, and for Arcanobacterium.

Epiglottitis

The epidemiology of epiglottitis has changed dramatically in children with the widespread use of the Haemophilus type B vaccine. This infection now is more prevalent in adults, and common causes include *S pneumoniae*, beta-hemolytic streptococci, *S aureus*, *M catarrhalis*, and both non-typeable and type B *H influenzae* [50]. Attempts to obtain cultures from the oropharynx in patients suspected of having epiglottitis may precipitate complete airway obstruction and should not be undertaken unless the patient's airway is secure. Blood cultures may be positive and always should be obtained.

Peritonsillar abscess (quinsy)

Peritonsillar abscess usually spreads from a contiguous focus in the tonsils or the peripharyngeal area. Again, bacterial causes include Streptococcus and Staphylococcus along with oral anaerobic organisms. Needle aspiration of any tonsillar mass or abscess is required for routine bacterial culture.

Mucositis and stomatitis

Patients who are immunocompromised because of malignancy or chemotherapy are at great risk for local or systemic infection because of the breakdown of the normal oropharyngeal mucosal barrier. The wide range of facultative and anaerobic organisms that normally colonize the oral cavity complicates the determination of specific infectious agents in this setting. Additionally, the patient's prior therapies and hospitalization may have resulted in colonization with enteric gram-negative bacteria that are not normally present in healthy individuals. Thus, swabs from the oral cavity for routine bacterial culture are not very helpful.

In patients who have acute ulcerative gingivitis ("trench mouth"), a Gram stain obtained from inflammatory exudates of local lesions may be more useful than cultures. The presence of long, slender, spindle-shaped gram-negative bacilli (fusiforms or Fusobacterium) in association with oral spirochetes is characteristic of this condition.

Candidal stomatitis is another entity in which the Gram stain provides useful information. White patches present in the oral cavity should be swabbed and cultured. If present, *Candida* spp will be identified by the presence of budding yeasts and pseudohyphae, which suggests active replication of organisms.

Other possible causes of ulcerative lesions in the oral cavity include HSV and VZV, Coxsackie virus, and enteroviruses. The base of these lesions should be scraped and sent for viral antigen detection and culture. Herpes viruses can be detected by the rapid antigen detection methods, but culture is required to determine the presence of other viruses such as coxsackie viruses, a common cause of herpangina and hand, foot, and mouth disease.

Mandibular osteomyelitis and actinomycosis

Mandibular osteomyelitis

Mandibular osteomyelitis secondary to odontogenic infections usually is caused by low-virulence bacteria from the normal oral flora, such as viridans streptococci, *Staphylococcus* spp, *Peptostreptococcus* spp, *Bacteroides* spp, and other oral anaerobes. Rarely, fungi and mycobacteria may be the causative agents. Specimens should include needle aspiration of loculated pus by an extraoral approach or bone biopsy using an open or closed procedure. These specimens should be submitted for routine microbiologic and histopathologic examination. Special requests for acid-fast mycobacteria and fungi may be warranted based on clinical suspicion.

Actinomycosis

Cervicofacial actinomycosis typically occurs following a dental infection or oromaxillofacial trauma. *A israeli* is the most common pathogen, but other species can be involved, including *A naeslundii*, *A odontolyticus*, *A viscosus*, *A meyeri*, and *A gerencseriae*. With the increasingly use of *16S* rRNA sequencing, the spectrum of *Actinomyces* spp in clinical disease has expanded to include species that have never before been described [51].

Actinomyces are small, non–spore-forming, gram-positive rods that grow in anaerobic or microaerophilic conditions. A key characteristic of actinomycosis is the finding of "sulfur granules" from clinical specimens. These granules are pigmented grains that appear macroscopically as sulfur granules but in fact are a conglomerate of bacteria. When sulfur granules are seen, they should be sent to the microbiology laboratory along with the tissue biopsy or fluid aspirate. The granules, crushed between two glass slides and Gram stained, can demonstrate beaded, branching gram-positive bacilli characteristic of Actinomyces. Sulfur granules also can be identified by histopathologic examination. Although other bacteria and fungi (particularly *Nocardia* spp and *Streptomyces madurae*) may produce similar granules at infected sites, these can be distinguished by the absence of peripheral clubs that are specific to *Actinomyces* spp.

Deep fascial space infections

Infections of deep fascial spaces

The microbiology of deep fascial space infections is usually polymicrobial, consisting of mixed anaerobic and facultative oral bacteria. Common pathogens include Bacteroides, Fusobacterium, Prevotella, Porphyromonas, anaerobic and microaerophilic streptococci, *Actinomyces* spp, and *Eikenella* spp [52–54]. Of note is the increasing resistance of oral *Bacteroides* spp to penicillin and of *Eikenella corrodens* to clindamycin. Fungal causes, such as histoplasmosis in susceptible hosts living in endemic areas, also can occur [55]. Tuberculosis needs to be considered in the microbiologic investigation of prevertebral space infection, as in Pott's disease. Diagnosis may be difficult because many patients have negative purified protein derivative skin tests, and cultures may be negative. Collection of appropriate specimens often is challenging because of the complex anatomy of the area. Blood cultures also may yield the causative organism and should be collected. In many instances, surgical drainage is required for definitive treatment, and microbiologic work-up is secondary, primarily for the detection of resistant microorganisms.

Necrotizing fasciitis

Necrotizing fasciitis in the head and neck region is a medical emergency requiring aggressive surgical débridement of necrotic tissues [56]. Again, the pathogens usually are polymicrobial and may include oral anaerobes, *Streptococcus* spp, and *S aureus*. For definitive microbiologic investigation, the spreading edge of necrotic tissues is the best specimen and should be obtained by aspiration or surgical débridement.

Lemierre's disease

Identification of *Fusobacterium necrophorum* from blood cultures in a septic patient should suggest the possibility of Lemierre's syndrome or suppurative jugular thrombophlebitis. Metastatic infection involving the lung, joints, bone, spleen, and meninges is common [57]. *F necrophorum* is the most virulent species of Fusobacterium, producing several virulence factors such as exotoxins, proteolytic enzymes, and hemolysin. Unlike *Fusobacterium nucleatum*, *F necrophorum* can be misinterpreted on Gram stain, because these bacteria often appear as pleomorphic, small, gram-negative bacilli rather than being spindle shaped. Species often can be identified by standard phenotypic methods using commercial systems. Other common causative agents that can cause Lemierre's disease include *Bacteroides* spp and *Prevotella* spp.

Cervical lymphadenitis

Infectious causes of cervical lymphadenitis are quite variable. The most common bacterial causes include *S aureus* and *Streptococcus pyogenes*.

Less common are other streptococci, *H influenzae*, *Corynebacterium* spp, *Actinomyces* spp, and other oral anaerobes. Bacteria with unique epidemiologic factors include *F tularensis*, *Yersinia* spp, *Brucella* spp, *Bartonella henselae*, and *Bacillus anthracis*. Viral causes include EBV, CMV, HSV, adenovirus, HIV, and human T-lymphotropic virus.

Mycobacteria, including *M tuberculosis*, *M avium-intracellulare* complex, *Mycobacterium scrofulaceum*, or other ubiquitous atypical mycobacteria, are particularly common in this setting. Additional causes include *B henselae*, the causative agent of cat-scratch disease, which can be detected by PCR. Fungal etiologies include Aspergillus, *C albicans*, *C neoformans,* Sporothrix, and Histoplasma. Parasitic causes include *T gondii*, which is ubiquitous, and in certain parts of the world, Leishmania, Trypanosoma, and Filaria. Aspirates from inflamed lymph nodes or excisional biopsies should be sent for culture of bacteria, mycobacteria, and fungi and for histopathologic examination. Serologic tests also may be useful, particularly in toxoplasmosis.

Summary

The microbiologic investigation of head and neck infections is challenging because of the anatomic complexity in this region and the difficulty in appropriate specimen sampling and collection. The majority of infections result from commensal organisms that are part of the normal flora of the oral cavity, upper respiratory tract, and the skin. Other pathogens such as *Mycobacterium* spp, invasive fungi, and a host of viruses also cause disease in this area. Key to successful laboratory diagnosis includes recognizing the likely causative agents, determining the best specimen type for investigation, avoiding contamination from commensal organisms during specimen collection, and communication with the clinical microbiology laboratory regarding specimen collection, transport, and testing for suspected pathogens.

Acknowledgment

The authors thank Dr. Eva Thomas, Children's & Women's Hospital, Vancouver, BC, for her review and suggestions regarding viral diagnostics.

References

[1] Mackowiak PA. The normal microbial flora. N Engl J Med 1982;307:83–93.
[2] Skinner FA, Carr JG, editors. The normal microbial flora of man. New York: Academic Press; 1974.
[3] Dewhirst FE, Tamer MA, Ericson RE, et al. The diversity of periodontal spirochaetes by 16s rRNA analysis. Oral Microbiol Immunol 2000;15:196–202.

[4] Hardie J. Microbial flora of the oral cavity. In: Schuster GS, editor. Oral microbiology and infectious disease. Baltimore (MD): Williams and Wilkins; 1983. p. 162.
[5] Ramirez-Ronda CH, Fuxench-Lopez Z, Nevarez M. Increased pharyngeal bacterial colonization during viral illness. Arch Intern Med 1981;141:1599–603.
[6] Wilson ML. General principles of specimen collection and transport. Clin Infect Dis 1996; 22:766–7.
[7] Gleaves CA, Rice DH, Lee CF. Evaluation of an enzyme immunoassay for the detection of herpes simplex virus antigen from clinical specimens in viral transport media. J Virol Methods 1990;28:133–9.
[8] Hageage GJ, Harrington BJ. Use of calcofluor white in clinical mycology. Lab Med 1984;15: 109–12.
[9] Perkins MD, Mirrett S, Reller LB. Rapid bacterial antigen detection is not clinically useful. J Clin Microbiol 1995;33:1486–91.
[10] Marr KA, Balajee SA, McLaughlin L, et al. Detection of Galactomannan antigenemia by enzyme immunoassay for the diagnosis of invasive aspergillosis: variables that affect performance. J Infect Dis 2004;190:641–9.
[11] Odabasi Z, Mattiuzzi G, Estey E. B-D-Glucan as a diagnostic adjunct for invasive fungal infections: validation, cutoff development, and performance in patients with acute myelogenous leukemia and myelodysplastic syndrome. Clin Infect Dis 2004;39:199–205.
[12] Musher B, Fredricks D, Leisenring W, et al. Aspergillus galactomannan enzyme immunoassay and quantitative PCR for diagnosis of invasive aspergillosis with bronchoalveolar lavage fluid. J Clin Microbiol 2004;42:5517–22.
[13] Verdaguer V, Walsh TJ, Hope W, et al. Galactomannan antigen detection in the diagnosis of invasive aspergillosis. Expert Rev Mol Diagn 2007;7:21–32.
[14] Kotilainen P, Heiro M, Jalava J, et al. Aetiological diagnosis of infective endocarditis by direct amplification of rRNA genes from surgically removed valve tissue. An 11-year experience in a Finnish teaching hospital. Ann Med 2006;38:263–73.
[15] Amann RI, Ludwig W, Schleifer K-H. Phylogenetic identification and *in situ* detection of individual microbial cells without cultivation. Microbiol Rev 1995;59:143–69.
[16] Zitterkopf NL, Leekha S, Espy MJ, et al. Relevance of influenza A virus detection by PCR, shell vial assay, and tube cell culture to rapid reporting procedures. J Clin Microbiol 2006;44: 3366–7.
[17] Public Health Agency of Canada. Proceedings of the National Microbiology Laboratory Pertussis Workshop. Canada Communicable Disease Report 2006;32:1–22.
[18] Kroes I, Lepp PW, Relman DA. Bacterial diversity within the human subgingival crevice. Proc Natl Acad Sci U S A 1999;96:14547–52.
[19] Clarridge JE 3rd. Impact of 16S rRNA gene sequence analysis for identification of bacteria on clinical microbiology and infectious diseases. Clin Microbiol Rev 2004;17:840–62.
[20] Whyte T, Hanahoe B, Collins T, et al. Evaluation of the BACTEC MGIT 960 and MB/BacT systems for routine detection of *Mycobacterium tuberculosis*. J Clin Microbiol 2000;38: 3131–2.
[21] Visvesvara GS, et al. Pathogenic and opportunistic free living amoebae. In: Patrick PR, Baron EJ, Jorgensen JH, et al, editors. Manual of clinical microbiology. 8th edition. Washington, DC: ASM Press; 2003. p. 1981–9.
[22] Clinical and Laboratory Standards Institute. Methods for dilution antimicrobial susceptibility tests for bacteria that grow aerobically [CLSI document M7–A7]. Wayne (PA): Clinical and Laboratory Standards Institute; 2006.
[23] Clinical and Laboratory Standards Institute. Performance standards for antimicrobial disk susceptibility tests. [CLSI document M2–A9]. Wayne (PA): Clinical and Laboratory Standards Institute; 2006.
[24] Clinical and Laboratory Standards Institute. Methods for antimicrobial susceptibility testing of anaerobic bacteria; approved standard. 7th edition. [CLSI document M11–A7]. Wayne (PA): Clinical and Laboratory Standards Institute; 2007.

[25] Clinical and Laboratory Standards Institute. Methods for antimicrobial dilution and disk susceptibility testing of infrequently isolated or fastidious bacteri. 1st edition. [CLSI document M45-A]. Wayne (PA): Clinical and Laboratory Standards Institute; 2006.
[26] Baker CN, Stocker SA, Culver DH, et al. Comparison of the E test to agar dilution, broth microdilution and agar diffusion susceptibility testing techniques by using a special challenge set of bacteria. J Clin Microbiol 1991;29:533–8.
[27] Huang M, Baker PN, Banerjee S, et al. Accuracy of the E test for determining antimicrobial susceptibilities of staphylococci, enterococci, Campylobacter jejuni, and gram negative bacteria resistant to antimicrobial agents. J Clin Microbiol 1992;30:3243–8.
[28] Koeth LM, Good CE, Appelbaum PC, et al. Surveillance of susceptibility patterns in 1297 European and US anaerobic and capnophilic isolates to co-amoxiclav and five other antimicrobial agents. J Antimicrob Chemother 2004;53:1039–44.
[29] Clinical and Laboratory Standards Institute. Reference method for broth dilution antifungal susceptibility testing of yeasts; approved standard. 2nd edition. [CLSI document M27-A2]. Wayne (PA): Clinical and Laboratory Standards Institute; 2002.
[30] Clinical and Laboratory Standards Institute. Method for antifungal disk diffusion susceptibility testing; approved standard. 1st edition. [CLSI document M44-A]. Wayne (PA): Clinical and Laboratory Standards Institute; 2004.
[31] Elnifro EM, Cooper RJ, Klapper PE, et al. Diagnosis of viral and chlamydial keratoconjunctivitis: which laboratory test? Br J Ophthalmol 1999;83:622–7.
[32] Hartikainen J, Lehtonen OP, Matti Saari K. Bacteriology of lacrimal duct obstruction in adults. Br J Ophthalmol 1997;81:37–40.
[33] Chow AW. Future and emerging treatments for microbial infections. In: Rootman J, editor. Proceedings of the Vancouver Orbital Symposium. New York: Marcel Dekker; 2005. p. 45–64.
[34] Tran THC, Rozenberg F, Cassoux N, et al. Polymerase chain reaction analysis of aqueous humour samples in necrotising retinitis. Br J Ophthalmol 2003;87:79–83.
[35] Salit IE, McNeely DJ, Chait. Invasive external otitis: review of 12 cases. Can Med Assoc J 1985;132:381–5.
[36] Brook I. Bacteriology of acute and chronic ethmoid sinusitis. J Clin Microbiol 2005;43: 3479–80.
[37] Brook I, Foote PA, Hausfeld JN. Frequency of recovery of pathogens causing acute maxillary sinusitis in adults before and after introduction of vaccination of children with the 7-valent pneumococcal vaccine. J Med Microbiol 2006;55(Pt 7):943–6.
[38] Huang WH, Hung PK. Methicillin-resistant *Staphylococcus aureus* infections in acute rhinosinusitis. Laryngoscope 2006;116:288–91.
[39] Chen DK, McGeer A, de Azavedo JC, et al. Decreased susceptibility of *Streptococcus pneumoniae* to fluoroquinolones in Canada. Canadian Bacterial Surveillance Network. N Engl J Med 1999;341:233–9.
[40] Welti M, Jaton K, Altwegg M, et al. Development of a multiplex real-time quantitative PCR assay to detect *Chlamydia pneumoniae*, *Legionella pneumophila* and *Mycoplasma pneumoniae* in respiratory tract secretions. Diagn Microbiol Infect Dis 2003;45:85–95.
[41] George DL, Falk PS, Meduri GU, et al. Nosocomial sinusitis in patients in the medical intensive care unit: a prospective epidemiological study. Clin Infect Dis 1998;27:463–70.
[42] Rouby J-J, Laurent P, Gosnach M, et al. Risk factors and clinical relevance of nosocomial maxillary sinusitis in the critically ill. Am J Respir Crit Care Med 1994;150:776–83.
[43] Brook I, Foote PA, Frazier EH. Microbiology of acute exacerbation of chronic sinusitis. Ann Otol Rhinol Laryngol 2005;114:573–6.
[44] Bisno AL. Acute pharyngitis. N Engl J Med 2001;344:205–11.
[45] Mackenzie A, Fuite LA, Chan FTH, et al. Incidence and pathogenicity of Arcanobacterium during a 2 year study in Ottawa. Clin Infect Dis 1995;21:177–81.
[46] Banck G, Nyman M. Tonsillitis and rash associated with *Corynebacterium haemolyticum*. J Infect Dis 1986;154:1037–40.

[47] Bourbeau PP. Role of the microbiology laboratory in diagnosis and management of pharyngitis. J Clin Microbiol 2003;41:3467–72.
[48] Gerber MA, Shulman ST. Rapid diagnosis of pharyngitis caused by group A streptococci. Clin Microbiol Rev 2004;17:571–80.
[49] Bisno AL, Gerber MA, Gwaltney JM, et al. Practice guidelines for the diagnosis and management of group A streptococcal pharyngitis. Clin Infect Dis 2002;35:113–25.
[50] Shah RK, Roberson DW, Jones DT. Epiglottitis in the *Haemophilus influenzae* type B vaccine era: changing trends. Laryngoscope 2004;114:557–60.
[51] Hall V, Talbot PR, Stubbs SL, et al. Identification of clinical isolates of Actinomyces species by amplified 16S ribosomal DNA restriction analysis. J Clin Microbiol 2001;39:3555–62.
[52] Baker AS, Montgomery WW. Oropharyngeal space infections. Curr Clin Top Infect Dis 1987;8:227–65.
[53] Gidley PW, Ghorayeb BY, Stiernberg CM. Contemporary management of deep neck space infections. Otolaryngol Head Neck Surg 1997;116:16–22.
[54] Sakaguchi M, Sato S, Ishiyama T, et al. Characterization and management of deep neck infections. Int J Oral Maxillofac Surg 1997;26:131–4.
[55] Ezzedine K, Accoceberry I, Malvy D. Oral histoplasmosis after radiation therapy for laryngeal squamous cell carcinoma. J Am Acad Dermatol 2006 Nov 16; [Epub ahead of print].
[56] Chattar-Cora D, Tulsyan N, Cudjoe EA, et al. Necrotizing fasciitis of the head and neck: a report of two patients and review. Head Neck 2002;24:497–501.
[57] Riordan T, Wilson M. Lemierre's syndrome: more than a historical curiosa. Postgrad Med J 2004;80:328–33.

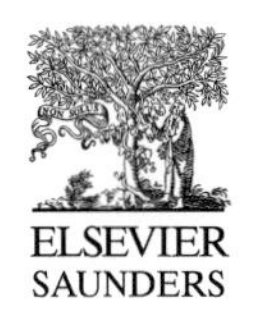
ELSEVIER
SAUNDERS

Infect Dis Clin N Am 21 (2007) 305–353

INFECTIOUS
DISEASE CLINICS
OF NORTH AMERICA

Imaging Studies for Head and Neck Infections

Michael C. Hurley, MRCPI, FRCR, FFR(RCSI), Manraj K.S. Heran, MD, FRCPC*

Division of Neuroradiology, Vancouver General Hospital, 899 West 12th Avenue, Vancouver, BC, Canada V5Z 1M9

Imaging techniques

Plain radiography, although easily accessible, rarely is helpful [1,2]. In limited circumstances, such as in confirming acute sinusitis, retropharyngeal swelling, or epiglottitis, conventional radiography may suffice. Even then, however, it rarely precludes more definitive imaging, which should not be delayed in the acutely unwell patient.

Ultrasound can characterize soft tissue neck masses and collections but is limited by its inability to penetrate bone or air-filled structures, its operator dependency, and variable reproducibility in serial imaging [3]. Ultrasound often is considered first-line imaging in the pediatric patient, whose smaller neck is more amenable to interrogation, and when avoiding radiation exposure is at a premium. Cross-sectional imaging, however, often is necessary for further evaluation.

Nuclear isotope studies can provide specific information. Examples of the usefulness of nuclear medicine imaging are ^{111}Indium-labeled leukocytes or ^{99m} Technetium (^{99m}Tc)-labeled antigranulocyte antibodies to confirm the diagnosis and location of infection and ^{99m}Tc-labeled methylene diphosphonate bone scan to detect early osteomyelitis [4].

The choice of a CT versus MRI examination depends on the region of interest and is discussed in each case. In general, CT gives higher spatial and temporal resolution. Multidetector CT scanning can generate isometric voxels, allowing multiplanar reformats with minimal artifact [2,5], negating the previous requirement for separate axial and coronal scans for the temporal bones, orbits, and paranasal sinuses [6]. Minimal slice thickness and

* Corresponding author.
E-mail address: manraj.heran@vch.ca (M.K.S. Heran).

doi:10.1016/j.idc.2007.04.001

pixel size is 0.5 mm to 0.75 mm, depending on the manufacturer, and allows resolution of structures as small as 1 mm if there is sufficient contrast, as in the temporal bone. Rapid data acquisition, over several seconds, minimizes motion artifact and patient discomfort and maximizes throughput, making CT the study of choice for acute and emergency cases. Timed intravenous contrast gives improved soft tissue resolution, although resolution may remain poor in cachectic patients, who usually lack adequate fat planes in the neck to allow regional analysis. CT gives excellent visualization of osseous structures, particularly of the temporal bones and paranasal sinuses, whereas bony anatomy usually is demonstrated poorly on MRI.

All intravenous (IV) iodine-based contrast agents now in general use are non-ionic and have a low osmolarity, with iso-osmolar agents such as iodixanol (Visipaque) also available. Even so, contrast-induced nephropathy currently is the third largest cause of admission to hospital with acute renal failure [7]. In patients who have pre-existing moderate (glomerular filtration rate [GFR] 30–60 mL/min) and severe (GFR $<$ 30 mL/min) renal impairment, precautions to prevent iodinated contrast-related nephrotoxicity include IV hydration, use of an iso-osmolar agent, oral acetylcysteine, and IV bicarbonate infusion [8,9]. The last two preventions, although widely in use, are not supported by strong evidence [10]. In addition, other imaging options, such as MRI, should be considered as alternative first-line investigative tools.

Developments in MRI include increased signal from multichannel technology (multiple receiver coils) and stronger magnetic fields (1.5T or 3T in clinical practice but 12T and higher in research facilities) [11]. New software exploits more efficient data acquisition by novel k-space filling to reduce scan times.

The great advantage of MRI is in soft tissue contrast resolution, with anatomy depicted well on T1-weighted images, and pathology on T2-weighted and after IV gadolinium–enhanced imaging. Signal from background fat, as can be abundant in the head and neck region, can be suppressed using a variety of techniques, including fat saturation or inversion recovery sequences. Diffusion-weighted imaging can help determine the complexity of fluid collections and the likelihood of abscess. Although MRI demonstrates cortical bone poorly, it has high sensitivity for medullary marrow disease, particularly useful in the assessment of infiltrating skull base lesions [12]. The advantage over CT in true multiplanar imaging has lessened somewhat with improvements in isometric CT reformatting.

Specific issues regarding MRI exist. Patients require screening for pacemakers and metallic implants, because these devices often are contraindications for MRI. Discomfort and claustrophobia can be problematic, because studies may take 30 minutes or longer, possibly requiring patient sedation. General anesthesia often is necessary in young children.

Although it is relatively safe, concerns have been raised regarding IV gadolinium–related nephrotoxicity at higher doses, such as for MR angiography (MRA) [9,13]. A widely used gadolinium-based agent, gadodiamide

(Omniscan), recently has been implicated as a cause of nephrogenic systemic fibrosis in patients who have renal impairment [14]. Confidence in the safety of MRI in pregnant patients continues to increase, although MRI is used with caution in these patients and generally is avoided in the first trimester [15,16].

Image-guided percutaneous procedures using modalities such as CT, ultrasound, or fluoroscopy can yield specimens for laboratory analysis. Therapeutic aspiration or catheter drainage may obviate the need for a more invasive open procedure [17].

Diagnostic issues

In general, the diagnosis of acute infection is heralded by the clinical and laboratory findings at presentation. The main role of imaging is to determine the source and extension of the lesion, not to determine the cause. Many features of inflammatory phlegmon or abscess overlap with those of an aggressive infiltrating/necrotic neoplasm. CT, MRI (including diffusion, perfusion and spectroscopy), and even positron emission tomography may give strongly suggestive, but not definitive, information in this regard. Indeed, infection may be a complication of an underlying benign or malignant neoplasm, as well as of certain developmental lesions. These issues are discussed in the appropriate sections.

Critical issues include compromise of the many vital structures that exist in the head and neck region, such as the airway, cervical vessels, orbits, intracranial space, and spinal canal. Fascial borders may be traversed by aggressive and prolonged inflammatory lesions, and key regions, such as the para- or retropharyngeal spaces and "danger spaces," render a predictable path for more extensive spread. Involvement of vessels, particularly emissary veins and lymphatics, also explains the pattern of disease and spread.

A key management issue is the progression of an inflammatory lesion from edematous fat stranding to a more homogenous phlegmonous mass with enhancement, eventually becoming more organized around a central liquefactive cavity; the last circumstance is an indication for drainage. Unfortunately, about one in four ring-enhancing lesions is not drainable at surgery [18]. Use of dual-phase imaging with a second, more delayed (several minutes) postcontrast scan may increase specificity by showing at least subtle central enhancement in a poorly liquefied lesion.

Imaging of head and neck infections

Unique aspects regarding imaging of various head and neck infections are discussed by region, including (1) oral cavity and salivary glands; (2) neck space infection; (3) cervical lymphadenopathy; (4) necrotizing fasciitis; (5) paranasal sinuses; (6) orbits; (7) temporal bones including middle ear and mastoid; and (8) intracranial suppuration.

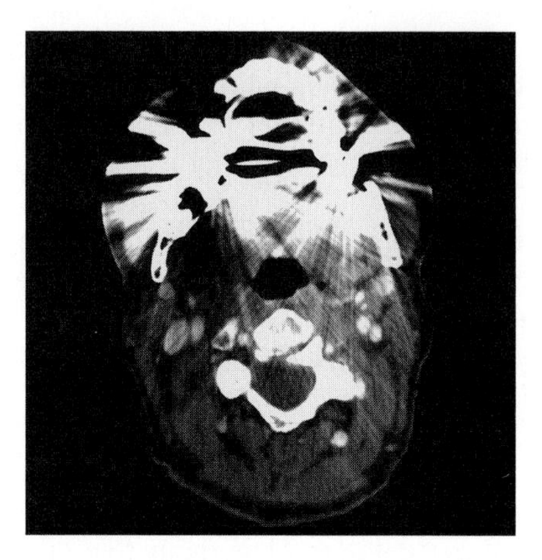

Fig. 1. CT metallic streak artifact caused by multiple dental amalgam fillings. The metallic attenuation far exceeds the dynamic range of the detector array. The masticator space and oral cavity are obscured.

Oral cavity and salivary glands

Oral cavity

The oral cavity comprises the dentition (the most common source of adult neck infections overall [19]) and the maxilla, mandible, oral mucosa, tongue, and submandibular and sublingual glands. CT remains the modality of choice for assessment of suspected infection [20]. Dental amalgam can cause CT metallic streak artifact, which may obscure the region of interest (Fig. 1) but seldom is significant on MRI [21].

Dental caries invading the dental pulp or gingival infection involving the periodontal space may extend to the root of a tooth, causing periapical

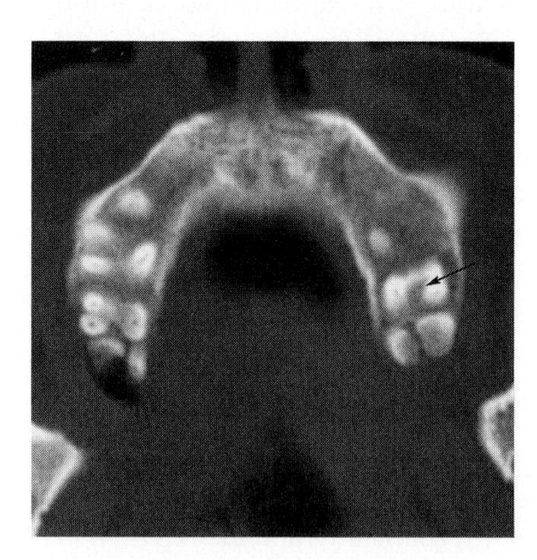

Fig. 2. Axial noncontrast CT of dental caries showing a small lytic lesion in the crown of a maxillary molar tooth (*arrow*).

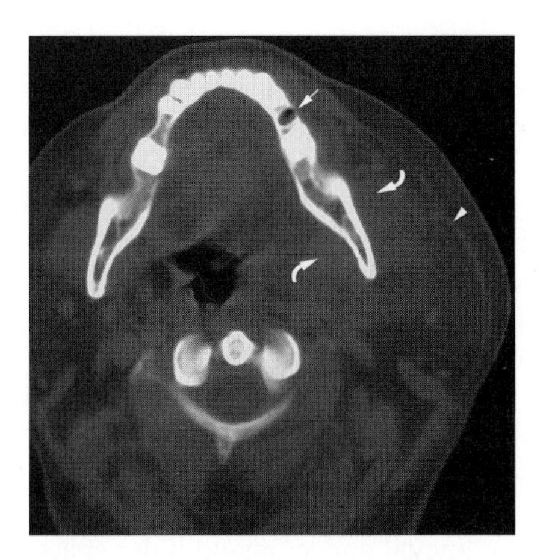

Fig. 3. Dental abscess extending to the sublingual space. CT at bone window setting showing infection arising from a gas-containing mandibular premolar periapical abscess (*arrow*) and involving the ipsilateral sublingual and masticator space (swollen masseter and pterygoid muscles) (*curved arrows*). Note fat stranding (edema) and thickening of the platysma muscle (*arrowhead*).

lucency on orthopantomography and CT (Fig. 2). This finding can develop into an acute alveolar or periapical abscess (Fig. 3) or chronic granuloma or can subside with residual periapical (radicular) cyst, a common incidental CT finding. Periapical abscess is suggested by its clinical presentation, as well as by widening or breech of the periodontal ligament or erosion of the lamina dura on imaging (Fig. 4). Destruction of alveolar bone, periosteal reaction (thickening and enhancement), and occasional subperiosteal abscess are hallmarks of osteomyelitis. Three-phase bone scintigraphy is more sensitive for

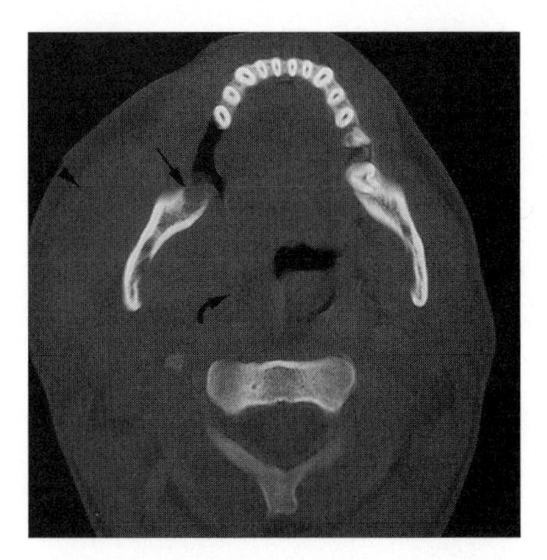

Fig. 4. Infection after dental extraction. CT showing a lytic abscess in the right retromolar trigone (*arrow*) that has breached the mandibular cortex to cause inflammation and swelling of the masticator space, indicated by swelling of the masseter muscle (*arrowhead*) and medial pterygoid muscle causing medial displacement of the parapharyngeal fat (*curved arrow*).

determining the extent of the lesion, and radiotracer-tagged white blood cell scanning gives increased specificity. CT is exquisitely sensitive to gas, which may indicate a gas-forming (often anaerobic) organism or complicating fistula, a predilection of actinomycosis. Chronic infection can incite adjacent condensing osteitis with focal sclerosis, and, if multiple foci coalesce, the appearance can mimic an osteoblastic neoplasm [22].

The pattern of extension of infection from the mandibular teeth is determined by the attachment of the mylohyoid muscle, which forms a posteriorly deficient floor of the mouth between the lingual and submandibular spaces [23]. The two most posterior mandibular molar teeth have roots below this line, and periapical infection can spread directly into the submandibular space (Fig. 5), whereas the rest of the teeth lie above the line and can directly extend to the lingual space (see Fig. 3). Respective secondary infective sialadenitis can ensue. The lingual and submandibular spaces communicate posteriorly with each other as well as the inferior parapharyngeal space.

Extension of infection from maxillary dentition may involve the maxillary antra, presenting with sinusitis, or the parotid gland, with associated painful mass. Orbital involvement has been reported through various routes, including maxillary sinus, premalar soft tissues, pterygopalatine fossa, inferior orbital fissure, or facial, angular, and ophthalmic veins [24]. The infected tooth usually requires extraction to achieve resolution, and its recognition may be delayed without an early CT examination [25].

Involvement of the tongue is unusual but can compromise the oropharyngeal airway. One should consider possible superinfection of a thyroglossal cyst, if midline (Fig. 6), or of an underlying ranula, if extending into the floor of the mouth.

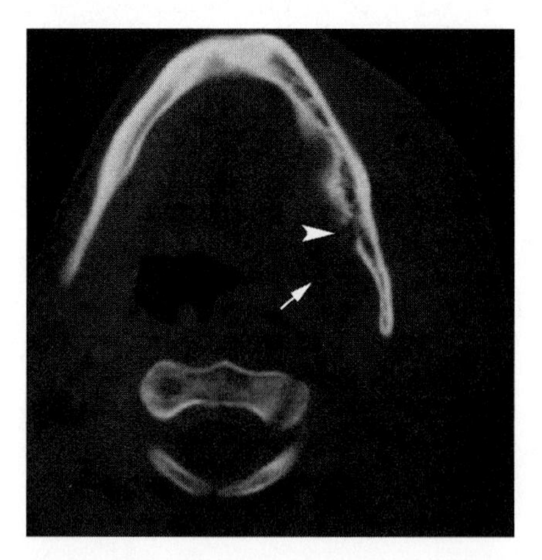

Fig. 5. Axial CT through the mandible, showing focal cortical erosion (*arrowhead*) and an odontogenic source of the rounded low attenuation lesion (*arrow*) deep to the mandible, displacing the mylohyoid muscle and oropharynx medially. Delayed postcontrast CT showed absent enhancement in the liquefied center of this abscess.

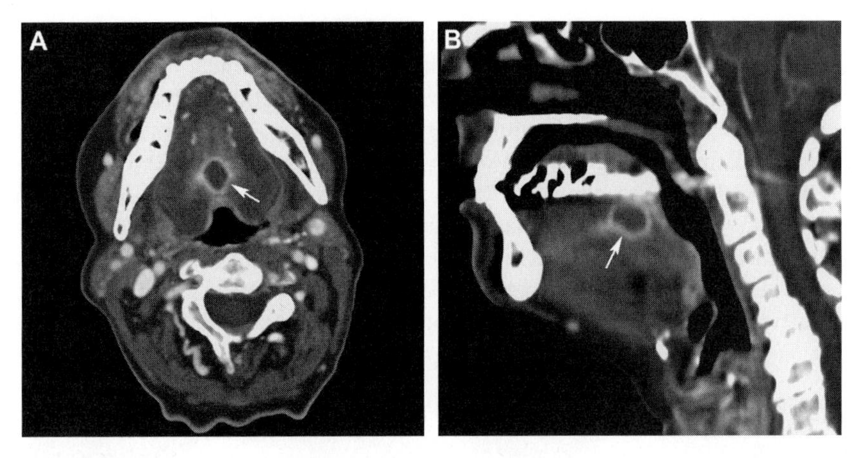

Fig. 6. Tongue abscess arising from an infected thyroglossal cyst. (*A*) Contrast-enhanced axial CT showing a thin and uniform ring-enhancing mass (*arrow*) with central low attenuation centered in the posterior midline tongue. (*B*) Reformatted sagittal CT showing relationship of the lesion (*arrow*) to the tongue and pharyngeal airway.

Salivary glands

Acute sialadenitis is characterized by diffuse salivary gland enlargement with hypoechogenic ultrasound texture and increased enhancement on CT (Fig. 7A). Bilateral involvement in children is most commonly viral (mumps) in cause. Bacterial infection is usually secondary to an obstructive calculus [26]. This infection can progress to nonenhancing central necrosis and a ring-enhancing granulating wall characteristic of abscess formation (Fig. 7B). The parotid space includes the parotid gland and traversing facial

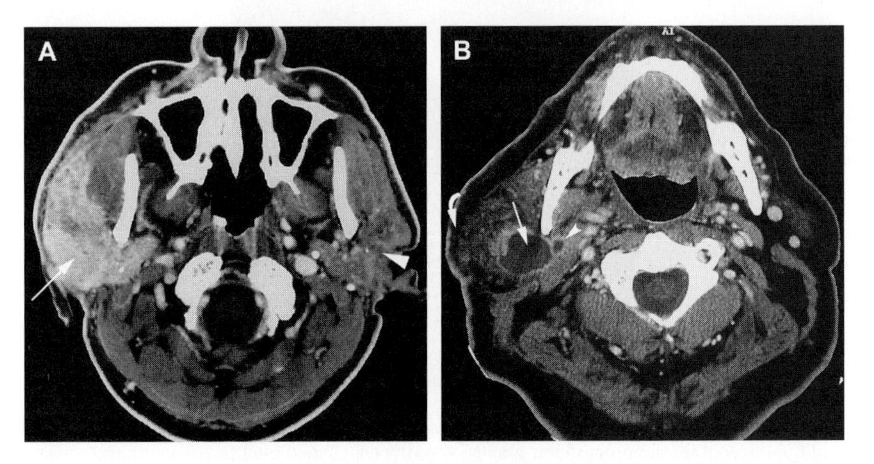

Fig. 7. Parotic involvement. Contrast-enhanced CT showing (*A*) diffuse enlargement and increased enhancement of the superficial and deep right parotid gland (*arrow*), in contrast to the normal side (*arrowhead*), and (*B*) mature right superficial and deep parotid abscess (*arrow*) with thin enhancing rim, a daughter abscess on its deep aspect (*arrowhead*), and stranding of superficial fat and thickening of the skin overlying the parotid (*curved arrow*).

nerve, vessels, and lymphatics/lymph nodes. One should be aware that reactive parotid lymphadenopathy may simulate a neoplasm.

Sialolithiasis may be associated with bacterial infection, often causing sialectasis and parenchymal atrophy over the long term. Calculi may occasionally be visualized along the path of the parotid (Stenson's) or submandibular (Wharton's) ducts on plain-film radiographs or more reliably on ultrasound and CT (Fig. 8). The superficial location of the parotid and submandibular glands makes them ideal for high-resolution ultrasound assessment [27,28], with calculi demonstrating characteristic echogenic surfaces and posterior acoustic shadowing. Calculi have far higher attenuation than enhancing

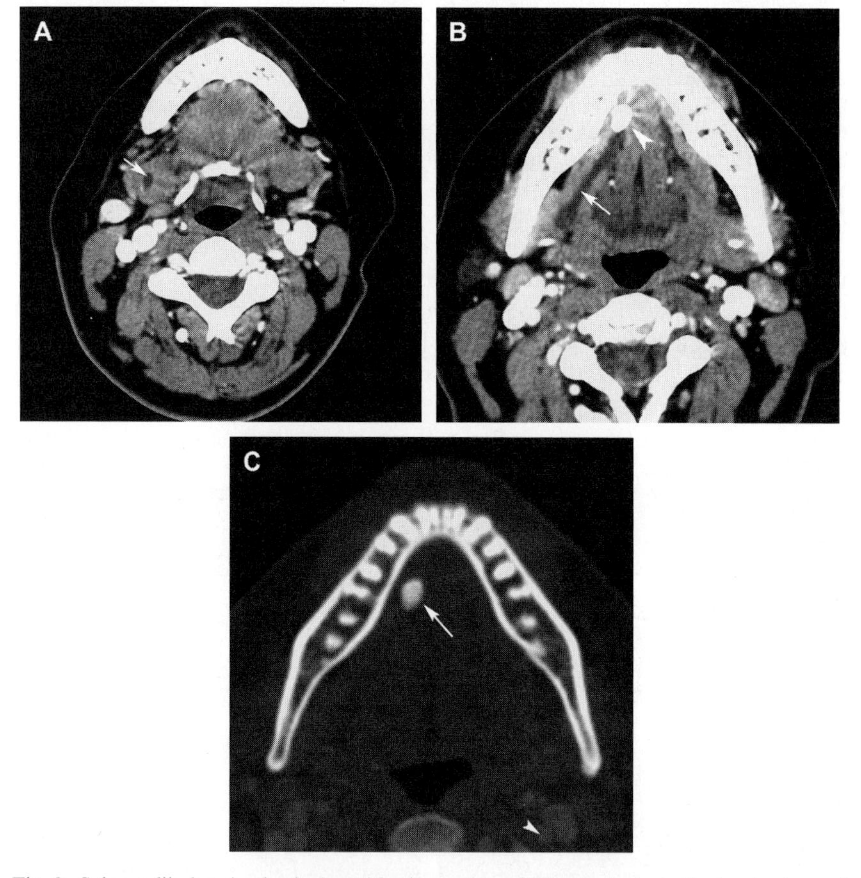

Fig. 8. Submandibular gland calculus with obstruction of Wharton's duct. Contrast-enhanced axial CT through the submandibular glands, showing (*A*) dilated duct (*arrow*) with well-defined fluid attenuation in the central right submandibular gland and no evidence of acute inflammation; (*B*) dilated duct (*arrow*) passing anteriorly to level of obstructing calculus (*arrowhead*) adjacent to the orifice; and (*C*) bone window setting, showing calculus (*arrow*), which has similar attenuation to cortical bone and is easily distinguished from lower-attenuation vascular contrast, as in the carotid artery (*arrowhead*).

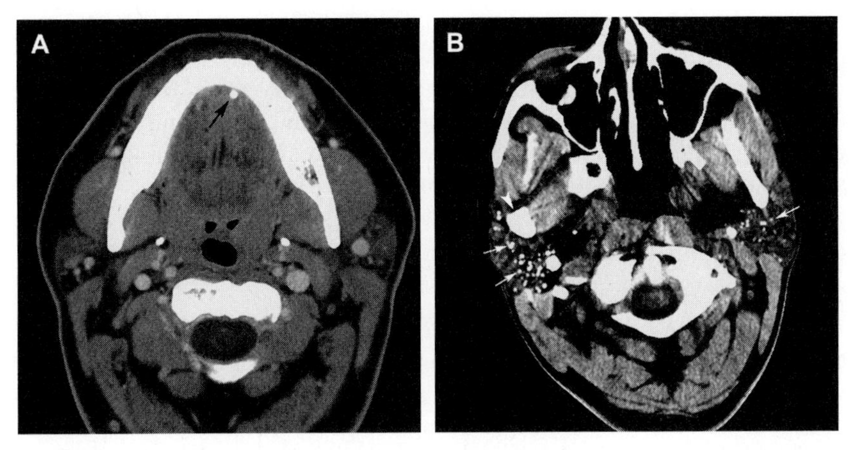

Fig. 9. Salivary gland calculi. (*A*) Contrast-enhanced axial CT showing tiny calculus at orifice of Wharton's duct (*arrow*) in characteristic location just deep to the mandible and to the left of midline, with no evidence of ductal dilatation or submandibular swelling on the other slices. (*B*) Noncontrast axial CT through the parotid glands, showing chronic bilateral parotid sialadenitis with multiple punctate calculi (*arrows*), with a large lesion in the right superficial parotid (*arrowhead*). The parotid glands are slightly reduced in size.

lesions or vessels, making a separate noncontrast CT unnecessary (Fig. 9A). Commonly the calculus is located close to the orifice opposite the second upper molar (Stenson's duct) or just posterior to the paramedian mental mandible (Wharton's duct). The presence of multiple calculi may indicate more

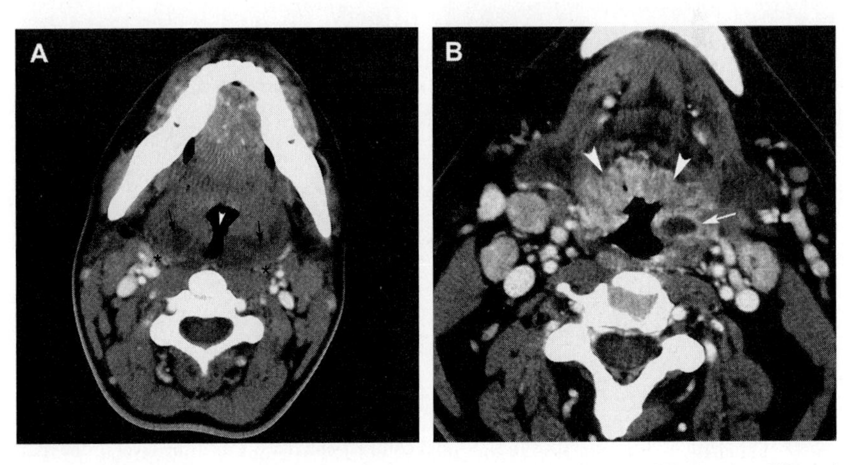

Fig. 10. Tonsillitis and tonsillar abscess. (*A*) Axial contrast-enhanced CT showing bilateral, swollen, low-heterogeneous palatine tonsils (*arrows*), with effacement of the parapharyngeal spaces (*) and posterior displacement of the carotid spaces. (*B*) Contrast-enhanced CT showing a ring-enhancing abscess in the left tonsil (*arrow*) with early pointing toward the oropharynx and reactive homogenous enhancement and prominence of the lingual and right pharyngeal tonsils (*arrowheads*).

extensive surgical management, including excision of the gland (Fig. 9B) [29].

Conventional direct fluoroscopic sialography is contraindicated in acute inflammation and has been largely replaced by MRI sialography, which can demonstrate normal ductal anatomy as well as pathologic changes such as sialectasis, especially with the use of modern surface array coils.

Neck space infection

The pharyngeal space

The pharyngeal space comprises the naso-, oro- and hypopharynx, which communicate anteriorly with the nasal space, oral cavity, and laryngeal vestibule, respectively. Lymphoid tissue in the adenoids, palatine, and lingual tonsils forms the Waldeyer's ring, normally prominent in childhood through adolescence and becoming diminutive in adulthood. Prominent lymphoid hypertrophy may be seen in response to common viral rhinitis, pharyngitis, and laryngitis or in reaction to adjacent infection. Chronic adenoidal prominence in adults is seen with HIV infection [30]. Swollen, reactive nasopharyngeal mucosa can obstruct the eustachian tube in the fossa of Rosenmueller causing a serous transudate to opacify the ipsilateral middle ear cavity; although in adults one should exclude nasopharyngeal carcinoma as a cause.

The tonsils are the most common site of oropharyngeal infection in children. The normal, highly convoluted, enhancing mucosal folds of the

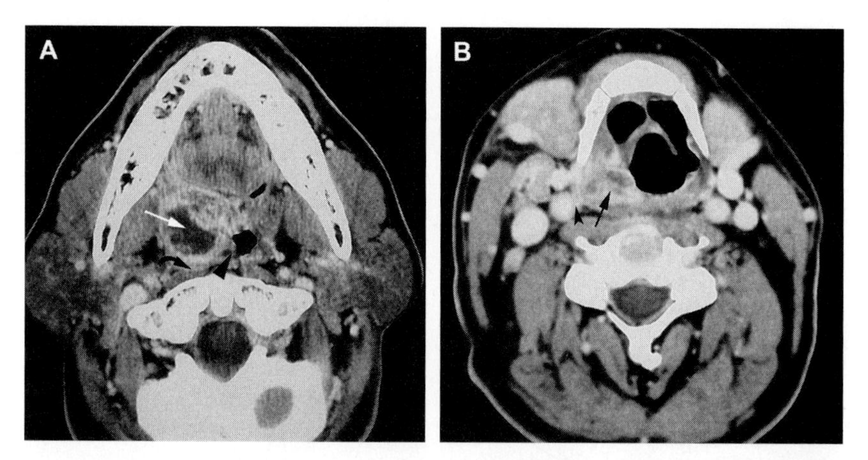

Fig. 11. Peritonsillar abscess (quinsy). (*A*) Axial contrast-enhanced CT at the level of the mandible showing a rounded, enhancing mass with necrotic center adjacent to the right pharyngeal tonsil (*arrow*), with medial displacement of the oropharynx (*arrowhead*) and flattening of the prevertebral longus colli muscle (*curved arrow*). (*B*) Axial contrast-enhanced CT at the level of the hyoid bone showing that the enhancing lesion extends inferiorly along the right hypopharyngeal mucosa (*arrow*), with an intimate relationship to the right internal carotid artery (*arrowhead*).

palatine tonsils should not be mistaken for disease. The tonsils often are swollen and edematous during an acute episode of tonsillitis (Fig. 10A) and, rarely, may progress to form a tonsillar abscess (Fig. 10B). Rounded, ring-enhancing swelling with central low attenuation is suggestive of an abscess, more often peritonsillar (quinsy) (Fig. 11) than tonsillar. Most cases of tonsillitis are self-limited; CT is reserved for complicated cases failing to respond to antibiotics. Plain-film lateral neck radiography may demonstrate airway compromise, and ultrasound can target a lesion requiring drainage. If CT is performed, noninfected reactive lymph nodes in the retropharyngeal space can demonstrate central low attenuation, spuriously simulating infectious suppuration.

Epiglottitis is now uncommon in developed countries with the widespread availability of antibiotics and the introduction of *Haemophilus influenzae*–conjugated vaccine. A high index of suspicion is required for prompt diagnosis and treatment [31]. Because precarious airway compromise may limit clinical examination, an erect lateral neck radiograph sometimes may be useful to confirm the diagnosis (Fig. 12). Further imaging that requires applied pressure (ultrasound) or in a supine patient (CT, MRI) usually is considered inappropriate and dangerous.

Retropharyngeal space

The retropharyngeal space extends from the base of the skull to the upper mediastinum. The level of the hyoid bone divides the space in two, with normal tissue content consisting of fat in both, and lymph nodes restricted to the suprahyoid compartment. Infection usually is caused by lymphatic

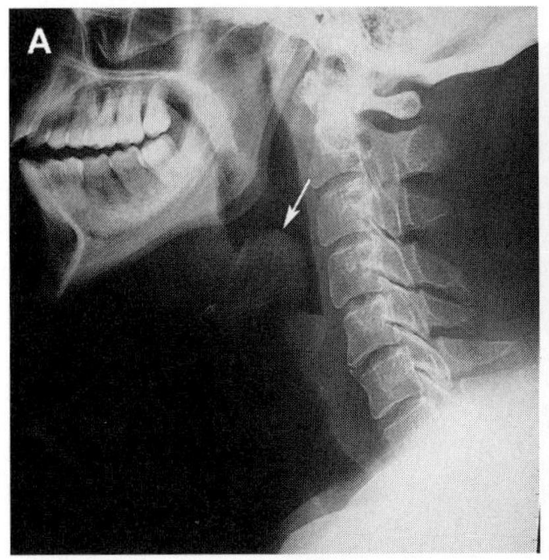

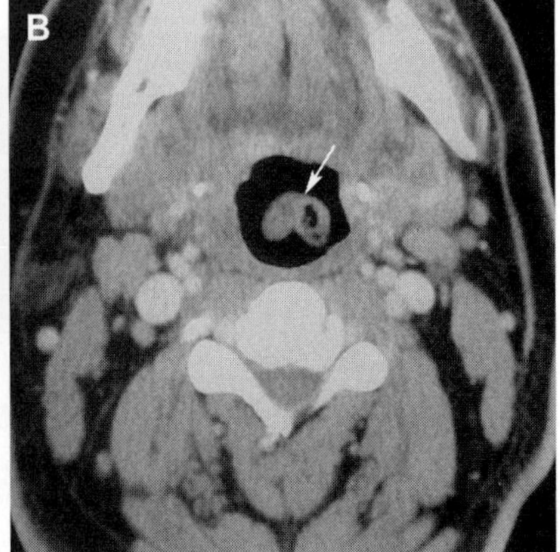

Fig. 12. Acute epiglottitis. (*A*) Lateral neck radiograph, showing a grossly swollen epiglottic silhouette with a bulbous contour (*arrow*). (*B*) Axial contrast-enhanced CT through the free edge of the epiglottis, confirming swelling of the epiglottis (*arrow*) and also revealing gas within the tip caused by gas-forming organisms or a mucosal laceration.

spread from the adjacent pharyngeal space (pharyngitis, tonsillitis) or prevertebral space (discitis, osteomyelitis), with the origin usually identifiable on clinical grounds but underestimated in extent [32]. Initial involvement of suprahyoid retropharyngeal nodes spreads to surrounding fat and then into the infrahyoid space.

Early imaging findings with CT may reflect reactive, nonsuppurative edema, mild fat stranding with discernable tissue planes, linear fluid, minimal mass effect, and no associated enhancement. Reactive, enlarged lymph nodes show mild, homogenous enhancement.

With frank retropharyngeal infection, necrotic nodes demonstrate central low attenuation and ring enhancement. Fat stranding evolves to enhancing inflammatory phlegmon and, with central breakdown and fluid collection, can lead to a ring-enhancing abscess. Significant collections tend to be biconvex with mass effect, flattening the prevertebral muscles, displacing the carotid space laterally and the parapharyngeal space anterolaterally (Fig. 13). Inflammatory stranding causes blurred fascial planes.

A lateral plain-film radiograph will show anterior displacement of the pharynx/upper airway by more than one half the width of the C4 vertebral body. Rarely, there can be gas within the mass. Contrast-enhanced CT demonstrates the extent well; however, if there is concern regarding extension into the spinal column (a rare complication), MRI should be performed to exclude an epidural abscess (Fig. 14). One also should evaluate for adjacent airway or vascular compromise (Fig. 15). Dense pus may mimic soft tissue phlegmon on CT, and if an unimpeded ultrasonic tissue window is available, properties such as low echogenicity, echo enhancement, and fluctuating contents on compression are strong predictors of success using percutaneous aspiration or open drainage.

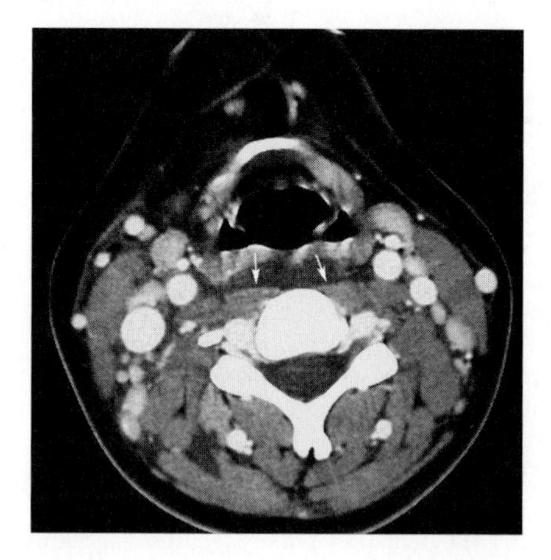

Fig. 13. Contrast-enhanced axial CT showing a retropharyngeal fluid collection (*arrows*) displacing the posterior oropharyngeal wall anteriorly and flattening the longus colli muscles posteriorly.

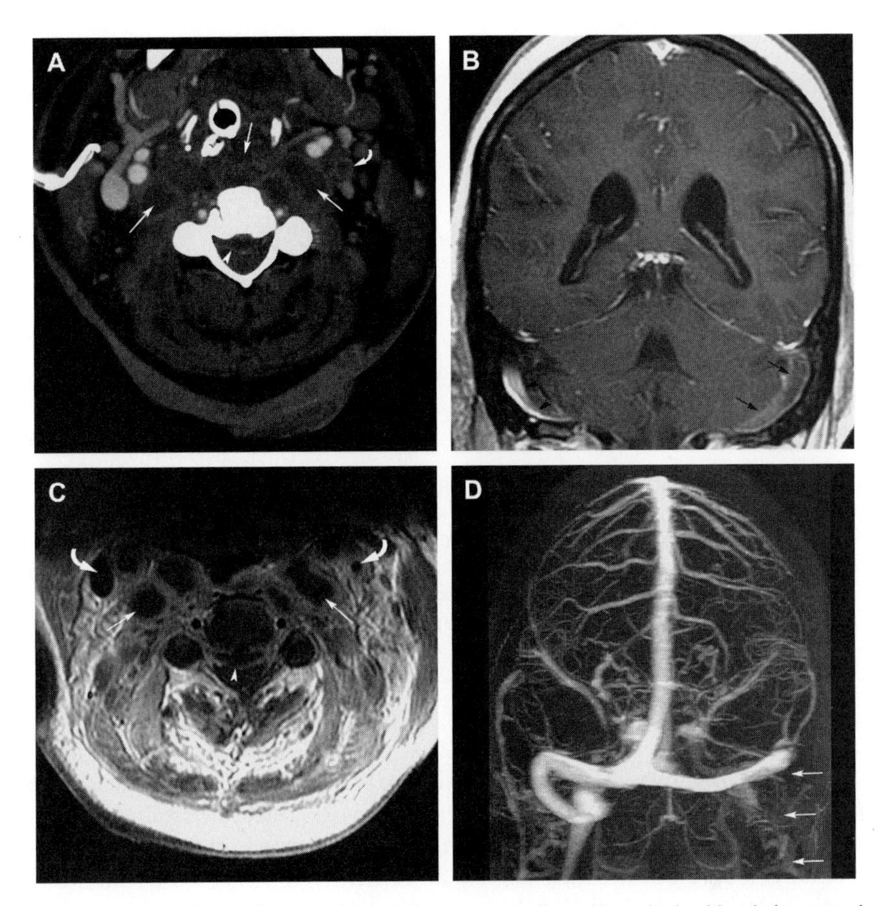

Fig. 14. Retro- and parapharyngeal space abscesses complicated by spinal epidural abscess and thrombosis of the left sigmoid sinus and internal jugular vein. (*A*) Contrast-enhanced CT showing multiloculated enhancing collections peripherally in the retropharyngeal and bilateral parapharyngeal spaces (*arrows*), with ring enhancement in the wall of the left internal jugular vein around the occluded nonenhancing lumen (*curved arrow*) and a peripherally enhancing collection in the anterior epidural space (*arrowhead*) consistent with abscess. (*B*) Coronal T1 postgadolinium MRI through the sigmoid sinuses showing occlusion of the left sigmoid sinus with enhancing dural wall around an intermediate signal indicating acute thrombus (*arrows*), in contrast to normal right side (*arrowhead*). (*C*) Axial T1 postgadolinium MRI showing the epidural abscess (*arrowhead*) more clearly than the CT examination and an enhancing phlegmon in the left carotid space (*arrows*) surrounding an attenuated left internal jugular vein with an isointense lumen (*curved arrows*) in comparison to the contralateral normal side. (*D*) MRI venography with timed contrast enhancement showing absent enhancement along expected course of the left sigmoid sinus and the superior left internal jugular vein (*arrows*), in contrast to normal flow on the right side.

Parapharyngeal space

The parapharyngeal space is composed predominantly of fat and provides a useful reference on axial imaging, becoming displaced by adjacent lesions in a predictable fashion. Infection can traverse the parapharyngeal

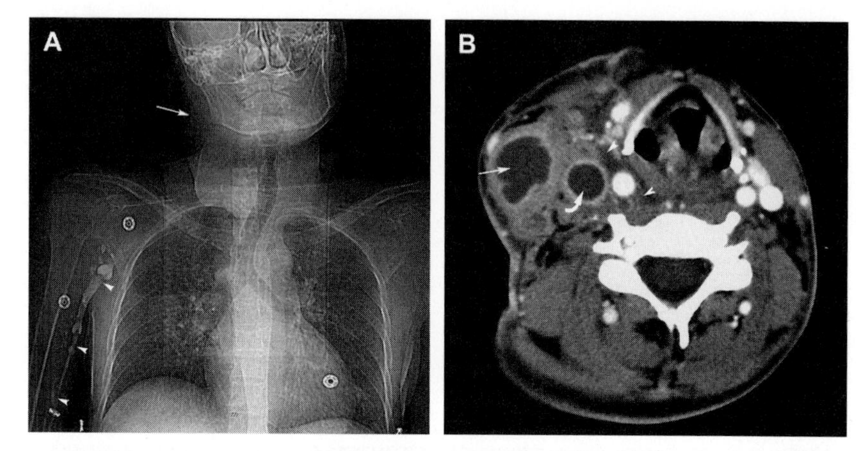

Fig. 15. Thrombosis of right internal jugular vein secondary to an abscess arising in the sternocleidomastoid muscle. (*A*) Frontal projection radiograph of the neck and chest, after IV contrast injection through a right upper limb venous access, showing right neck swelling (*arrow*) and stasis of contrast in the right upper limb basilic vein (*arrowheads*). (*B*) Contrast-enhanced CT of the neck, showing a ring-enhancing abscess within the right sternocleidomastoid muscle (*arrow*); the adjacent internal jugular vein is expanded with an enhancing wall around an occluded, nonenhancing lumen (*curved arrow*). Note edema, which causes fat stranding in the inferior parapharyngeal space (*arrowheads*).

space to the neurovascular bundle in the carotid sheath and may necessitate CT angiography or MRA/MR venography (MRA/MRV) examination.

Lemierre syndrome of jugular vein thrombosis secondary to anaerobic infection is a rare but dreaded disease and often is complicated by bland or septic pulmonary emboli [33]. Mycotic carotid artery aneurysms can occur within a few days of developing postinfective vasculitis. Although noninvasive vascular imaging techniques have largely replaced catheter angiography, conventional angiography occasionally may be necessary for preoperative work-up or endovascular management of complications.

Prevertebral space

Extension of infection from the spine through the prevertebral space most often arises from infectious discitis. In developed countries staphylococcus is more common than tuberculosis. Associated irregular vertebral end plate erosion should be visible on plain-film radiographs and CT (best seen on sagittal reformats) by this stage. MRI including fat-saturated, contrast-enhanced T1 sequences should be performed to detect epidural phlegmon or drainable empyema (Fig. 16). Advanced cases may show spinal cord congestion, edema, or even intramedullary abscess (Fig. 17). Tuberculosis, the most common infection worldwide, develops insidiously and may have large paravertebral collections and deforming vertebral destruction (gibbus deformity) at presentation.

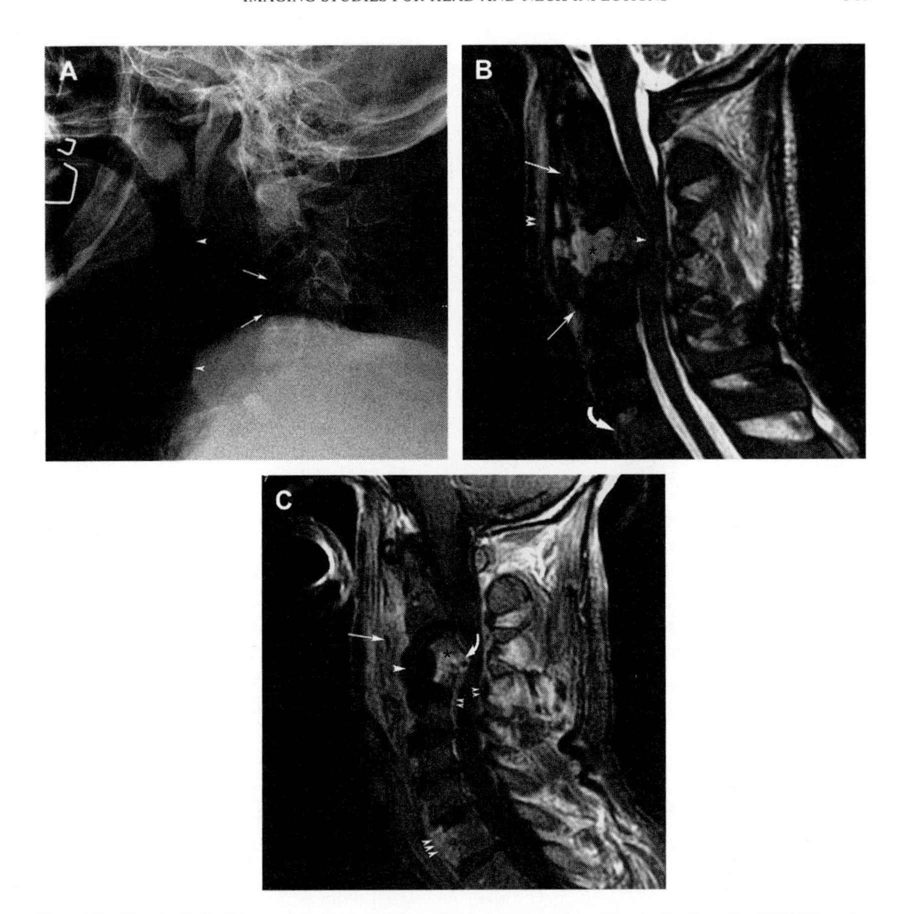

Fig. 16. Cervical discitis and osteomyelitis. (*A*) Lateral neck radiograph showing C3/C4 vertebral body lucency and cortical destruction (*arrows*) with collapse and kyphotic deformity and prevertebral and retropharyngeal swelling causing anterior displacement of the pharyngeal airway (*arrowheads*). (*B*) Cervical sagittal T2 MRI showing complete loss of the C3/C4 disc interspace, posterior prolapse of T2 hyperintense edematous vertebral material into the anterior spinal canal causing cord compression (*arrowhead*), and a more homogenous T2 hyperintense lesion (*) extending from the anterior vertebrae into the prevertebral space (*arrows*), with reactive edema in the adjacent retropharyngeal space (*double arrowheads*). A second, less advanced lesion is present at the C7/T1 level, with disc hyperintensity, end-plate destruction (*curved arrow*), and T1-vertebral hyperintensity consistent with vertebritis. (*C*) Cervical sagittal T1 postgadolinium MRI with fat saturation showing nonenhancement of the frankly necrotic lesion in the anterior vertebral bodies (*arrowhead*) and adjacent enhancing vertebritis (*), epidural phlegmon (*double arrowheads*), a small epidural abscess (*curved arrow*), and heterogeneously enhancing phlegmon in the prevertebral space (*arrow*), as well as enhancing phlegmon and vertebra at the second C7/T1 discitis (*triple arrowheads*).

Calcific tendonitis is a noninfectious, idiopathic inflammation of the longus colli tendon insertions, causing retropharyngeal effusion and swelling. Because of its clinical presentation and plain-film appearance, it may be mistaken for infection, but cross-sectional imaging allows the correct diagnosis

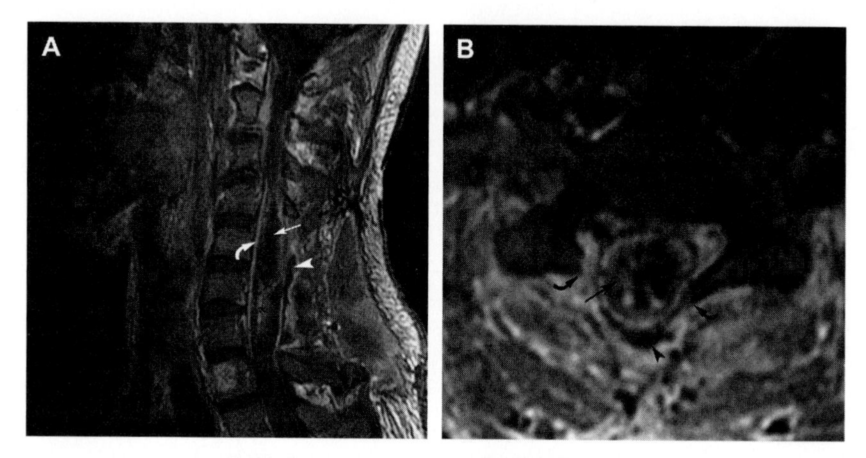

Fig. 17. Cervical cord abscess and recurrent epidural abscess after previous surgical decompression and drainage. (*A*) Sagittal T1 postgadolinium MRI of the cervical spine showing an irregular ring-enhancing lesion (*arrow*) expanding the cord centrally from C2 to C3, with noncavitating enhancement inferiorly (*), a posterior peripherally enhancing epidural abscess (*arrowhead*), anterior epidural enhancement possibly caused by inflammatory phlegmon/exudate or venous compression, and a superficial postsurgical collection caused by extensive posterior spinal decompression. (*B*) Axial CT at C3 level showing an irregular, centrally necrotic, ring-enhancing mass (*arrow*) causing the cord to bulge through the decompressing surgical laminectomy (*curved arrows*) and a posterior epidural abscess (*arrowhead*).

[34]. CT may show calcification in the tendon (Fig. 18); MRI best demonstrates the elliptical prevertebral effusion extending from C1 to C6.

Visceral space

The visceral space in the infrahyoid neck includes the thyroid gland, trachea, and esophagus. Infectious suppurative thyroiditis (Fig. 19) is rare and may be associated with a congenital piriform sinus fistula [35]. The visceral space communicates with the mediastinum below, allowing spread of infection into the chest (Fig. 20).

Cervical lymphadenopathy

Suppurative cervical lymphadenitis may be unilateral or bilateral and manifests radiographically as enlarged, enhancing lymph nodes on CT, with central low attenuation if necrotic. There typically is extensive surrounding fat stranding caused by inflammatory edema. Tuberculosis and nontuberculous mycobacterial lymphadenitis is associated with more gradual nodal enlargement, often appearing as conglomerate masses [36]. Typical imaging features of these nodal masses include thick peripheral enhancement, central low attenuation, and a relative lack of fat stranding and effacement (Fig. 21) [37]. The presence of calcification strongly suggests

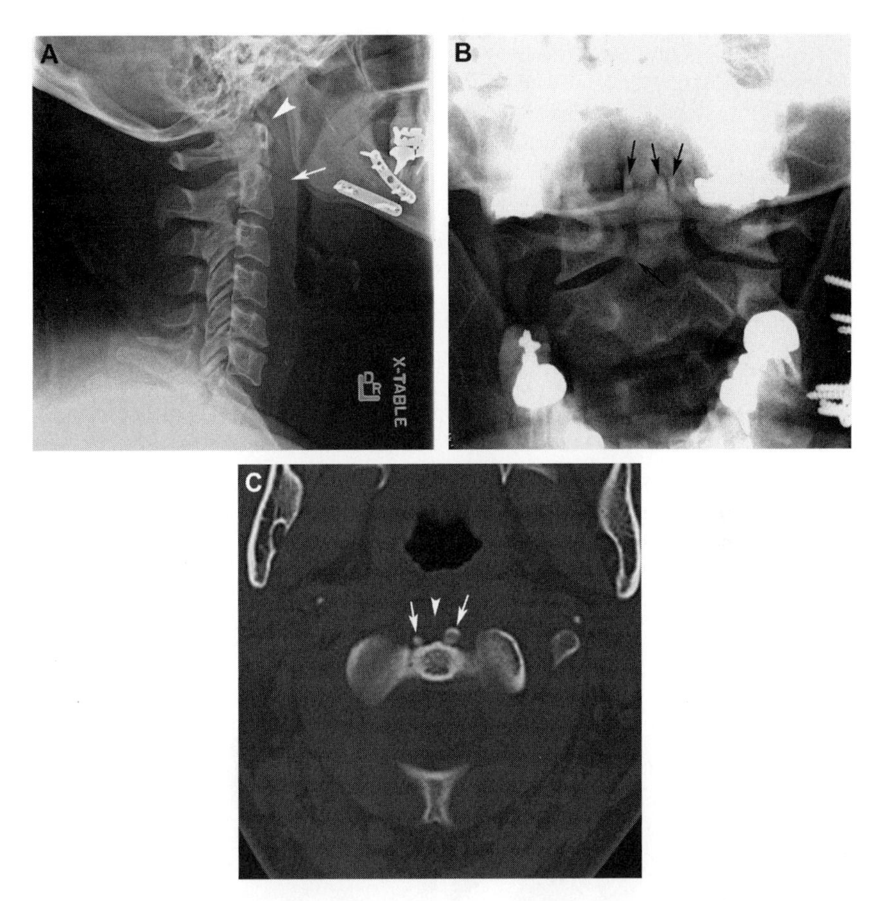

Fig. 18. Calcific tendinitis of the longus colli simulating retropharyngeal infection. (*A*) Plain radiograph of the lateral neck showing widening of the retropharyngeal space (*arrow*) and poorly visualized, subtle calcification adjacent to the anterior C1 arch (*arrowhead*). (*B*) Anteroposterior radiograph of the dens through the open mouth, showing discrete, punctate foci of calcification (*arrows*) projecting over the midline at the level of C1 and C2. (*C*) Noncontrast CT with bone window setting demonstrating foci of calcification at the insertion of the longus colli onto the anterior surface of C2 (*arrows*), with prevertebral edema (*arrowhead*).

the diagnosis. Patients who have tuberculosis tend to be more systemically unwell than those who have nontuberculous mycobacteriosis [38].

Not to be mistaken for nodal disease, infected branchial cleft cysts must be recognized by their characteristic locations. Appropriate management consists of delayed resection after the acute infection has subsided (Fig. 22).

Necrotizing fasciitis

Cellulitis may be recognized by diffuse inflammatory stranding through the subcutaneous fat and thickening of the skin. Infectious necrotizing fasciitis is characterized by thickening of the superficial and deep fascial planes

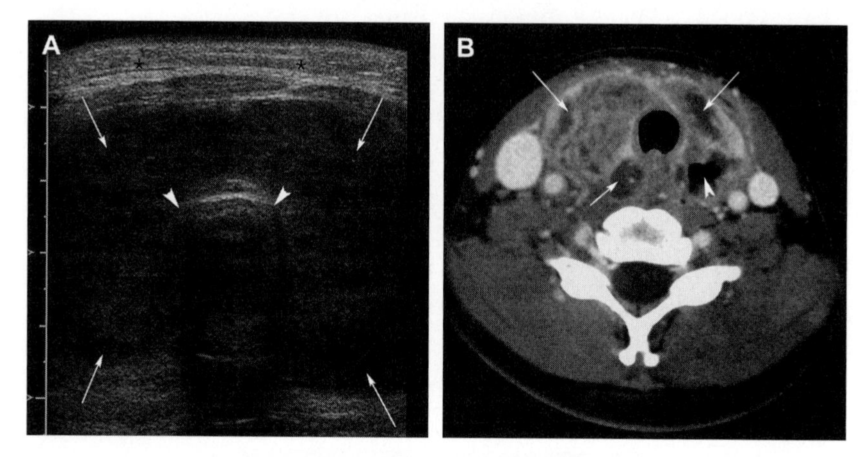

Fig. 19. Purulent thyroiditis. (*A*) Ultrasound examination (axial plane), showing a diffusely swollen, echo-poor thyroid gland (*arrows*) with mild swelling of the subcutaneous tissue and strap muscles (*) and normal acoustic shadowing from the tracheal cartilage (*arrowheads*). (*B*) Axial contrast-enhanced CT of the neck showing gross swelling of the thyroid with multifocal, necrotic areas (abscesses) (*arrows*), including one that has generated gas (*arrowhead*). The patient had not undergone instrumentation.

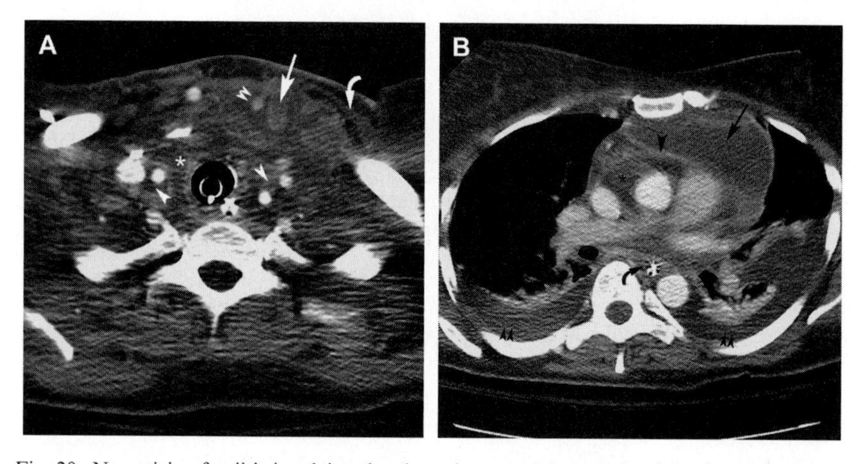

Fig. 20. Necrotizing fasciitis involving the visceral space with extension into the mediastinum. (*A*) Contrast-enhanced CT through the lower neck and chest showing a diffuse pattern of inflammatory fat stranding, predominantly in both the anterior cervical space (with swollen sternocleidomastoid and strap muscles) (*arrow*), thickened platysma (*curved arrow*), and attenuated anterior jugular vein (*double arrowheads*), and the visceral space (*), infiltrating the thyroid gland and extending around the trachea into the carotid spaces (*arrowheads*).(*B*) Continuation of inflammatory process through the visceral (paratracheal) space to form fluid collections in the anterior mediastinum (*arrow*) and posterior mediastinum (*curved arrow*) adjacent to the esophagus and nasogastric tube. A pericardial effusion (*) has developed as the result of a secondary pericarditis, with thickened pericardium (*arrowhead*) outlined by fluid on both sides and bilateral pleural effusions (*double arrowheads*).

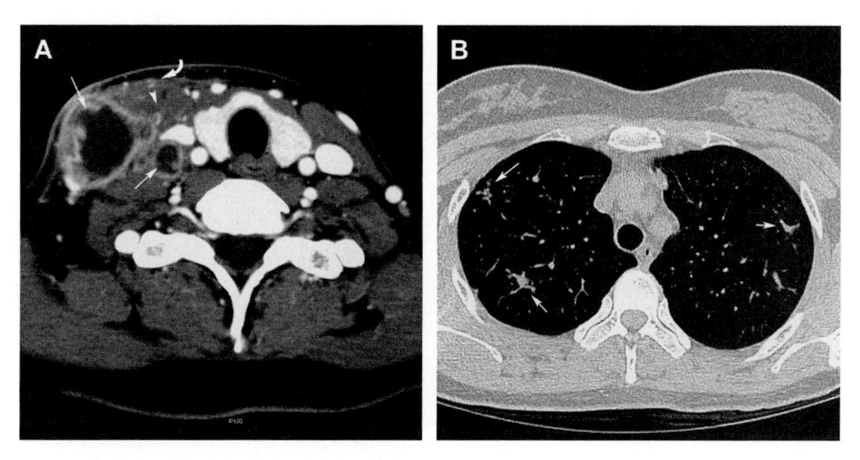

Fig. 21. Tuberculous cervical adenitis. (*A*) Contrast-enhanced CT of the neck showing multiple, peripherally enhancing mass lesions with irregular walls (*arrows*), enlarged and displaced right sternocleidomastoid (*arrowhead*) with small foci of enhancement, thickened and enhancing right platysma muscle (*curved arrow*), and anteromedial displacement of the carotid sheath. (*B*) High-resolution chest CT showing "tree-in-bud" pattern characteristic of bronchoalveolar tuberculosis (*arrows*).

(fasciitis), and muscles (myositis) (Fig. 23). It may form neck space collections with pockets of gas and can spread to the mediastinum. Once believed to only be of dental origin (Ludwig's angina), numerous cases arising from the pharynx, sinuses, and other locations now have been described [39].

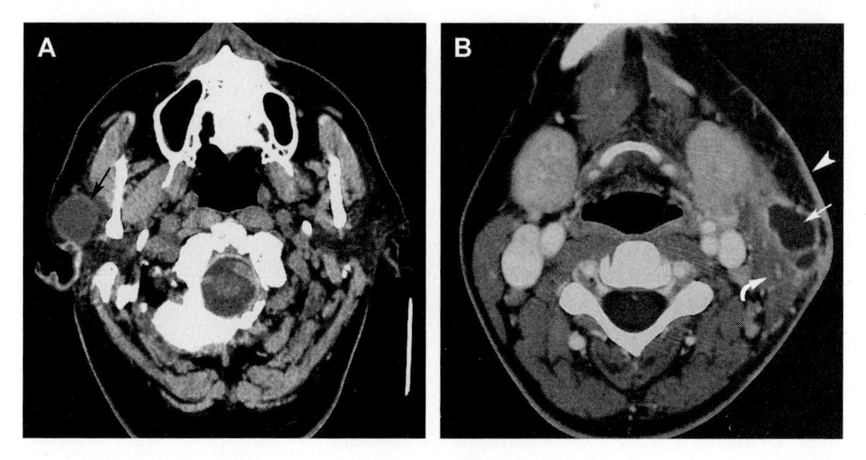

Fig. 22. Infected branchial cleft cysts. (*A*) An incidental, well-defined, uniformly thin-walled lesion of the first branchial cleft cyst (*arrow*), without enhancement or surrounding edema. (*B*) Multiloculated, ring-enhancing lesion (*arrow*) with edema of the overlying skin and subcutaneous tissues (*arrowhead*) arising from an infected congenital second branchial cleft cyst in a characteristic location adjacent to the anterior surface of the sternocleidomastoid muscle, which is swollen and edematous (*curved arrow*), and lateral to the submandibular gland, which is displaced medially.

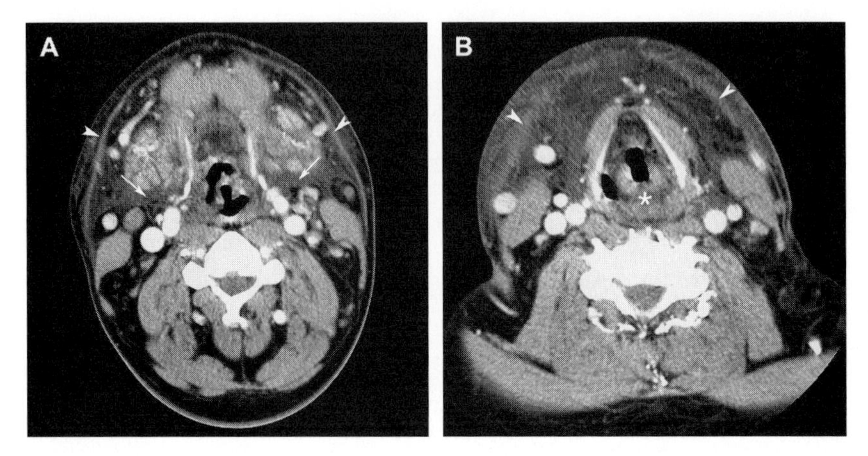

Fig. 23. Necrotizing fasciitis. (*A*) Contrast-enhanced CT of the neck showing marked edema of the subcutaneous and anterior cervical spaces, causing stranding of fat through the parapharyngeal spaces (*arrows*), the submandibular space, and on both sides of a thickened platysma muscle (*arrowhead*). (*B*) Gross swelling of the anterior neck space and the platysma muscles (*arrowheads*), with fat stranding and mass effect of the visceral space (*).

Paranasal sinuses

Most cases of acute rhinosinusitis are secondary to the common cold (rhinovirus), and imaging studies seldom are required. Plain radiography may support the diagnosis if an air–fluid level is observed, most often seen in the maxillary antrum on a Water's (OM30) view. The ethmoid and sphenoid sinuses are not well assessed on plain-film radiographs [40].

CT should be reserved for recurrent or complicated episodes when a predisposing cause is sought [41]. Imaging findings usually are nonspecific as to allergic or infectious origin; rather, the usefulness of imaging is in gauging disease location and extent. Axial multidetector CT with coronal reconstruction avoids artifact from dental amalgam, which frequently affects direct coronal acquisitions. Free sinus fluid may obscure the osteomeatal complex, limiting interpretation. This obscuring is less likely to occur in the prone, head-extended position than with traditional supine imaging.

A fluid level implies sinus obstruction and is more specific for acute infectious sinusitis than incidental mucosal thickening. Contrast-enhanced CT demonstrates enhancing mucosa (Fig. 24) around nonenhancing fluid and is useful to exclude a possible underlying obstructive mass. MRI may show T1 hyperintensity depending on the protein concentration of the fluid, which usually is hyperintense on T2-weighted imaging. Very dark T2 signal or signal void, other than air or cortical bone, should raise the possibility of fungal infection (Fig. 25). MRI is particularly useful for assessing possible spread of infection intracranially, and vascular complications such as cavernous sinus thrombosis (Fig. 26) should be considered in all situations where this is suspected [42].

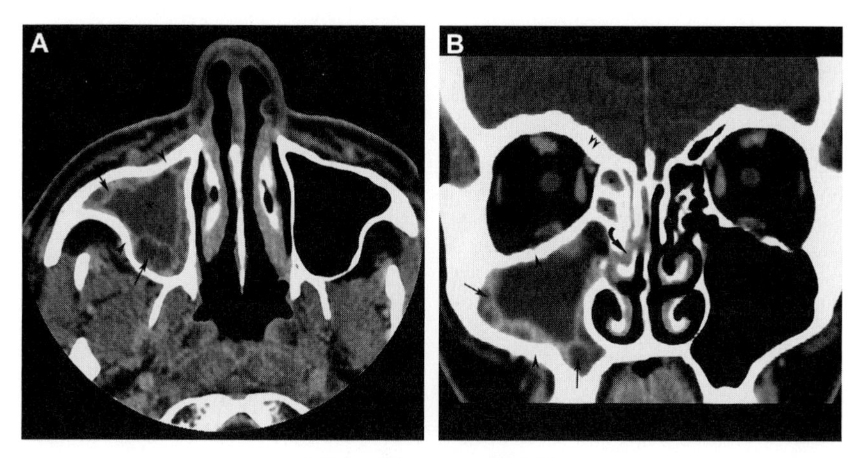

Fig. 24. Chronic sinusitis. (*A*) Axial noncontrast sinus CT showing cobblestone thickening of edematous mucosa (*arrows*) in the right maxillary antrum with associated low attenuation secretions (*) and chronic bony wall thickening (*arrowheads*). (*B*) Coronal reformatted CT showing edematous mucosa (*arrows*) and wall thickening (*arrowheads*) that obstruct the right osteomeatal complex (*curved arrow*), opacification of the right ethmoid sinus (*), and nonaerated right frontal sinus (*double arrowhead*).

Infectious sinusitis tends to spread to adjacent sinuses and is asymmetrical, in contradistinction to hypersensitive sinusitis. Posttrauma patients can have fluid levels caused by hemorrhage (typically appearing as hyperattenuating fluid), cerebrospinal fluid (CSF) leak, or nasogastric intubation with prolonged bed rest in a supine position. In chronic sinusitis, prominent

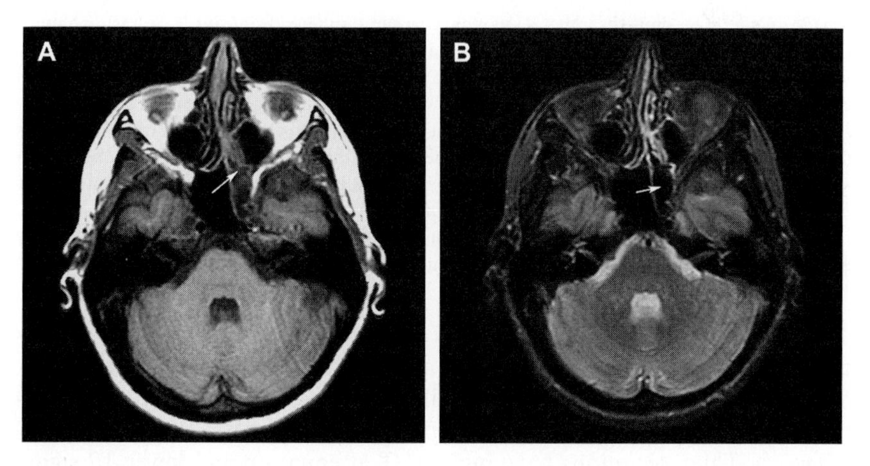

Fig. 25. MRI appearances of fungal sinusitis. (*A*) Axial T1 noncontrast MRI, showing abnormal isointense signal in the left sphenoid and posterior ethmoid sinuses (*arrow*). (*B*) Axial T2-weighted MRI showing the lesion as signal void (*arrow*) and indistinguishable from the surrounding sinus air. This finding is characteristic of fungal sinusitis.

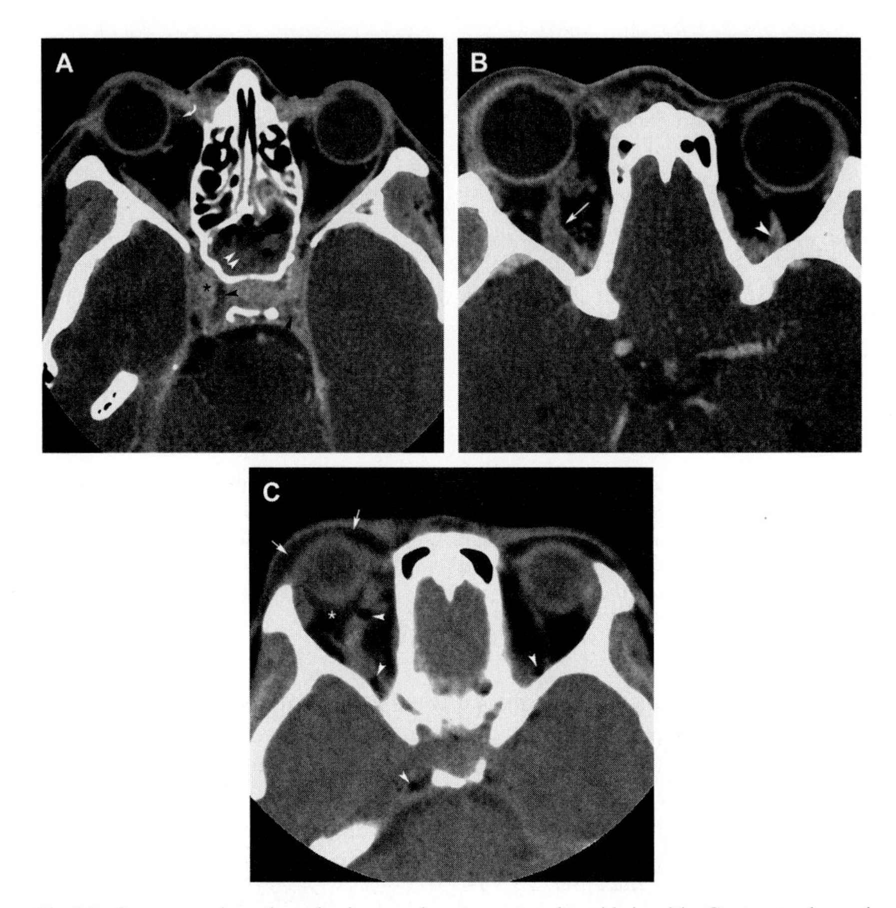

Fig. 26. Cavernous sinus thrombosis secondary to acute sphenoid sinusitis. Contrast-enhanced CT of the orbits showing (*A*) inspissated material with gas bubbles in the sphenoid sinus (*double arrowhead*), fat stranding reflecting right intraorbital edema (*curved arrow*), lack of normal enhancement in the right cavernous sinus (*arrowhead*) around the right cavernous carotid artery (*), and heterogeneous enhancement in the left cavernous sinus caused by partial thrombosis (*arrow*); (*B*) expansion of thrombosed right superior ophthalmic vein (*arrow*), with a nonocclusive filling defect representing partial thrombosis of the left superior ophthalmic vein (*arrowhead*). (*C*) Repeat postcontrast CT several days later shows increased edema in the right preseptal (*arrows*) and retro-orbital fat (*); gas is visible now in the right and left superior ophthalmic veins and in the right cavernous sinus (*arrowheads*).

mucosa, bony sinus wall thickening, and sclerosis are observed. Occasionally reduced sinus volume in the maxillary antrum can cause a reciprocal increase in orbital volume to cause enophthalmos (the silent sinus syndrome) (Fig. 27). Thick secretions have higher CT attenuation and lower T2 signal intensity. Mucosal calcification may occur.

Paranasal sinus infection can cause osteomyelitis or spread through emissary veins, more common in chronic and acute sinusitis, respectively.

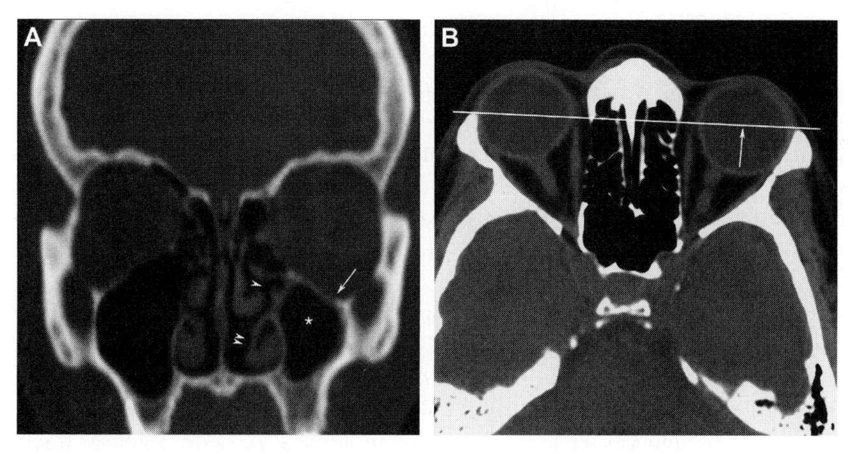

Fig. 27. Silent sinus syndrome. (*A*) Coronal reformatted noncontrast CT of the sinuses showing reduced size (atelectasis) of the left maxillary antrum (*), causing inferior retraction of the orbital floor (*arrow*) with enlarged left meatus (*arrowhead*) and nasal airway (*double arrowhead*). (*B*) Axial noncontrast CT through the orbits showing left sided enophthalmus (*arrow*).

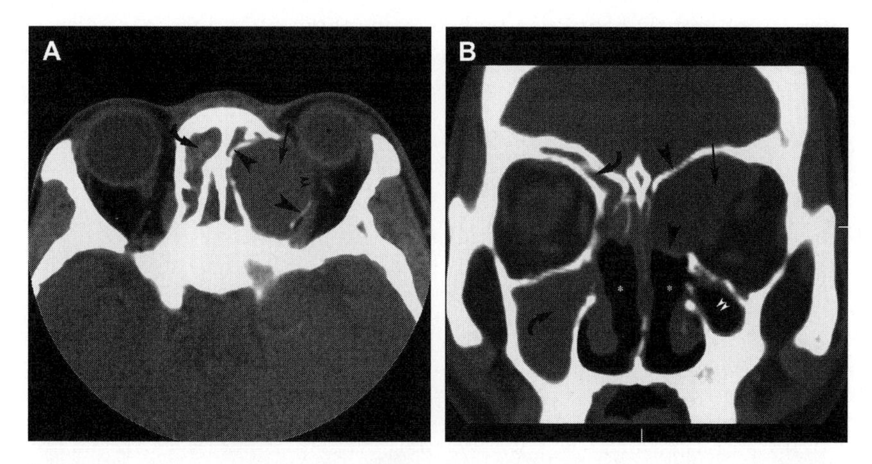

Fig. 28. Frontal sinus mucocele. (*A*) Axial noncontrast CT through the orbits showing a homogeneous, rounded fluid-attenuation mass (*arrow*) that expands the left frontal sinus with bowing of the inferomedial and inferolateral walls (*arrowheads*) and encroachment on the orbit causing a left proptosis (*). The lateral wall is incompletely visualized because of marked thinning beyond the scan resolution (*double arrowhead*). There is mucosal thickening and secretions in the ethmoid sinuses (*curved arrow*). (*B*) Coronal reformats of the axial CT with better demonstration of the relationship of the mass (*arrow*) to the frontal sinus, showing extension into the ethmoid sinus, which also is expanded. The orbital roof and floor is thinned (*arrowheads*), and part of the orbital roof is nonvisualized. Mucosal thickening and secretions fill the right frontal and maxillary sinuses (*curved arrows*), with bony wall thickening consistent with chronic sinusitis without expansion. The middle turbinates (*) were resected from previous surgery, and the small left maxillary sinus (*double arrowhead*) is the result of previous chronic obstruction without mucocele.

Extension from the ethmoid air cells through emissary veins passing through the lamina papyracea can result in a peripherally enhancing subperiosteal abscess along the medial orbit. Frontal sinus infection can extend anteriorly through the bone into the adjacent extracranial soft tissues. This involvement can lead to the development of a subgaleal abscess, also known as "Pott's puffy tumor." Intracranial extension can cause an epidural abscess or subdural empyema. Sphenoid disease can cause cavernous sinus thrombosis. These entities are discussed in greater detail in the section dealing with intracranial infection. Chronic obstruction of a sinus can cause retained secretions to expand the sinus gradually, resulting in a mucocele (Fig. 28).

Paranasal fungal disease presents differently depending on the immune status of the patient [41]. Chronic colonization of a sinus in the immunocompetent patient causes granulomatous inflammation with mucosal thickening and bony sclerosis, indistinguishable from chronic rhinosinusitis (Fig. 29). Fungus balls (mycetoma or aspergilloma) are more commonly hyperattenuating on CT, because of the tightly packed hyphae, and may be heavily calcified. Profoundly low signal on T2 imaging may mimic normal sinus air and is relatively specific if recognized (see Fig. 25).

Acute invasive fungal sinusitis usually is limited to immunocompromised patients and poorly controlled diabetics, in whom often fulminant disease infiltrates surrounding soft tissues with an angioinvasive propensity and

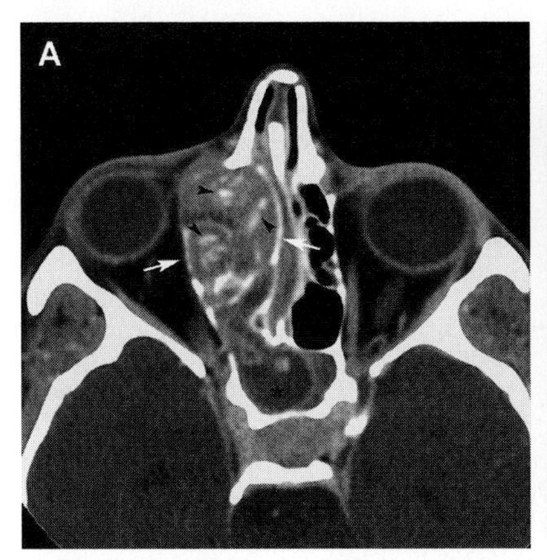

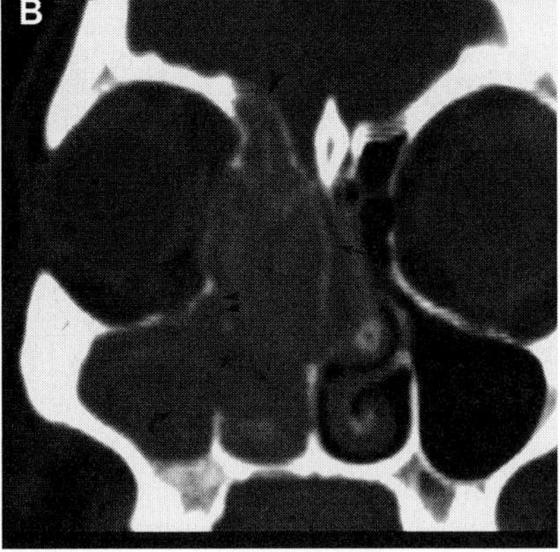

Fig. 29. Chronic fungal sinusitis. (*A*) Postcontrast axial CT showing mixed attenuation material containing multiple foci of calcification (*arrowheads*) expanding the ethmoid sinuses and extending through the sphenoethmoidal recess into the sphenoid sinus (*), causing lateral bowing of the lamina papyracea into the orbit and medial bowing of the right middle turbinate (*arrows*). (*B*) Coronal reformats showing the full extent of the lesion from the maxillary antrum (*curved arrow*) to the frontal sinus (*arrowhead*) with marginal bowing (*arrows*) and filling and expansion of the right osteomeatal complex compared with the left (*double arrowhead*). There is no bony destruction or spread beyond the sinuses, and the right uncinate process is markedly thinned and poorly visualized (*) but probably is present.

possible early orbital or intracranial spread. Again, CT is best at detecting early bony erosion (Fig. 30), and post-Gadolinium MRI is best for detecting spread beyond the sinus. MRA or CT angiography may demonstrate vascular invasion, thrombosis, and, rarely, mycotic aneurysm [2,43]. Chronic fungal infection in diabetics causes nongranulomatous inflammation but has no specific imaging features to distinguish it from the granulomatous type, although it does have greater potential for spread to surrounding structures such as the orbit.

Last, allergic fungal sinusitis caused by an atopic, IgE-mediated hypersensitivity to environmental fungal antigens presents as severe rhinosinusitis with multiple sinus involvement, hyperattenuating, heterogeneous material with sinus expansion, and possible bony erosion. T2 hypointensity may be observed and aids in making the diagnosis.

Orbits

Orbital infection most often is secondary to spread from an adjacent sinusitis, where it complicates 3% of cases. Other sources are skin/conjunctiva or hematogenous seeding, with an odontogenic origin being rare [44]. Most patients have clinically apparent periorbital cellulitis, and the role of imaging is to evaluate the degree of orbital or retroorbital involvement.

Contrast-enhanced CT often is preferred as the primary imaging modality because it is acquired rapidly, usually avoids motion artifact caused by

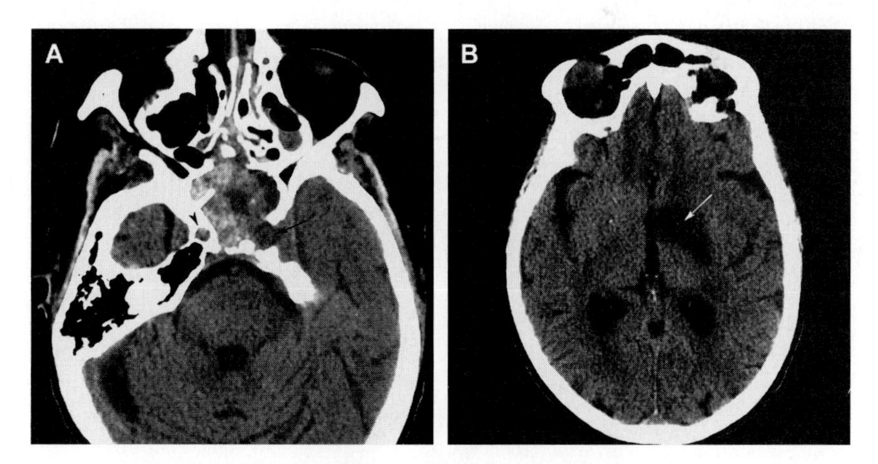

Fig. 30. Fungal sphenoid sinusitis directly invading the left internal carotid artery resulting in left lenticulostriate infarction. Axial noncontrast CT of the head showing (*A*) hyperattenuating material in the sphenoid sinus (*) with erosion through the left superoposterior sphenoid roof to surround the left petrous/intracavernous internal carotid artery (*arrow*), in contrast to normal appearance of the right carotid canal (*arrowhead*); (*B*) focal low-attenuation lenticulostriate territory infarction of the left lentiform nucleus, capsular genu, and posterior head of caudate nucleus (*arrow*).

eye movements, and can be performed in the axial plane with coronal reconstruction to avoid or minimize dental artifact. Low-attenuation orbital fat provides intrinsic tissue contrast, outlining the soft tissue structures of concern. Also, bone detail and assessment of the adjacent sinuses are optimal.

MRI is subject to motion artifact in the nonsedated patient and to susceptibility artifact from bone and air interfaces [45]. Fat saturation or inversion recovery techniques are essential to assess inflammatory involvement of orbital fat or to allow lesion discrimination, because fat and inflammatory edema can have similar signal characteristics. These sequences, however, prolong acquisition time. Although MRI is more sensitive than CT for myositis or optic neuritis, it may be possible to detect early findings such as orbital fat edema, blurring of adjacent planes, and enhancement by CT (Fig. 31).

Most infection is limited to preseptal or periorbital cellulitis. CT demonstrates swelling and stranding of involved fat. The orbital septum usually is well defined by surrounding fat as it arises from the periorbital marginal periosteum and inserts into the tarsal plates of the eyelids; however, it may become obscured if there is extensive fatty edema (Fig. 32). Retro-orbital extension requires cross-sectional imaging for adequate assessment [46], because the disease may be both intra- and extraconal. Inflammatory fat stranding is demonstrated, with possible myositis or optic neuritis, by abnormal enlargement, enhancement, and poorly defined contours. Involvement of the orbital apex compromises the optic nerve and increases the risk of intracranial extension (Fig. 33). Higher grades of infection are characterized by subperiosteal (usually medial wall secondary to adjacent ethmoid infection) or orbital abscess. IV contrast is required to differentiate ring-enhancing abscess from more homogeneously enhancing inflammatory

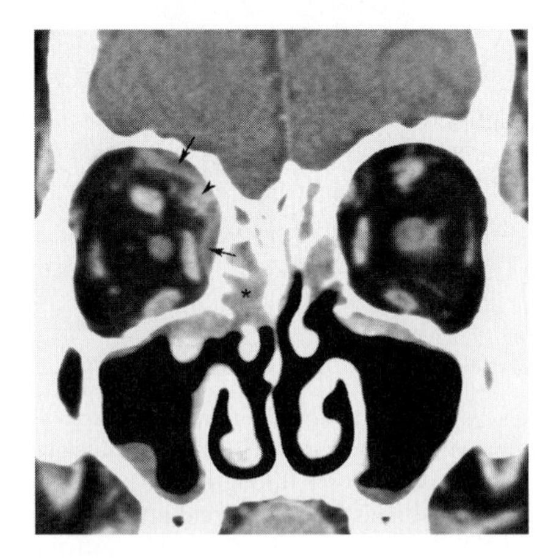

Fig. 31. Coronal contrast-enhanced CT through the orbits, showing an orbital subperiosteal abscess (*arrowhead*) arising from the ethmoidal sinusitis (*), causing orbital fat edema (*arrows*).

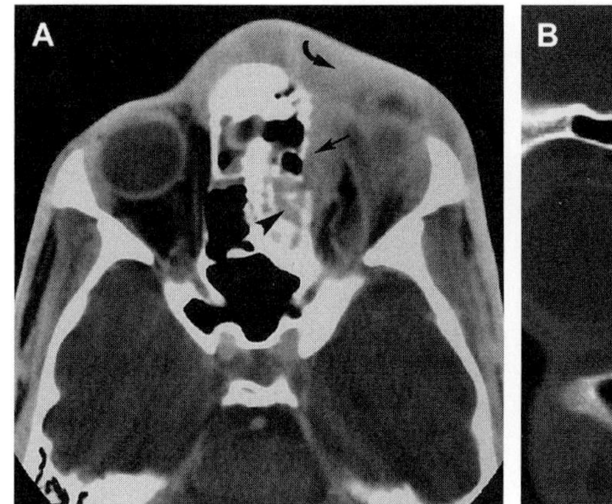

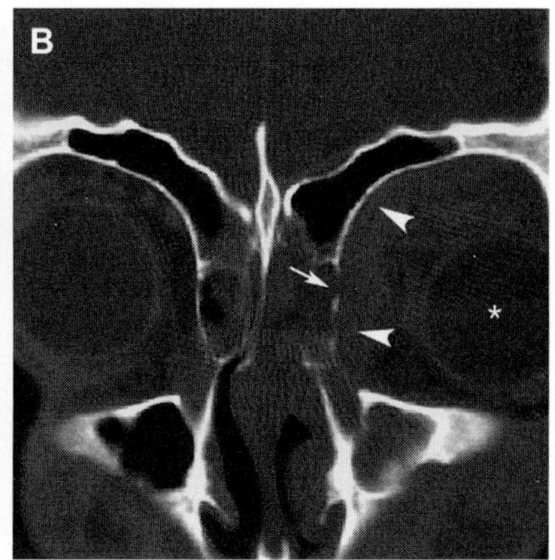

Fig. 32. Orbital subperiosteal abscess. (*A*) Axial contrast-enhanced CT showing enhancing material arising from the ethmoid sinus (*arrowhead*), which has eroded and traversed the left lamina papyracea to form a medial wall subperiosteal phlegmon (*arrow*) displacing the medial rectus muscle laterally and causing proptosis and extensive preseptal cellulitis with enhancement and swelling (*curved arrow*) in a plane indistinguishable between it and the intraorbital space; (*B*) direct coronal CT with bone window of the orbits showing erosion of the lamina papyracea (*arrow*), subperiosteal enhancing phlegmon (*arrowheads*), and adjacent inflammatory fat stranding that displaces the orbit inferolaterally (*).

phlegmon on CT and MRI. Orbital ultrasound may demonstrate lower echogenicity in a liquefying abscess [47].

Mass effect from abscess or inflamed tissues may cause proptosis with associated straightening of the optic nerve, potentially progressing to traction deformity of the posterior globe. This latter appearance probably indicates an emergency surgical decompression to preserve vision. Abnormal distension of the superior ophthalmic vein and/or intraluminal filling defects seen on postcontrast imaging, raise the specter of cavernous sinus thrombosis, a rare but highly morbid complication. Orbital CT always should include the cavernous sinus in the imaging field of view; its asymmetrical enhancement and enlargement support the diagnosis (see Fig. 26). On MRI, T1 noncontrast imaging may show increased signal because of associated venous thrombosis; however, this finding may be spurious and also can arise from normal slow venous flow or fat in the wall of the cavernous sinus. Loss of T2 flow signal void and heterogeneous enhancement should be observed.

Temporal bones

The temporal bones can be divided into the external auditory canal, middle ear, mastoid, petrous apex, inner ear, and internal auditory canal. CT and MRI provide complementary information. High-resolution (0.5–1.5 mm)

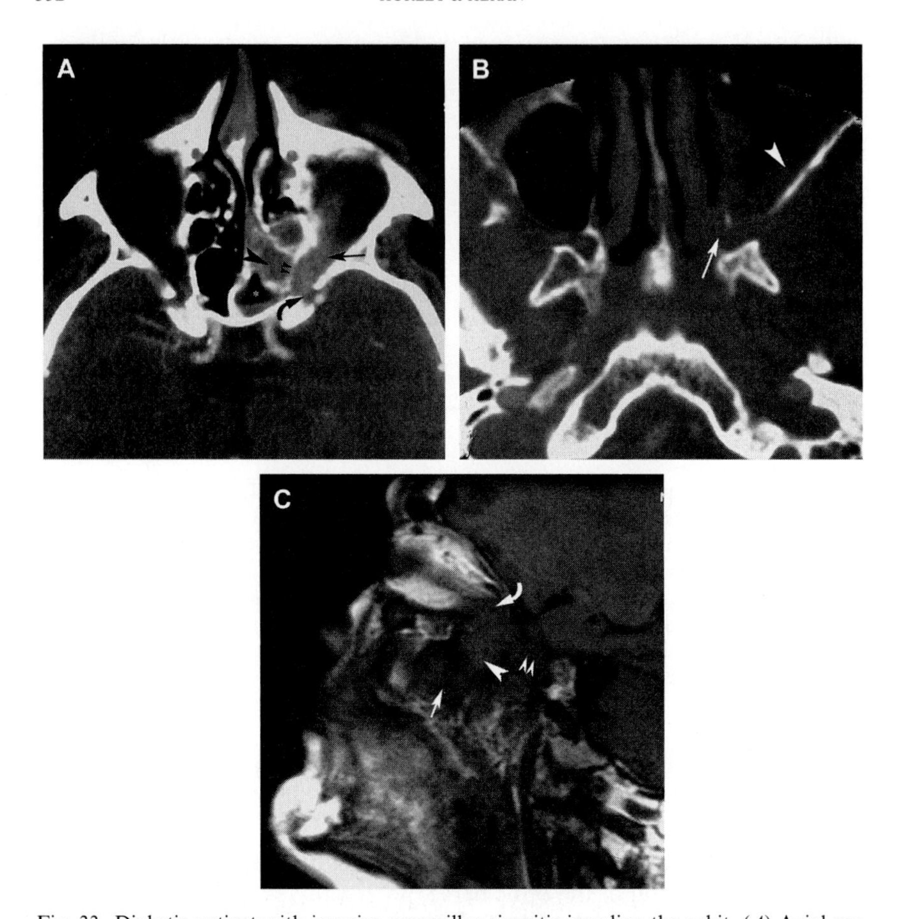

Fig. 33. Diabetic patient with invasive aspergillus sinusitis invading the orbit. (*A*) Axial contrast-enhanced CT showing enhancing inflammatory material in the left sphenoid (*) and ethmoid sinus (*arrowhead*) eroding through the medial wall (*double arrowhead*) and the orbital apex (*arrow*) to the level of the superior orbital fissure (*curved arrow*). (*B*) Axial contrast-enhanced CT showing mucosal thickening of the antrum (*arrowhead*) with extension of inflammatory material to cause erosive widening of the left pterygopalatine fossa at the level of the sphenopalatine foramen (*arrow*). (*C*) Sagittal noncontrast T1 MRI showing an isointense lesion extending from the left sphenopalatine foramen inferiorly (*arrow*) through the pterygopalatine fossa (*arrowhead*), across the inferior orbital fissure (*curved arrow*) into the orbital apex, and posteriorly from the pterygopalatine foramen into the foramen rotundum (*double arrowhead*), another potential route of intracranial spread.

axial CT with coronal reconstruction elegantly demonstrates the detailed bony anatomy. Soft tissue contrast is poor, however, and postcontrast enhancement often is undetectable adjacent to the high-attenuation bone. MRI of the temporal bone normally shows signal void (black bone against black air) on all sequences and is largely featureless apart from the endolymph-containing labyrinthine structures (cochlea, vestibule, and semicircular canals) that have intermediate T1 and high T2 signal. Post-Gadolinium scans are sensitive to subtle enhancement of pathologic processes against the signal-devoid background. Multiplanar imaging augmented by MRA/MRV aids in the recognition of intracranial extension and possible vascular complications, such as dural venous thrombosis.

External auditory canal

Necrotizing external otitis, previously termed "malignant otitis externa" because of its morbidity, difficult treatment, and high recurrence rate (20%), is a severe, often fulminant cellulitis and osteomyelitis arising from the external auditory canal (Fig. 34). It characteristically occurs in the diabetic patient secondary to *Pseudomonas aeruginosa* infection, introduced by cotton wool buds or other manipulations [48]. The early CT findings are characterized by mucosal thickening and enhancement beginning at the junction of the bony and cartilaginous canal. These findings eventually are supplemented by the hallmark of bone erosion, consistent with osteomyelitis, and spread of the lesion to adjacent regions: inferiorly through the fissures of Santorini to the masticator space, medially across the tympanic membrane to the middle ear, posteriorly to the mastoid, anteriorly to the temporomandibular joint, or superiorly to the intracranial space. MRI post-Gadolinium contrast administration should be performed to assess intracranial complications, and fat-saturated sequences should be performed to evaluate extension to or involvement of the skull base.

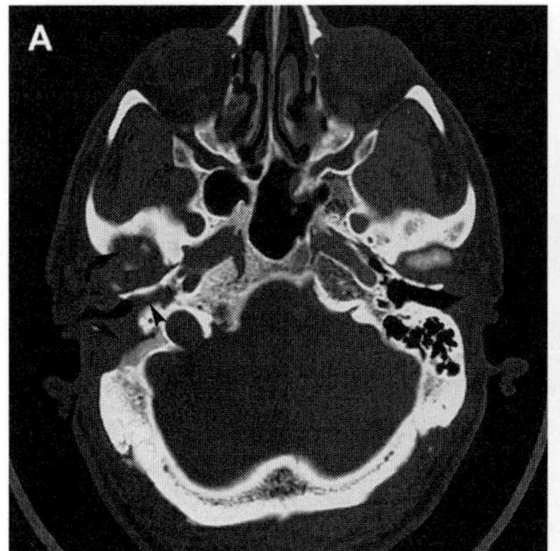

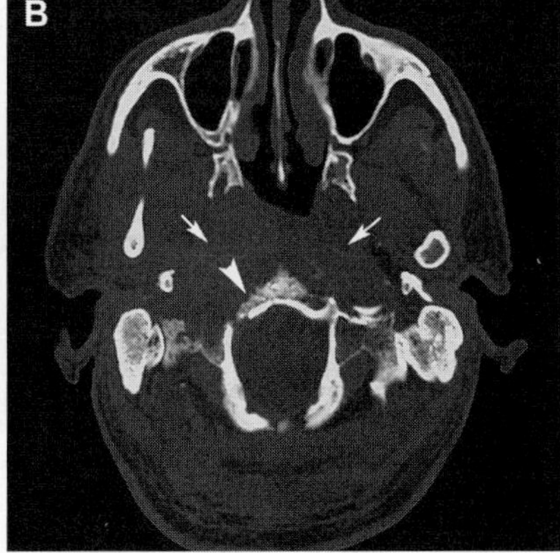

Fig. 34. Necrotizing (malignant) otitis externa. (*A*) Contrast-enhanced CT at bone window settings showing postauricular soft tissue edema representing cellulitis (*arrow*), soft tissue attenuation material occupying the right external auditory canal (*arrowhead*) and middle ear, with adjacent bony erosion consistent with osteomyelitis. Infection has extended anteriorly into the right temporomandibular joint (*curved arrow*). (*B*) Contrast-enhanced CT at bone window settings showing extension of bone erosion to the clivus at the base of the external skull (*arrowhead*), with extensive prevertebral and retropharyngeal soft tissue mass (*arrows*).

Osteomyelitis may be demonstrated earlier on a nuclear medicine study, such as ^{99m}Tc- methylene diphosphonate bone scans, ^{111}Indium-labeled white blood cell scans, or gallium citrate (Ga-67) scans. This condition usually requires surgical débridement, in addition to antibiotic therapy, for effective treatment.

Middle ear

The eustachian tube maintains equalized pressure and aeration of the middle ear. It also can provide a conduit for infection from the upper respiratory tract, particularly in children. Middle ear opacification results from any form of eustachian tube dysfunction/obstruction and is termed "serous otitis" or "otitis media with effusion." It is commonly caused by reactive adenoidal hypertrophy in children; in adults, however, a nasopharyngeal neoplasm should be excluded. Acute otitis media is clinically obvious and may be associated with air–fluid levels on imaging (Fig. 35). Most cases are self-limited and respond to antibiotics. A small number may be complicated by the development of acute mastoiditis.

Acquired cholesteatoma may be a complication of repeated or chronic otitis media. It can cause retraction of keratinizing stratified squamous epithelium from the external canal through a defect in the tympanic membrane, almost always in the pars flaccida superiorly. The continued active production and intralesional shedding of keratin causes expansion and erosion of adjacent bony structures, usually starting with the adjacent scutum, then filling Prussak's space. Further progression can involve the ossicular chain. In advanced cases, the lesion can extend into the bony labyrinth, along the skull base, and even intracranially. The hallmark of bony erosion is well demonstrated on CT (Fig. 36). On MRI, the lesion has heterogeneous

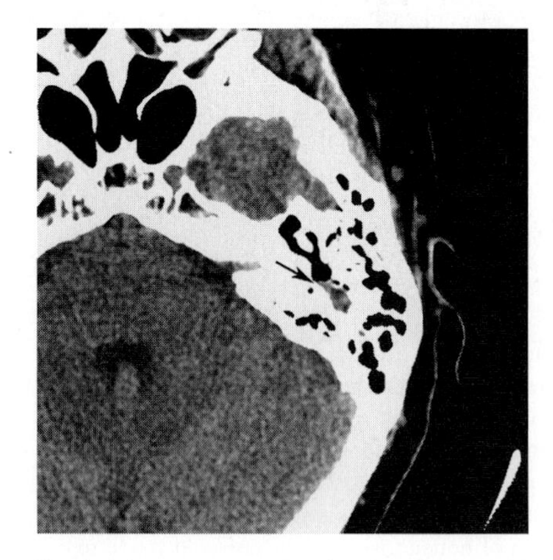

Fig. 35. Acute otitis media. Axial noncontrast CT showing fluid level in the middle ear (*arrow*).

T2 hyperintensity and has a T1 signal that is slightly higher than intracranial CSF. Suppression on diffusion-weighted imaging reflects the complex macromolecular keratinous content. Characteristically, the lesion does not enhance postcontrast, although rare cases of subtle enhancement have been reported, perhaps secondary to infection or repeated rupture and inflammation [49]. The lesion can recur late and in unusual locations (Fig. 37). Treatment is surgical, requiring total excision to prevent recurrence.

Other sequelae of chronic otitis include middle ear granulation tissue, a relatively common finding differentiated from cholesteatoma by lack of bony destruction on CT and intense enhancement on contrast-enhanced MRI. Tympanosclerosis is caused by dystrophic calcification or new bone formation occurring within scar tissue. It can involve the ossicular chain from the tympanic membrane to the oval window and is well demonstrated on CT. New bone formation obliterating the normal air spaces is a common response to chronic inflammation in other parts of the temporal bone, such as mastoid and petrous apex (Fig. 38).

Mastoid

Suspected acute mastoiditis should be assessed by CT to distinguish the low-grade, antibiotic-responsive incipient subtype from the aggressive coalescent subtype. Incipient mastoiditis has a CT appearance limited to mastoid air-cell opacification (Fig. 39) caused by exudative mucosal

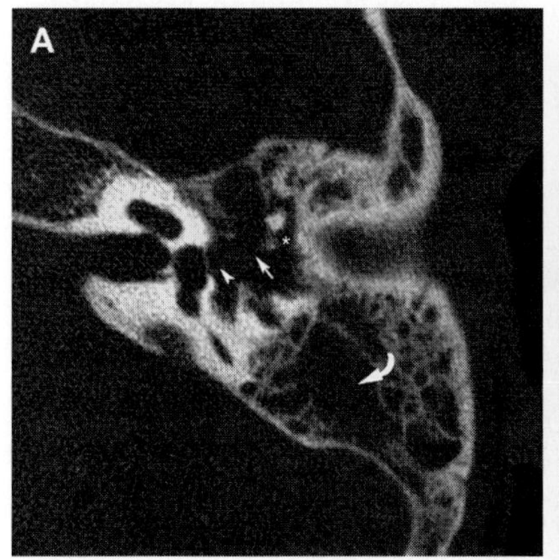

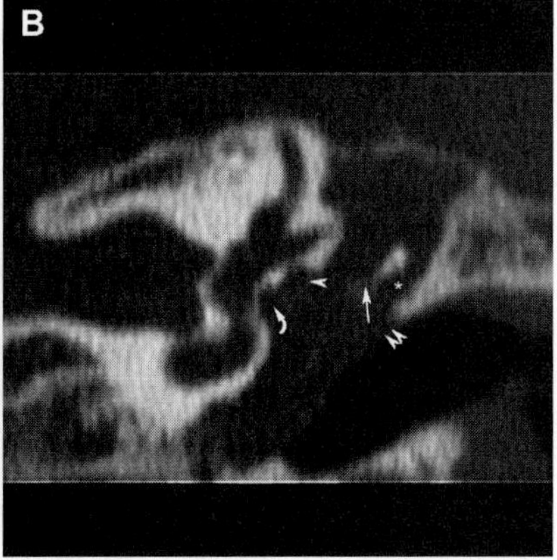

Fig. 36. Acquired middle ear cholesteatoma. (*A*) Axial 1.25-mm CT through the left temporal bone showing complete opacification of the middle ear and mastoid with erosion of the mastoid septa (*curved arrow*), long process of incus (*arrow*), and stapes (*arrowhead*). Note location of the Prussak's space (*). (*B*) Coronal reformats of axial CT showing truncated scutum (*double arrowhead*), opacification of Prussak's space (*), and erosion of the ossicular chain, all hallmarks of acquired cholesteatoma. Erosion of the long process of incus (*arrow*) and stapes extending to the round window (*curved arrow*) is noted, as well as erosion of the inferior wall of the tympanic facial nerve canal (*arrowhead*).

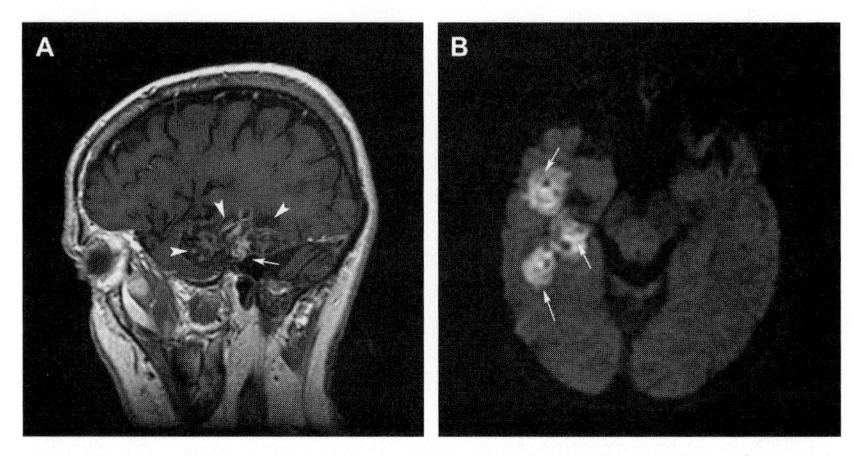

Fig. 37. Pathologically confirmed case of recurrent, acquired cholesteatoma with intracranial localization. (*A*) Sagittal T1 postgadolinium MRI showing predominantly low-signal mass lesion (*arrowheads*) centered above the temporal bone (*arrow*) and displacing the temporal lobe, demonstrating central strands of enhancement (unusual for cholesteatoma). (*B*) Diffusion-weighted MRI, showing increased signal in the lesion (*arrows*), suggesting diffusion restriction characteristic of cholesteatoma.

thickening and usually responds to antibiotic therapy alone. Coalescent mastoiditis demonstrates septal destruction and periostitis consistent with osteomyelitis [50]. Erosion of the cortical plate overlying the sigmoid sinus is a relatively sensitive and specific sign (Fig. 40) [51]. This morbid condition has become more prevalent because of increasing antibiotic resistance [2]

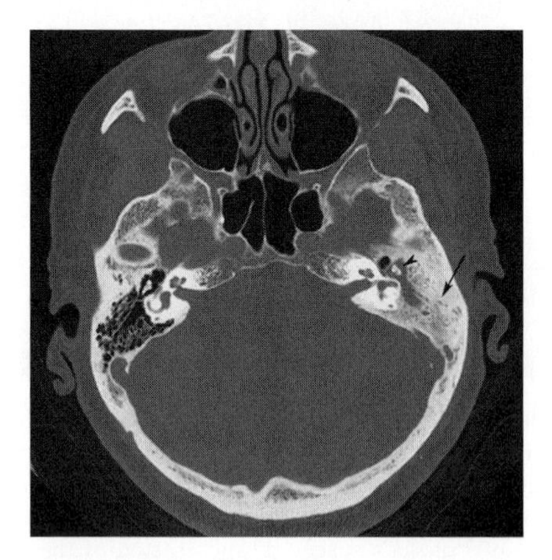

Fig. 38. New bone formation in chronic mastoiditis. Axial CT at bone windows setting showing replacement of the mastoid air cells predominantly by sclerotic bone (*arrow*). Low-attenuation material in the middle ear was suspicious for a cholesteatoma (*arrowhead*).

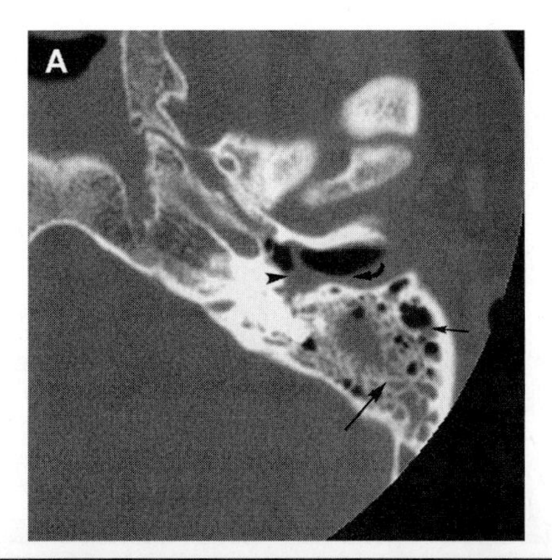

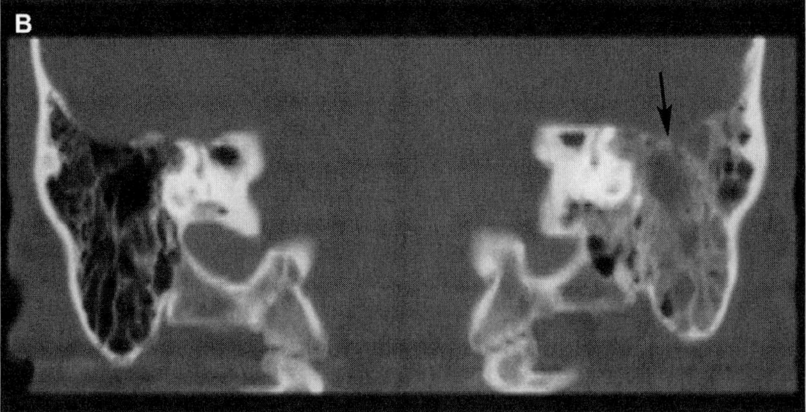

Fig. 39. Acute incipient mastoiditis and otitis media. (*A*) Axial CT showing opacification and multiple air–fluid levels in the left mastoid air cells (*arrows*), middle ear (*arrowhead*), and external meatus (*curved arrow*) but no septal bone erosion evident (compared with the normal right side). (*B*) Coronal reformatted CT showing opacification of the left mastoid air cells with extension to the tegmen tympani, which appears thin but intact (*arrow*). The image plane is parallel to the fluid levels, which therefore are not visible.

and often requires surgical intervention in combination with antibiotic therapy.

Direct spread of infection into the middle ear can lead to spontaneous decompression through the tympanic membrane. The additus ad antrum usually is obstructed, however, and alternative routes of spread, either directly or by emissary veins, may occur: laterally to produce a subperiosteal abscess, inferiorly through an aerated mastoid tip to cause a soft tissue neck abscess (Bezold abscess), posteriorly to form an abscess around the sigmoid sinus, and superiorly to cause a petrous apicitis. Labyrinthitis and facial nerve involvement (usually tympanic or mastoid segments) are best demonstrated by abnormal enhancement on MRI. Intracranial complications, also

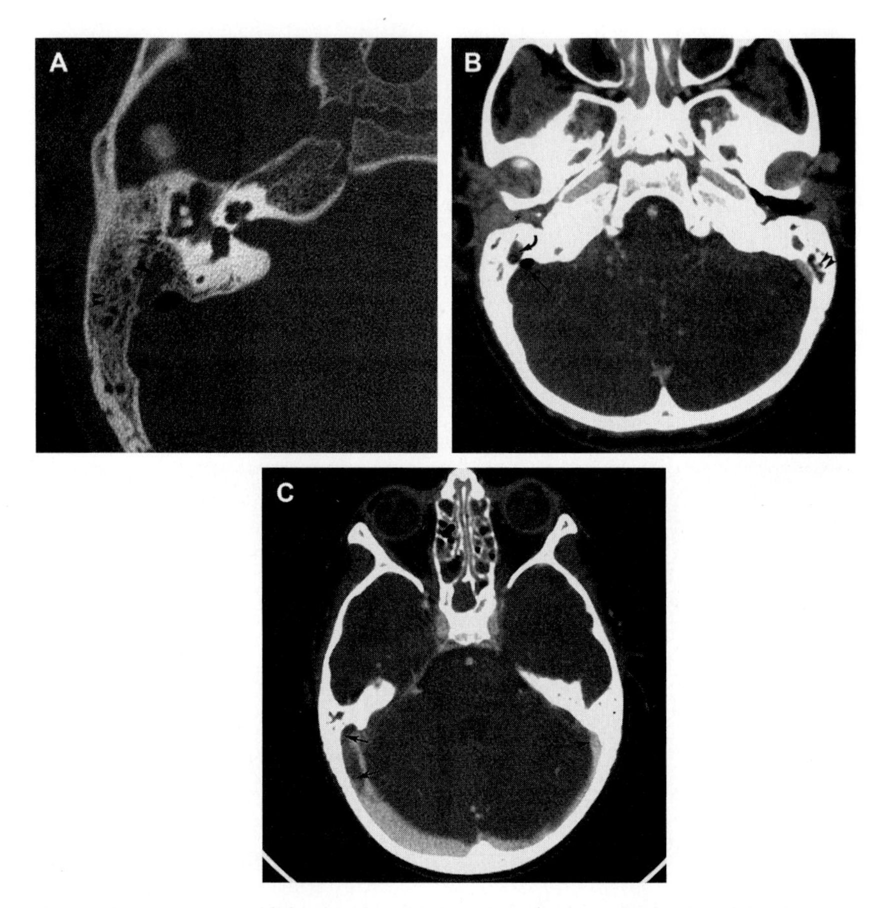

Fig. 40. Coalescent mastoiditis with sigmoid sinus thrombosis. (*A*) Axial CT of the right temporal bone showing opacification of the mastoid air cell (*double arrowhead*) and middle ear (*), focal septal erosion (*arrowhead*) consistent with coalescent mastoiditis, and erosion of the cortical plate over the sigmoid sinus with adjoining intracranial gas (*arrow*). (*B*) Axial contrast-enhanced CT, showing bilateral mastoid opacification (*curved arrow on right, double arrowhead on left*), normal enhancement of sigmoid sinus on the left (*arrowhead*), but nonenhancement of thrombosed right sigmoid sinus with adjacent gas bubble (*arrow*). (*C*) Axial contrast-enhanced CT at a more superior level showing enhancing dural wall around an occlusive filling defect in the right sigmoid sinus (*arrows*). The left sigmoid sinus (*arrowhead*) is nondominant (as is often the case) but otherwise is normal.

best demonstrated on MRI, include subdural empyema, epidural abscess, and associated cerebritis or cerebral abscess in advanced cases. Dural sinus thrombosis may occur secondary to adjacent empyema or osteothrombophlebitis. These entities are discussed in the final section dealing with intracranial infection.

Incidental mastoid fluid and mucosal thickening, without clinical signs of infection, was noted in a series of patients who had transverse sinus thrombosis and presumably was caused by impaired venous drainage mimicking an incipient mastoiditis [52].

Petrous apex

Spread of infection to the petrous apex probably requires the presence of an aerated apex (30% of population). CT with coronal reformats may show erosion of the apical bone. Coronal Gadolinium-enhanced MRI detects possible adjacent dural enhancement, often associated with inflammatory involvement of the closely related trigeminal Gasserian ganglion in the Meckel's cave, and abducens nerve in the Dorrelo canal, giving the clinical triad of Gradenigo's syndrome (ipsilateral trigeminal neuralgia, lateral rectus palsy, and ear discharge). Gallium single-photon emission CT scanning is useful to monitor response to antibiotic therapy and to decide when surgical intervention is required [53].

Complications include cholesterol granuloma (Fig. 41) and the less common petrous apex mucocele. Both show expansion of the petrous apex and associated septal erosion, but cholesterol granuloma appears as a characteristic hyperintense lesion on noncontrast T1 imaging, and as hypointense blood products in T2 imaging because of lipid-laden macrophages.

Labyrinth

Labyrinthitis, most commonly caused by a viral infection, and less often caused by bacterial or noninfectious inflammation, is identified by abnormal postgadolinium MRI enhancement of the endolymphatic channel resulting from breakdown of the blood–endolymph barrier. Precontrast T1 imaging is useful to exclude blood products (caused by methemoglobin) or

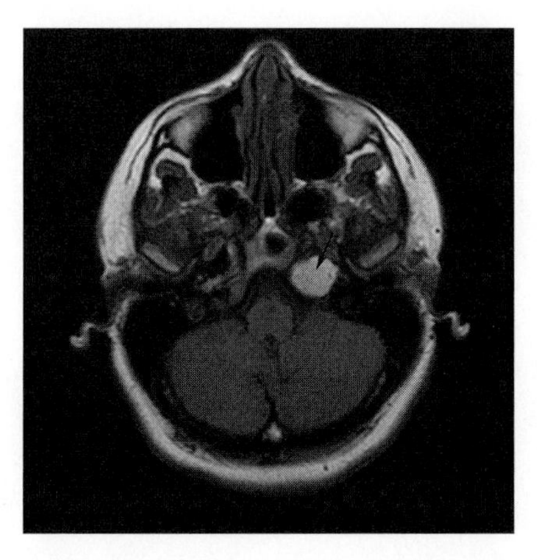

Fig. 41. Axial T1 noncontrast MRI, showing a bright, expansile lesion in the left petrous apex (*arrow*) characteristic of a cholesterol cyst.

proteinaceous fluid as a cause of hyperintensity that may be mistaken for enhancement on the postcontrast study.

Postinfectious labyrinthitis may undergo healing by an intense fibroblastic infiltration and subsequent neo-ossification (labyrinthine ossificans), recognized by diminution or complete loss of the normal fluid-attenuation membranous labyrinth. The scala tympanum in the basal cochlea adjacent to the round window is the site most commonly affected. Ossification is seen well on CT (Fig. 42), and there may be a labyrinthine "white-out" in severe cases. MRI demonstrates replacement of the normal endolymphatic T2 hyperintensity by signal void.

Intracranial suppuration

This section deals with the intracranial complications of ear, nose, and throat infections. Primary CNS infections are manifold and are beyond the scope of this article, as is the constellation of HIV-related neurologic disorders. Cavernous sinus thrombosis has been discussed previously.

Extra-axial space infection may arise by direct extension, as is typical in epidural abscess and subdural empyema. Epidural abscess is a more focal, inwardly convex lesion, being tightly bound by the dura to the inner skull surface and therefore unable to cross the cranial sutures. Unlike subdural empyema, it can cross the midline, being external to the interhemispheric falx and dural sinuses (Fig. 43). Subdural empyema is a more insidious, thin-layered process, which can insinuate itself more freely over a broad area (Fig. 44). It can track over the tentorium or adjacent to the midline falx, which forms a barrier to its passage across the midline (Fig. 45). These thin collections may be of similar attenuation to brain parenchyma, given their thick purulence, and may be missed on noncontrast CT. Even with IV contrast, additional coronal CT reformats are advised to detect small

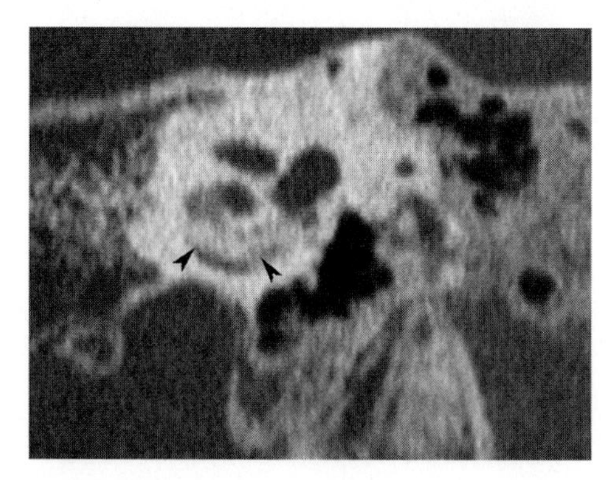

Fig. 42. Postinfectious labyrinthine ossificans. Oblique reformatted CT image through the cochlea showing new bone formation in the scala tympani of the basal cochlea (*arrowheads*).

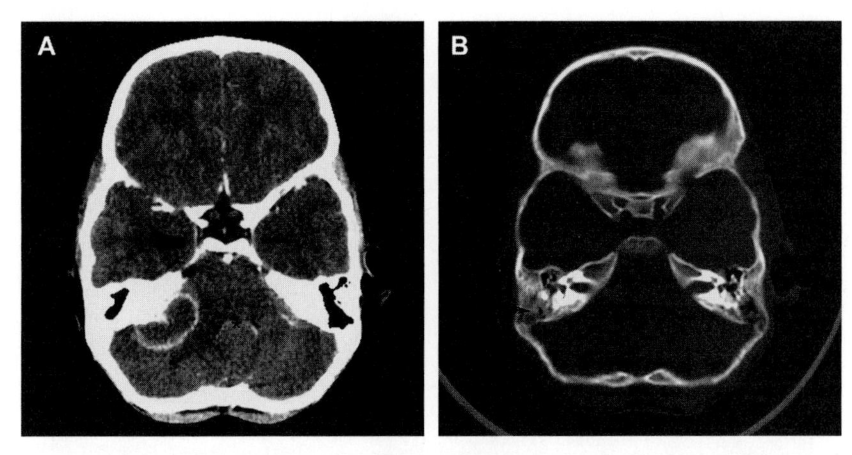

Fig. 43. Intracranial epidural abscess arising from coalescent mastoiditis. (*A*) Axial postcontrast CT of the head showing uniform peripheral enhancement of a large focal epidural abscess (*arrow*) extending into the right cerebellopontine angle with adjacent cerebellar edema (*arrowhead*) and displacement of the fourth ventricle (*) across the midline. (*B*) CT of the head with bone window showing opacification of the right mastoid air cells with septal destruction (*arrow*) and loss of defined cortical contour of the posterior petrous bone (*arrowhead*).

lesions, and postgadolinium MRI is recommended as the criterion standard [54]. Often, there is intense reactive edema in the adjacent brain parenchyma. Complications such as venous thrombosis always should be considered in this setting.

Leptomeningitis (bacterial meningitis) usually is blood borne in sepsis and involves the pia/arachnoid as well as subarachnoid CSF. Contrast-enhanced CT (Fig. 46) and post-Gadolinium MRI demonstrate enhancing leptomeninges within the sulci, MRI being more sensitive. T2-weighted fluid attenuated inverse recovery is exquisitely sensitive to proteinaceous material or CSF, appearing as increased signal intensity. Complications include cerebral edema, obstructive hydrocephalus, sinus thrombosis, arterial infarction, and involvement of the labyrinthine scala tympani, leading to labyrinthine ossificans (see Fig. 42) and deafness. Rarely, cerebral or epidural abscess and subdural empyema can ensue.

Tuberculosis tends to involve the dura, causing a basal pachymeningitis. Presentation typically is delayed, with possible symptoms related to vascular narrowing and ischemia, or a gradual extension over the basal dura (Fig. 47) resulting in sequential cranial neuropathies. Thick, enhancing exudates are seen in the basilar cisterns and sylvian fissures. Large, rounded tuberculomas can simulate dural-based tumors such as meningioma (Fig. 48). Hydrocephalus is common. Parenchymal tuberculomas may complicate miliary disease. They tend to have more irregular and thick, enhancing walls compared with a typical bacterial abscess [55].

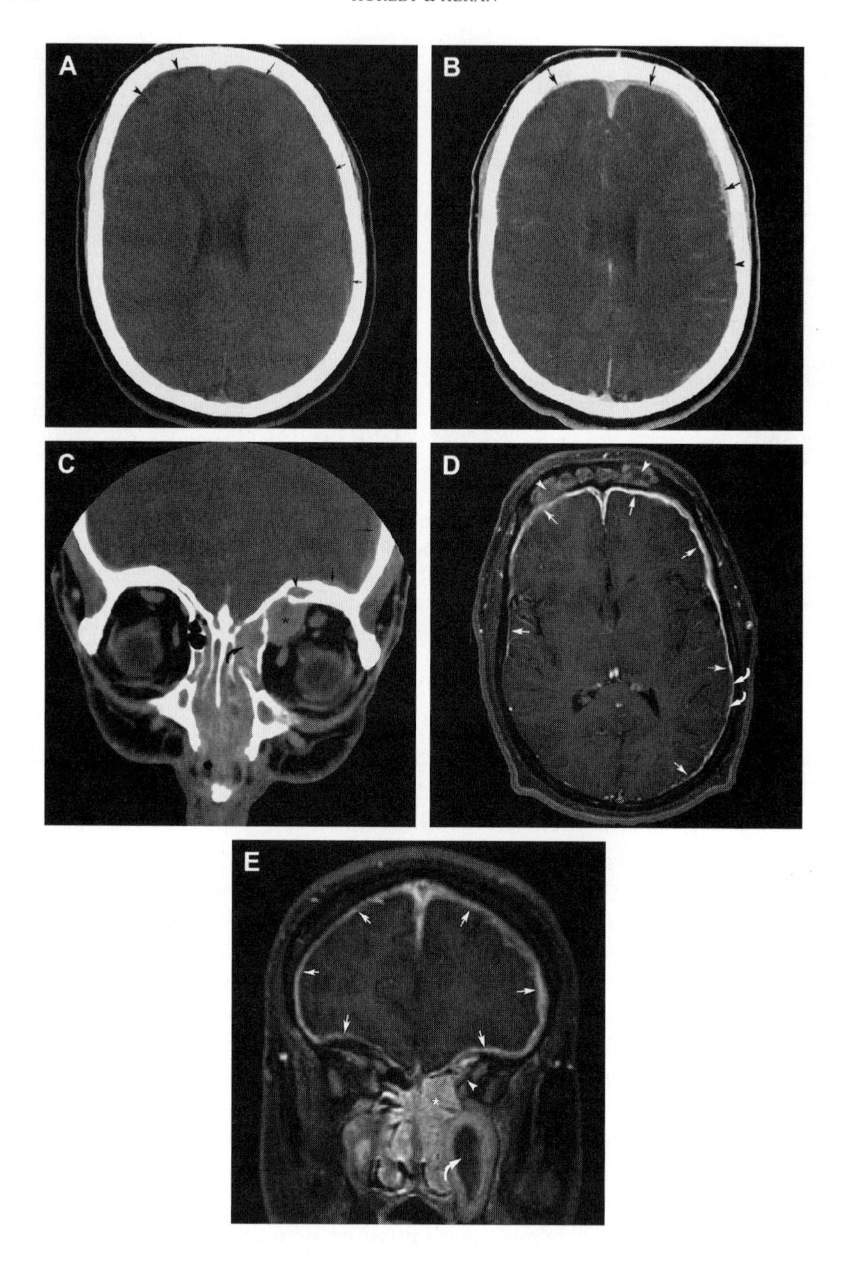

Bacterial infection of the cerebral parenchyma may result from a contiguous extra-axial lesion or, more commonly, from hematogenous seeding. Early inflammation and subsequent organization are described in four phases. Early cerebritis (1–3 days) is characterized by mild edema, swelling, and faint, patchy enhancement, which progresses to a more obvious, central

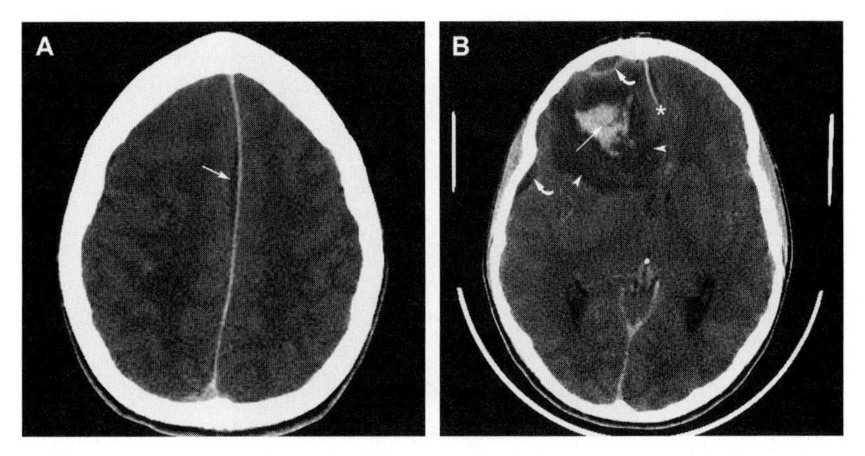

Fig. 45. Subdural empyema progressing to cause venous infarction. (*A*) Postcontrast CT of the head showing thin low attenuation collection (*arrow*) adjacent to and displacing the enhancing dural falx. (*B*) Postcontrast CT showing paramedian, right frontal, low-attenuation infarct extending to the head of the caudate (*arrowheads*), with central hyperattenuating hemorrhage (*arrow*) and peripherally enhancing subdural empyema over the frontal hemisphere (*curved arrows*). Increased midline shift to the left (*) threatens to cause subfalcine herniation.

low attenuation with poorly defined peripheral enhancement (late cerebritis, 3–10 days) (Fig. 49). The periphery matures into a granulating membrane in an attempt to wall off the focus of infection, forming a well-defined enhancing wall and a low-attenuation liquefactive center by 10 to 14 days, referred to as the "early capsule phase." In the late capsule phase the wall matures and thickens with reduction in size of the necrotic center [56].

The stereotypical cerebral abscess is a well-defined, uniformly ring-enhancing lesion on axial postcontrast imaging (Fig. 50). If caused by hematogenous seeding, it usually forms at the gray/white junction, which is

Fig. 44. Intracranial subdural empyema secondary to frontoethmoidal sinusitis. (*A*) Axial noncontrast CT of the head showing low to isoattenuating, bilateral subdural collections (*arrows* and *arrowheads*) with effacement of the underlying sulci particularly in the left frontal lobe. (*B*) Postcontrast CT showing enhancing thickened dura (*arrows*) and nonenhancing purulent subdural fluid (*arrowhead*) of higher attenuation than CSF. (*C*) Coronal reformatted postcontrast CT showing enhancing material in the sinuses bilaterally, a superomedial left orbital subperiosteal abscess (*) secondary to extension from the ethmoid (*curved arrow*) and frontal (*arrowhead*) sinuses, and subdural enhancement tracking superiorly from the left supraorbital surface (*arrows*). (*D*) Axial T1 postgadolinium MRI with fat saturation showing avidly enhancing bilateral subdural phlegmon (*arrows*) with purulent foci of ring enhancement (*curved arrows*) and enhancing mucosa and inflammatory debris in the frontal sinuses (*arrowheads*). (*E*) Coronal T1 postgadolinium MRI with fat saturation showing bilateral enhancing dura (*arrows*) extending into the interhemispheric falx, an enhancing ethmoid lesion (*) with intraorbital extension (*arrowhead*), and mucosal thickening and enhancement in the left maxillary antrum (*curved arrow*).

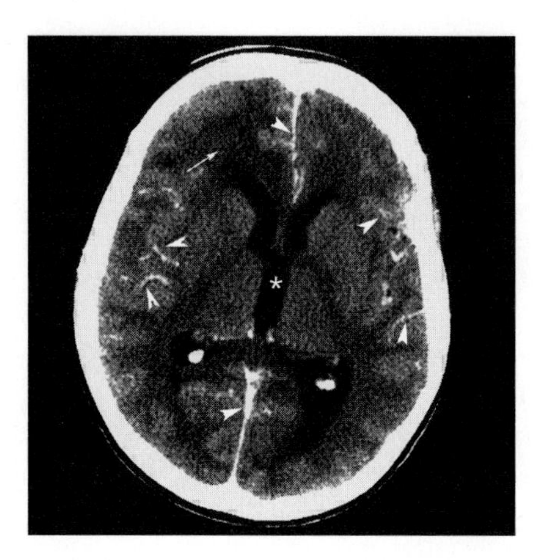

Fig. 46. Acute bacterial meningitis. Contrast-enhanced CT, showing leptomeningeal enhancement extending into the subarachnoid cerebral sulcal spaces (*arrowheads*), moderate hydrocephalus (*), and right frontal edema (*arrow*) probably related to cortical venous compromise.

relatively vascular. Likewise, most cerebral abscesses are situated supratentorially in the middle cerebral artery distribution, that being the territory receiving most blood flow. Avid enhancement of the granulating abscess wall is caused by disruption of the blood–brain barrier, and its permeability also results in florid vasogenic edema. The main differential is an aggressive, necrotic glioblastoma or metastasis. An abscess tends to have a thinner, more uniform wall and daughter (satellite) lesions.

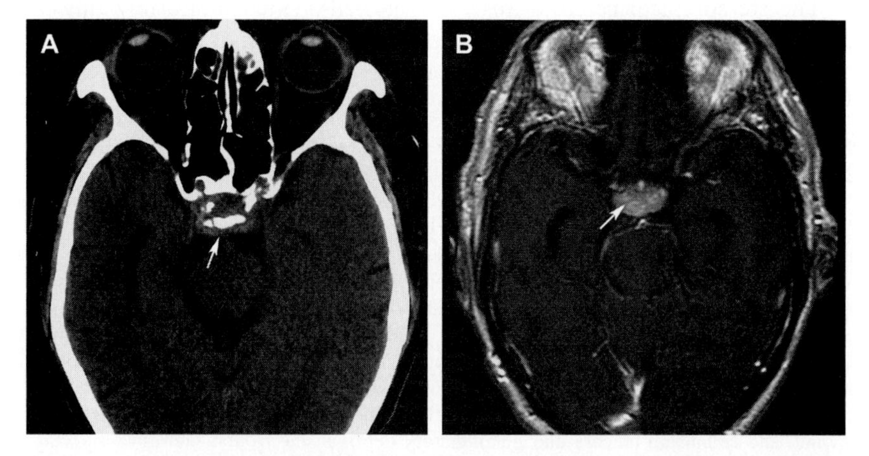

Fig. 47. Basal tuberculous pachymeningitis. (*A*) Noncontrast CT of the head showing focal dural thickening overlying the clivus/dorsum sellae (*arrow*), but no bone destruction. (*B*) T1 postgadolinium MRI, showing homogeneous enhancement of the lesion (*arrow*) and normal enhancing pituitary infundibulum anteriorly.

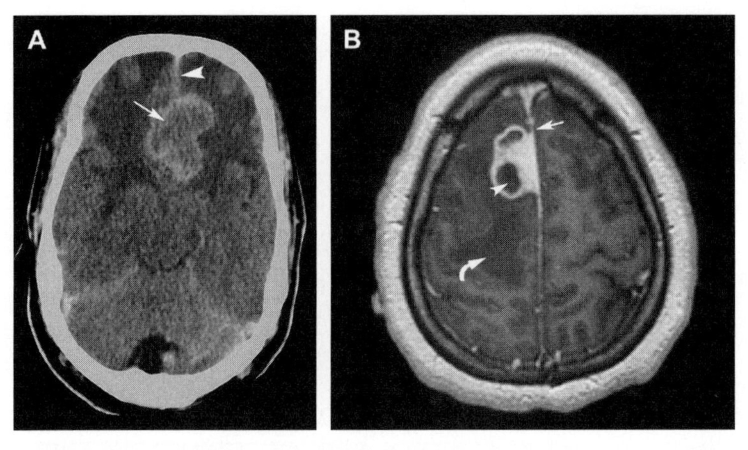

Fig. 48. Intracranial tuberculoma. (*A*) Contrast-enhanced CT showing a lobular, faintly ring enhancing mass (*arrow*) intimately related to the dura of the anterior falx (*arrowhead*) and extensive surrounding vasogenic edema. (*B*) Postgadolinium 1 MRI in another patient, showing a dural tail (*arrow*) as well as heterogeneous mass (*arrowhead*) and vasogenic edema (*curved arrow*).

On MRI, relatively low T2 signal in the abscess wall is speculated to represent abundant free oxygen radicals. Restricted diffusion on diffusion-weighted MRI typically is seen in the center of an abscess (appearing bright on diffusion-weighted MRI, dark on an apparent diffusion coefficient map) is thought to reflect the complex debris contents (see Fig. 50). These features help, but exceptions to the rule do occur, such

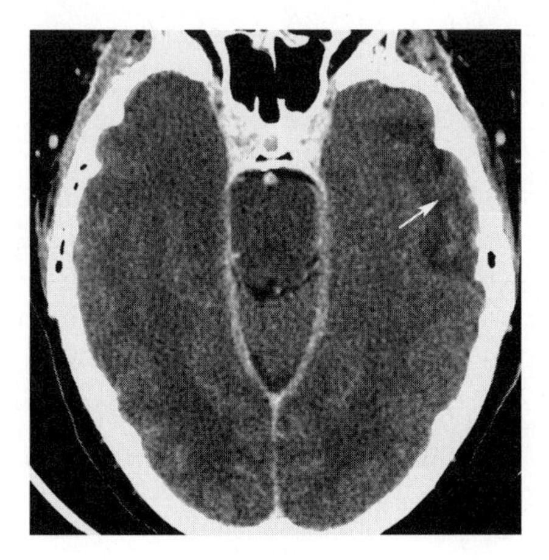

Fig. 49. Contrast-enhanced CT of the head, showing late cerebritis with low attenuation and mild mass effect involving subcortical white and gray matter (*arrow*) but no ring enhancement or frank homogeneous necrotic focus.

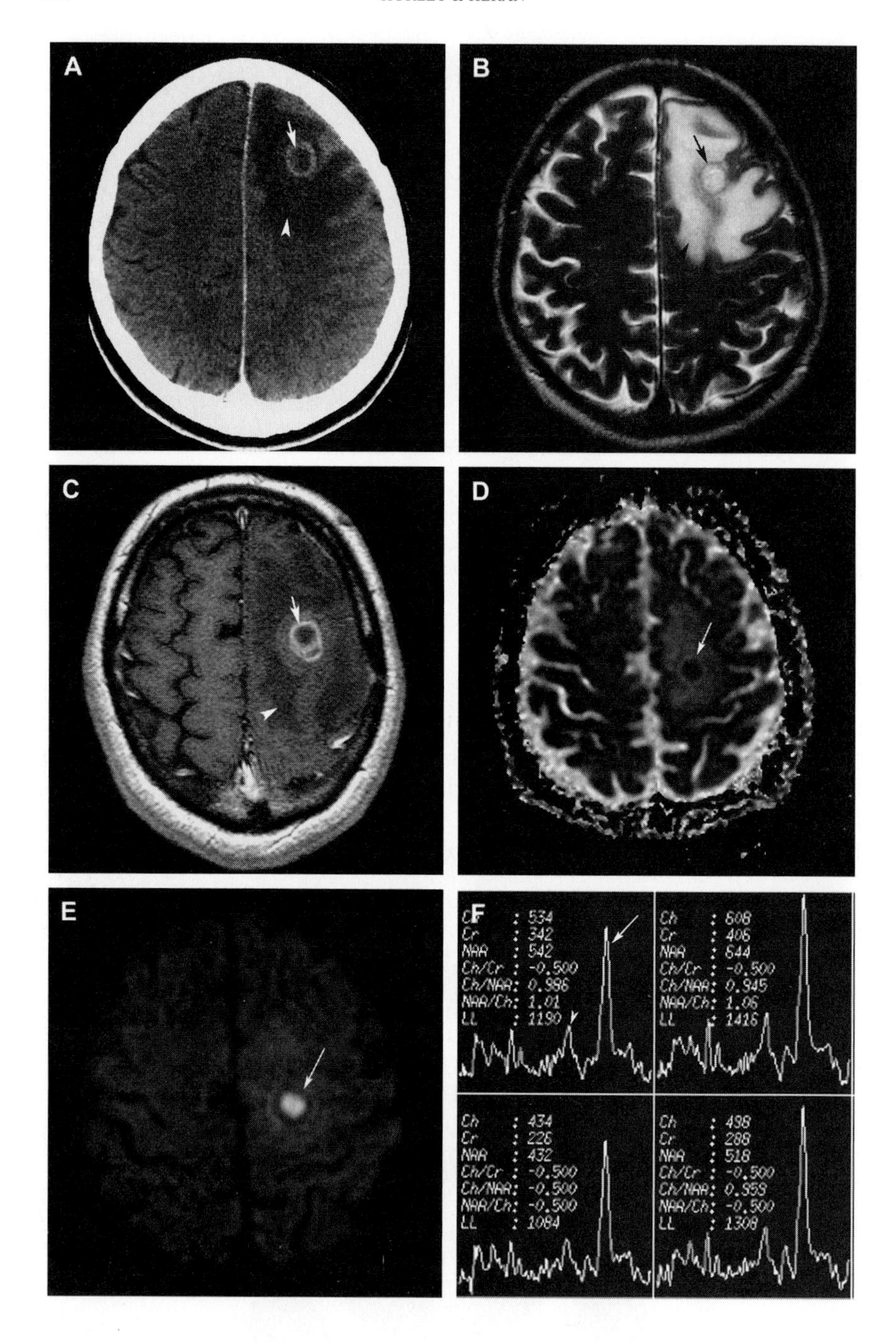
A
B
C
D
E
F
Ch : 534
Cr : 342
NAA : 542
Ch/Cr : -0.500
Ch/NAA: 0.986
NAA/Ch: 1.01
LL : 1190
Ch : 608
Cr : 406
NAA : 644
Ch/Cr : -0.500
Ch/NAA: 0.945
NAA/Ch: 1.06
LL : 1416
Ch : 434
Cr : 226
NAA : 432
Ch/Cr : -0.500
Ch/NAA: -0.500
NAA/Ch: -0.500
LL : 1084
Ch : 498
Cr : 288
NAA : 518
Ch/Cr : -0.500
Ch/NAA: 0.959
NAA/Ch: -0.500
LL : 1308

as restricted diffusion in a highly cellular lymphoma, primitive neuroectodermal tumors, or keratin-filled epidermoid tumors. Likewise, MRI spectroscopy of the abscess core may demonstrate the presence of multiple metabolites rather than a solitary lactate peak of a necrotic tumor [57]. This MRI spectroscopy differentiation often poses significant challenges in day-to-day clinical practice.

Cerebral abscesses can rupture into the ventricles, resulting in ependymitis/ventriculitis and possibly hydrocephalus. Visualized debris within the ventricle is a more common finding than hydrocephalus or ependymal enhancement [58]. Mycotic aneurysms tend to be peripheral and associated with parenchymal hemorrhage. Usually a conventional cerebral angiogram is required to visualize these entities, because they typically occur distal to the circle of Willis.

Dural sinus thrombosis is caused most commonly by paranasal sinus infection but also can complicate mastoiditis or, less commonly, neck space infection tracking up to the skull base. It may be asymptomatic if restricted to the transverse and sigmoid sinuses but can propagate to other sinuses, potentially resulting in local or diffuse cerebral edema, venous infarction, or hemorrhage (Fig. 51), all caused by intracranial venous hypertension. The involved dural sinus also can become a source of septic pulmonary emboli. These complications result in high morbidity and mortality.

Dural sinus hyperattenuation on noncontrast CT and postcontrast enhancement of the inflamed sinus wall around nonenhancing thrombus (empty delta sign) (Fig. 52A) may not be obvious, and MRI (Fig. 52B) is more sensitive for direct visualization of thrombus, especially with gradient imaging techniques. Both CT venography and MRV demonstrate an irregular, attenuated, or occluded sinus (Fig. 52C).

Imaging pitfalls include common anatomic variations such as a small, nondominant, usually left-sided transverse sinus and arachnoid granulations causing prominent intrasinus filling defects [59]. Two-dimensional time-of-flight MRV is particularly prone to flow-related artifacts [60]. These

Fig. 50. Cerebral abscess. (*A*) Contrast-enhanced CT of the head showing uniformly ring-enhancing mass in the subcortical frontal white matter (*arrow*) and extensive surrounding vasogenic edema (*arrowhead*) consistent with an abscess. Differential diagnosis includes metastasis and aggressive glioblastoma; however, the latter usually has a more irregular appearance. (*B*) T2-weighted MRI showing that the abscess has a characteristic hypointense rim (*arrow*), possibly caused by the presence of free radicals, and T2-hyperintense vasogenic edema (*arrowhead*). (*C*) T1-weighted postgadolinium MRI showing slightly more complex enhancing appearance of the abscess (*arrow*) with a single septation and vasogenic edema sparing the gray matter (*arrowhead*). (*D*) Apparent diffusion coefficient map showing true diffusion restriction in the abscess (*arrow*) with persistent high signal edema (unrestricted). (*E*) Diffusion-weighted MR image showing high signal intensity in the lesion (*arrow*) and less intense surrounding edema (T2 shine through). (*F*) Spectroscopic analysis of voxels taken from the lesion, showing multiple metabolites including elevated lactate (*arrow*) and reduced n-acetyl aspartate (*arrowhead*), a nonspecific finding in necrotic cerebral lesions.

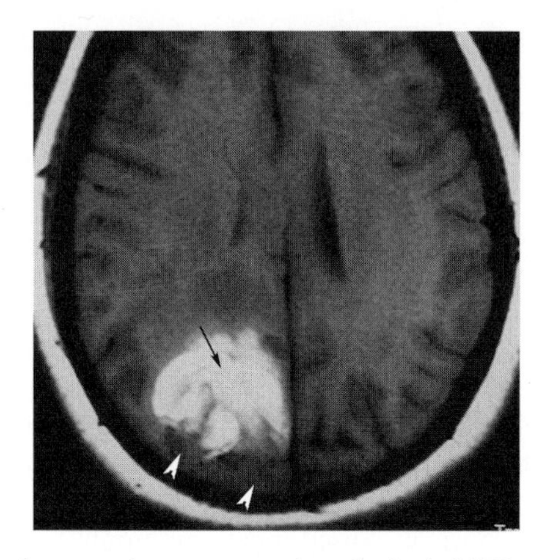

Fig. 51. Venous infarction secondary to venous thrombosis. Axial T1 noncontrast MRI showing a hyperintense lesion in the paramedian, subcortical left parietal lobe (*arrow*) that effaces but spares most of the adjacent sulci (*arrowheads*).

artifacts are not an issue with current contrast-enhanced volumetric MRV techniques. Early thrombus (1–3 days) can have a confusing MRI appearance, with very low signal deoxyhemoglobin mimicking normal flow void on T2 imaging and intermediate signal on T1 imaging (Fig. 53), similar to adjacent parenchyma, before it degrades into more obvious T1 and T2 hyperintense extracellular methemoglobin (3–30 days). As a result, sequences such as T2*-weighted scans, which are sensitive to magnetic field perturbations resulting from these blood products, are mandatory for identification of early venous thrombosis.

Summary

Multidetector CT is the established imaging modality for the assessment of suspected acute infections of the head and neck, with the additional utility of single-breathhold and full volumetric data acquisitions that allow post-processing at exquisite spatial resolutions. MRI remains a secondary modality in imaging of acute infections in the neck, paranasal sinuses, orbits, and temporal bones because of inferior demonstration of cortical bone and logistical issues such as accessibility, scan times, and magnetic field compatibility. MRI becomes mandatory, however, in cases of suspected intracranial or spinal canal involvement, where its superior soft tissue contrast is critical. Both CT angiography and MRA can be used to assess vascular complications, replacing the need for conventional angiography in many cases.

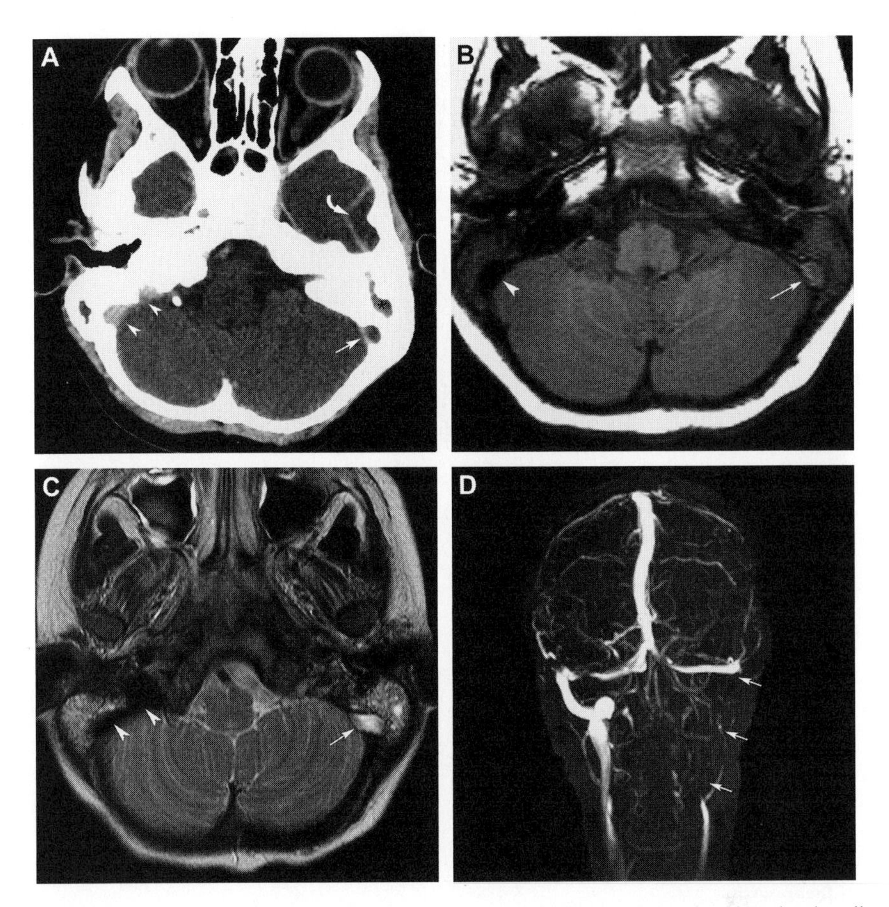

Fig. 52. Dural sinus thrombosis. (*A*) Contrast-enhanced CT showing enhancing dural wall around nonenhancing thrombus in the left sigmoid sinus (*arrow*), in contrast to the normal right side (*arrowheads*), and the primary source of infection from coalescent mastoiditis (*) and secondary subdural empyema (*curved arrow*). (*B*) Axial T1 noncontrast MRI, showing hyperintense signal in the left sigmoid sinus (*arrow*) adjacent to a mastoiditis, and normal flow void on the right (*arrowhead*). (*C*) Axial T2 noncontrast MRI showing more clearly the lesions shown in the T1 noncontrast MRI. (*D*) Three-dimensional gadolinium-enhanced MRV showing nonflow in the left sigmoid sinus and jugular vein to the mid neck (*arrows*).

In the acute setting, clinical signs guide the diagnosis of an infectious cause. On axial imaging, characteristic features are demonstrated, but none are pathognomic for infectious versus other inflammatory conditions or neoplasia. Isotope leukocyte studies are specific but take several days to perform.

The role of the initial axial imaging remains the assessment of the origin, extent, and associated complications of the pathologic process.

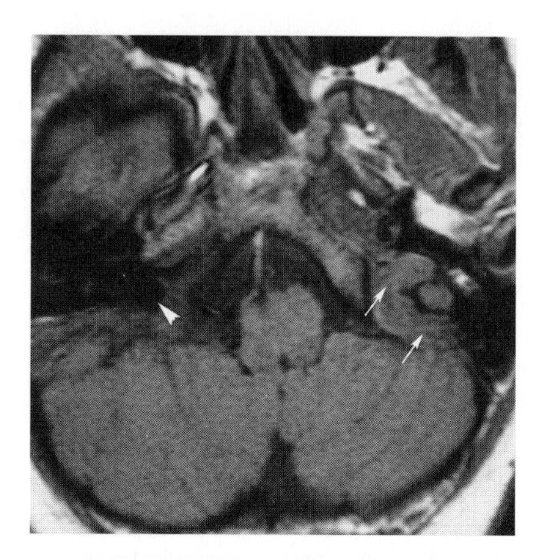

Fig. 53. Early (< 3 days) dural thrombus. Axial T1 noncontrast MRI, showing intermediate signal in the thrombosed sigmoid sinus (*arrows*) with similar signal intensity as in the cerebellar parenchyma, in contrast to normal signal void on the right side (*arrowhead*).

Acknowledgments

The authors acknowledge Drs. Ashu Jhamb, Robert A. Nugent, and William D. Robertson, all from the Division of Neuroradiology at Vancouver General Hospital, for their valuable contributions in completing this article.

References

[1] Nagy M, Backstrom J. Comparison of the sensitivity of lateral neck radiographs and computed tomography scanning in pediatric deep-neck infections. Laryngoscope 1999;109(5): 775–9.

[2] Zapalac JS, Billings KR, Schwade ND, et al. Suppurative complications of acute otitis media in the era of antibiotic resistance. Arch Otolaryngol Head Neck Surg 2002;128:660–3.

[3] Douglas SA, Jennings S, Owen VMF, et al. Is ultrasound useful for evaluating paediatric inflammatory neck masses? Clin Otolaryngol 2005;30:526–9.

[4] Palestro CJ, Kipper SL, Weiland FL, et al. Osteomyelitis: diagnosis with 99mTc-labeled antigranulocyte antibodies compared with diagnosis with 111in-labeled leukocytes—initial experience. Radiology 2002;223:758–64.

[5] Lewis MA. Multislice CT: opportunities and challenges. Br J Radiol 2001;74(885):779–81.

[6] Imhof H, Czerny C, Dirisamer A. Head and neck imaging with MDCT. Eur J Radiol 2003; 45(Suppl 1):s23–31.

[7] Nash K, Hafeez A, Hou S. Hospital acquired renal insufficiency. Am J Kidney Dis 2002; 39(5):930–6.

[8] Benko A, Fraser-Hill M, Magner P, et al. Canadian Association of Radiologists: guidelines for the prevention of contrast induced nephropathy. Can Assoc Radiol J 2007;58(2):79–87.

[9] Thomsen HS. How to avoid CIN: guidelines from the European Society of Urogenital Radiology. Nephrol Dial Transplant 2005;20(Suppl 1):18–22.

[10] Barrett BJ, Parfrey PS. Preventing nephropathy induced by contrast medium. N Engl J Med 2006;354(4):379–86.
[11] Glockner JF, Hu HH, Stanley DW, et al. Parallel MR imaging: a users guide. Radiographics 2005;25:1279–97.
[12] Chong VFH, Khoo JBK, Fan YFF. Imaging of the nasopharynx and skull base. Magn Reson Imaging Clin N Am 2002;10:547–71.
[13] Ergun I, Kevin K, Uruc I, et al. The safety of gadolinium in patients with stage 3 and 4 renal failure. Nephrol Dial Transplant 2006;21(3):697–700.
[14] Thomsen HS. Nephrogenic systemic fibrosis: a serious late adverse reaction to gadodiamide. Eur Radiol 2006;16(12):2619–21.
[15] De Wilde JP, Rivers AW, Price DL. A review of the current use of magnetic resonance imaging in pregnancy and safety implications for the fetus. Prog Biophys Mol Biol 2005; 87(2–3):335–53.
[16] Webb JA, Thomsen HS, Morcos SK, and the Members of Contrast Media Safety Committee of European Society of Urogenital Radiology (ESUR). The use of iodinated and gadolinium contrast media during pregnancy and lactation. Eur Radiol 2005;15(6):1234–40.
[17] Kee-Min Yeow, Chun-Ta Liao, Shen-Po Hao. US-guided needle aspiration and catheter drainage as an alternative to open surgical drainage for uniloculated neck abscesses. J Vasc Interv Radiol 2001;12(5):589–94.
[18] Lazor JB, Cunningham MJ, Eavey RD, et al. Comparison of computed tomography and surgical findings in deep neck infections. Otolaryngol Head Neck Surg 1994;111:746–50.
[19] Parhiscar A, Har-El G. Deep neck abscess: a retrospective review of 210 cases. Ann Otol Rhinol Laryngol 2001;110(11):1051–4.
[20] Branstetter BF, Weissman JL. Infection of the facial area, oral cavity, oropharynx, and retropharynx. Neuroimaging Clin N Am 2003;13:393–410.
[21] Eggers G, Rieker M, Kress B, et al. Artefacts in magnetic resonance imaging caused by dental material. MAGMA 2005;18(2):103–11.
[22] Abrahams JJ, Berger SB. Inflammatory disease of the jaw. AJR Am J Roentgenol 1998; 170(4):1085–91.
[23] Chow AW. Infections of the oral cavity, head and neck. In: Mandell GL, Douglas RG, Bennett JE, editors. Mandell, Douglas and Bennett's principles and practice of infectious diseases. 4th edition. New York: Churchill Livingstone; 1995. p. 593–605.
[24] Stubinger S, Leiggener C, Sader R, et al. Intraorbital abscess. A rare complication after maxillary molar extraction. J Am Dent Assoc 2005;136:921–5.
[25] Caruso PA, Watkins LM, Suwansaard P, et al. Odontogenic orbital inflammation. Radiology 2006;239(1):187–94.
[26] Howlett DC, Kesse KW, Hughes DV, et al. The role of imaging in the evaluation of parotid disease. Clin Radiol 2007;57:692–701.
[27] Alyas F, Lewis K, Williams M, et al. Diseases of the submandibular gland as demonstrated using high resolution ultrasound. Br J Radiol 2005;78(928):362–9.
[28] Madani G, Beale T. Inflammatory conditions of the salivary glands. Semin Ultrasound CT MR 2006;27(6):440–51.
[29] Avrahami E, Englender M, Chen E, et al. CT of submandibular gland sialolithiasis. Neuroradiology 1996;38(3):287–90.
[30] Yousem DM, Loevner LA, Geckle RJ, et al. Adenoidal width and HIV factors. AJNR Am J Neuroradiol 1997;20(6):1186–7.
[31] Rotta AT, Wiryawan B. Respiratory emergencies in children. Respir Care 2003;48(3): 248–58.
[32] Crespo AN, Chone CT, Fonesca AS, et al. Clinical versus computed tomography evaluation in the diagnosis and management of deep neck infecion. Sao Paulo Med J 2004;122(6): 259–63.
[33] O'Brien WT, Lattin GE, Thompson AK. Lemierre syndrome: an all-but-forgotten disease. AJR Am J Roentgenol 2006;187:W324.

[34] Eastwood JD, Hudgins PA, Malone D. Retropharyngeal effusion in acute calcific prevertebral tendinitis: diagnosis with CT and MR imaging. AJNR Am J Neuroradiol 1998;19(9): 1789–92.

[35] Park SW, Han MH, Sung MH, et al. Neck infection associated with pyriform sinus fistula: imaging findings. AJNR Am J Neuroradiol 2000;21(5):817–22.

[36] Moon WK, Han MH, Chang KH, et al. CT and MR imaging of head and neck tuberculosis. Radiographics 1997;17(2):391–402.

[37] Hanck C, Fleisch F, Katz G. Imaging appearance of nontuberculous mycobacterial infection of the neck. AJNR Am J Neuroradiol 2004;25(2):349–50.

[38] Robson CD, Hazra R, Barnes PD, et al. Nontuberculous mycobacterial infection of the head and neck in immunocompetent children: CT and MR findings. AJNR Am J Neuroradiol 1999;20:1829–35.

[39] Djupesland P. Necrotizing fasciitis of the head and neck: report of three cases and review of the literature. Acta Otolaryngol 2000;543(Suppl 543):186–9.

[40] Som PM, Brandwein MS. Sinonasal cavities. Inflammatory diseases. In: Som PM, Curtin HD, editors. Head and neck imaging. 4th edition. St. Louis (MO): Mosby; 2003. p. 196–200.

[41] Yoshimi A, Bevan Y. Imaging evaluation of sinusitis: diagnostic performance and impact on health outcome. Neuroimaging Clin N Am 2003;13:251–63.

[42] Herrmann BW, Forsen JW Jr. Simultaneous intracranial and orbital complications of acute rhinosinusitis in children. Int J Pediatr Otorhinolaryngol 2004;68(5):619–25.

[43] Hurst RW, Judkins A, Bolger W, et al. Mycotic aneurysm and cerebral infarction resulting from fungal sinusitis: imaging and pathologic correlation. AJNR Am J Neuroradiol 2001; 22(5):858–63.

[44] Blake FA, Siegert J, Wedl J, et al. The acute orbit: etiology, diagnosis, and therapy. J Oral Maxillofac Surg 2006;64(1):87–93.

[45] Belden CJ, Zinreich SJ. Orbital imaging techniques. Semin Ultrasound CT MR 1997;18(6): 413–22.

[46] Howe L, Jones NS. Guidelines for the management of periorbital cellulitis/abscess. Clin Otolaryngol Allied Sci 2004;29(6):725–8.

[47] Mair MH, Geley T, Jufmaier W, et al. Usin orbital sonography to diagnose and monitor treatment of acute swelling of the eyelids in pediatric patients. AJR Am J Roentgenol 2002;179:1529–34.

[48] Handzel O, Halperin D. Necrotizing (malignant) external otitis. Am Fam Physician 2003; 68(2):309–12.

[49] Rutherford SA, Leach PA, King AT. Early recurrence of an intracranial epidermoid cyst due to low-grade infection: case report. Skull Base 2006;16(2):109–15.

[50] Vazquez E, Castellote A, Piqueras J, et al. Imaging of complications of acute mastoiditis in children. Radiographics 2003;23:359–72.

[51] Antonelli PJ, Garside JA, Mancuso AA, et al. Computed tomography and the diagnosis of coalescent mastoiditis. Otolaryngol Head Neck Surg 1999;120(3):350–4.

[52] Fink JN, McAuley DL. Mastoid air sinus abnormalities associated with lateral venous sinus thrombosis: cause or consequence? Stroke 2002;33:290–2.

[53] Lee YH, Lee NJ, Kim JH, et al. CT, MRI and gallium SPECT in the diagnosis and treatment of petrous apicitis presenting as multiple cranial neuropathies. Br J Radiol 2005;78(934): 948–51.

[54] Adame N, Hedlund G, Byington CL. Sinogenic intracranial empyema in children. Pediatrics 2005;116:461–7.

[55] Garg RK. Classic diseases revisited: tuberculosis of the central nervous system. Postgrad Med J 1999;75(881):133–40.

[56] Grossman RI, Yousem DM. Infectious and noninfectious inflammatory diseases of the brain. In: Grossman GI, Youssem DM, editors. Neuroradiology. The requisites. 2nd edition. St. Louis (MO): Mosby; 2003. p. 273–330.

[57] Chang KH, Song IC, Kim SH, et al. In vivo single-voxel proton MR spectroscopy in intracranial cystic masses. AJNR Am J Neuroradiol 1998;19:401–5.
[58] Fukui MB, Williams RL, Mudigonda S. CT and MR imaging features of pyogenic ventriculitis. AJNR Am J Neuroradiol 2001;22:1510–6.
[59] Liang L, Korogi Y, Sugahara T, et al. Normal structures in the intracranial dural sinuses: delineation with 3D contrast-enhanced magnetization prepared rapid acquisition gradient-echo imaging sequence. AJNR Am J Neuroradiol 2002;23:1739–46.
[60] Ayanzen RH, Bird CR, Keller PJ, et al. Cerebral MR venography: normal anatomy and potential diagnostic pitfalls. AJNR Am J Neuroradiol 2000;21:74–8.

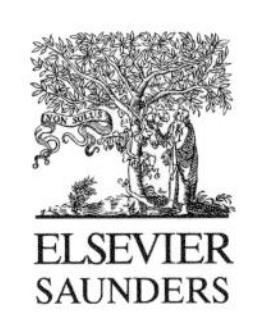

ELSEVIER
SAUNDERS

INFECTIOUS
DISEASE CLINICS
OF NORTH AMERICA

Infect Dis Clin N Am 21 (2007) 355–391

Microbiology and Principles of Antimicrobial Therapy for Head and Neck Infections

Itzhak Brook, MD, MSc

Department of Pediatrics and Medicine, Georgetown University School of Medicine, 4431 Albemarle St. NW, Washington, DC 20016, USA

The predominant aerobic and anaerobic bacteria in head and neck infections and their resistance to antimicrobial agents

The predominant aerobic and anaerobic bacteria isolated in common head and neck infections are summarized in Table 1. The major aerobic pathogens recovered in acute upper respiratory tract infections (URTI) are *Streptococcus pneumoniae, Haemophilus influenzae*, and *Moraxella catarrhalis*. Antimicrobial resistance among these micro-organisms has increased significantly in the past 2 decades. Anaerobic bacteria also are common in chronic head and neck infections that are serious and life threatening. The source of anaerobes in these infections is often the oropharynx. Because of their fastidiousness, these organisms are difficult to culture and often are overlooked. Their exact role in health and disease often is difficult to ascertain from the medical literature because of the inconsistent methodologies used for their isolation and identification [1]. Treatment of anaerobic infection is complicated by the slow growth of these organisms, their polymicrobial nature, and increasing antimicrobial resistance.

An important mechanism of antibiotic resistance of both aerobic bacteria (*Staphylococcus aureus, H influenzae*, and *M catarrhalis*) and anaerobic gram-native bacilli (AGNB) is the production of the enzyme β-lactamase. β-Lactamase–producing bacteria (BLPB) can be involved directly in the infection and protect themselves and other penicillin-susceptible organisms in the vicinity from β-lactam antibiotics. This protection can occur when the enzyme is secreted into the infected tissue or abscess fluid in sufficient

E-mail address: ib6@georgetown.edu

doi:10.1016/j.idc.2007.03.014

Table 1
Aerobic and anaerobic bacteria isolated in selected head and neck infections

Type of infection	Aerobic and facultative organisms	Anaerobic organism
Otitis media, acute	*S pneumoniae* *H influenzae*[a] *M catarrhalis*[a]	*Peptostreptococcus* spp
Otitis media and mastoiditis, chronic	*S aureus*[a] *E coli*[a] *K pneumoniae*[a] *P aeruginosa*[a]	Pigmented *Prevotella* and *Porphyromonas* spp *Bacteroides* spp[a] *Fusobacterium* spp[a] *Peptostreptococcus* spp
Peritonsillar and peripharyngeal abscess	*S pyogenes* *S aureus*[a] *S pneumoniae*	*Fusobacterium* spp[a] Pigmented *Prevotella* and *Porphyromonas* spp[a]
Suppurative thyroiditis	*S pyogenes* *S aureus*[a]	Pigmented *Prevotella* and *Porphyromonas* spp[a]
Sinusitis, acute	*H influenzae*[a] *S pneumoniae* *M catarrhalis*[a]	*Peptostreptococcus* spp
Sinusitis, chronic	*S aureus*[a] *S pneumoniae* *H influenzae*	*Fusobacterium* spp[a] Pigmented *Prevotella* and *Porphyromonas* spp[a]
Cervical lymphadenitis	*S aureus*[a] *Mycobacterium* spp	Pigmeted *Prevotella* and *Porphyromonas* spp[a] *Peptostreptococcus* spp
Postoperative infection disrupting oral mucosa	*Staphylococcus* spp[a] Enterobacgeriaceae[a]	*Fusobacterium* spp[a] *Bacteroides* spp[a] Pigmented *Prevotella* and *Porphyromonas* spp[a] *Peptostreptococcus* spp
Odontogenic and deep neck infections	*Streptococcus* spp *Staphylococcus* spp[a]	Pigmented *Prevotella* and *Porphyromonas* spp[a] *Bacteroides* spp[a] *Fusobacterium* spp[a] *Peptostreptococcus* spp
Necrotizing ulcerative gingivitis, or Vincent's angina	*Streptococcus* spp *Staphylococcus* spp[a]	*Fusobacterium necrophorum*[a] Spirochetes, *P intermedia*

[a] Organisms that have the potential of producing β-lactamase.

quantities to degrade the β-lactam ring of penicillin or cephalosporin before it can kill the susceptible bacteria [2].

Streptococcus pneumoniae

There are 90 antigenically distinct capsular serotypes in 42 distinct serogroups of *S pneumoniae*. Seven serotypes, 14, 6B, 19F, 18C, 23F, 4, and 9V (in order of decreasing prevalence), accounted for 78% of clinical isolates obtained from children in the United States [3]. These seven serotypes constitute the heptavalent conjugated pneumococcal vaccine currently in use in the United States. Antimicrobial resistance is present mainly in serotypes 6A, 6B, 9, 14, 19F, and 23F, whereas serotypes 1, 3, 4, 5, 7, 11, 15, and 18 are rarely resistant [4].

Resistance to β-lactams occurs following stepwise alterations in penicillin-binding proteins (PBPs) leading to decreased binding affinities for β-lactam antibiotics. Different degrees of resistance to penicillin and other β-lactams emerge because changes can occur in multiple PBPs to change their affinity for β-lactams. There are six known PBPs in *S pneumoniae* (1a, 1b, 2b, 2x, 2z, and 3), and alterations in 1a, 2b, and 2x are most often associated with resistance to penicillin [5]. Isolates with penicillin minimal inhibitory concentrations (MICs) of 0.06 μg/mL or less are defined as penicillin-susceptible, whereas penicillin-intermediate strains have MICs of 0.12 to 1.0 μg/mL, and penicillin-resistant isolates have MICs of 2 μg/mL or higher. The latter two groups are also referred to as "penicillin-nonsusceptible." Multidrug-resistant *S pneumoniae* are defined as organisms resistant to three or more classes of antibiotics.

The increasing prevalence of penicillin-nonsusceptible *S pneumoniae* (MICs of $\geq$ 0.12 μg/mL) in the United States has been a major concern. The Alexander Project is a worldwide surveillance study that collects respiratory tract isolates from community-based physicians and uses pharmacokinetic/pharmacodynamic (PK/PD) susceptibility breakpoints to evaluate the in vitro activity of various antimicrobial agents [6]. Data from the United States portion of the Alexander Project from 1998 to 2000 showed that 12% of isolates were penicillin-intermediate, and 25% were penicillin-resistant. Approximately 26% of *S pneumoniae* isolates were resistant to penicillin and two other classes of agents, and about 16% were resistant to any four classes of agents [7]. The prevalence of penicillin nonsusceptibility peaked in 2001 and since has decreased to 32.7% in 2004 [8]. Resistance to other antimicrobial classes also has decreased. This trend may be the result of several factors, including widespread use of heptavalent protein-polysaccharide pneumococcal conjugate vaccine in children since 2000 as well as less antimicrobial use overall.

Increased use of macrolides, particularly azithromycin, is responsible for the recent increase in macrolide-resistant *S pneumoniae*. Resistance to macrolides is mediated primarily by two genes: *erm*, which encodes for a ribosomal methylase, and *mef*, which encodes for the efflux mechanism [9,10]. The efflux mechanism conveys a relatively moderate degree of resistance, compared with the high-level resistance associated with altered ribosomal methylation. The efflux mechanism is more common in the United States but is relatively rare in most other parts of the world. Ribosomal methylase also confers cross-resistance to clindamycin.

Resistance to fluoroquinolones results from mutations in two target binding sites of these agents, DNA gyrase and topoisomerase IV. Mutations in either the *parC* gene encoding for topoisomerase IV or in the *gyrA* gene encoding for the Gyr A subunit of DNA gyrase result in low-level quinolone resistance. Mutations in both genes result in high-level quinolone resistance. Even though cross-resistance usually occurs among the fluoroquinolones, the newest agents often remain active against some strains that have become resistant to the older ones. The respiratory fluoroquinolones (ie, levofloxacin, gatifloxacin, moxifloxacin, and gemifloxacin) remain active against *S pneumoniae*, with less than 3% of all isolates showing resistance [6]. A fluoroquinolone efflux mechanism (*pmrA*) also has been described for *S pneumoniae* [11].

Resistance to trimethoprim (TMP) and sulfonamides results from mutations in the target binding sites of these agents, dihydropteroate synthase and dihydrofolate reductase. The prevalence rates of resistance to trimethoprim/sulfamethoxazole (TMP/SMX), macrolides, doxycycline, and clindamycin were 37%, 29%, 21%, and 10%, respectively [6]. Resistance to these antimicrobial agents generally is higher among penicillin-nonsusceptible isolates [6].

Haemophilus influenzae

The nontypeable strains, which have not been affected by the use of *H influenzae* type b vaccines, are typically the major cause of URTI. The main mechanism of resistance to β-lactams is through the production of β-lactamases [12]. Alterations in PBPs also have been reported in 5% to 10% of *H influenzae* isolates, and these strains are referred to as "β–lactamase-negative ampicillin-resistant" (BLNAR). Resistance among BLNAR *H influenzae* strains is attributable to alterations in PBPs 3a and 3b [13]. The prevalence of β-lactamase–producing *H influenzae* ranges from 30% to 40% [6,14]. All *H influenzae* isolates with the exception of BLNAR strains are susceptible to high-dose amoxicillin-clavulanate [6]. BLNAR strains are rarer in the United States than in other countries [6].

β-Lactamase inhibitors (ie, clavulanic acid, sulbactam, tazobactam) block the effects of β-lactamase–mediated resistance. Third-generation cephalosporins (eg, ceftriaxone and cefixime) are stable in the presence of β-lactamases. Combinations of β-lactams and β-lactamase inhibitors (eg, amoxicillin-clavulanic acid) are generally effective in the treatment of many infections caused by BLPB, including *H influenzae, M catarrhalis*, and AGNB.

H influenzae has an effective efflux pump that is chromosomally mediated by *acrAB* genes and is responsible for removing macrolides and azalides from the bacteria. As a result, these agents have intrinsically poor activity against *H influenzae* [15]. Based on PK/PD susceptibility breakpoints, less than 3% of *H influenzae* isolates were susceptible to erythromycin, clarithromycin, and azithromycin [6]. Approximately 22% of recent *H influenzae* isolates from the United States were resistant to TMP/SMX.

Moraxella catarrhalis

The main mechanism of β-lactam resistance by *M catarrhalis* is β-lactamase production. Because these enzymes are different from those produced by *H influenzae*, some agents (eg, cefpodoxime proxetil, cefuroxime axetil) are less active against *M catarrhalis* than against *H influenzae*. The Alexander Project found that 92% of *M catarrhalis* isolates produced β-lactamases [6]. *M catarrhalis* also is intrinsically resistant to trimethoprim [6,12].

Anaerobic bacteria

The predominant oropharyngeal anaerobes include gram-negative bacilli (*Bacteroides*, *Prevotella*, *Porphyromonas*, *Fusobacterium*, *Bilophila*, and *Sutterella* spp), gram-positive cocci (primarily *Peptostreptococcus* spp), gram-positive spore-forming bacilli (*Clostridium* spp) and non–spore-forming bacilli (*Actinomyces, Propionibacterium, Eubacterium, Lactobacillus,* and *Bifidobacterium* spp), and gram-negative cocci (mainly *Veillonella* spp) [1]. All with the exception of *Clostridium* spp can be recovered from head and neck infections (Table 2). Most of the infections caused by anaerobes are polymicrobial involving both aerobic and anaerobic organisms [1]. Pigmented *Prevotella* (*P melaninogenica* and *P intermedia*), *Porphyromonas asaccharolytica,* nonpigmented *Prevotella,* and *Fusobacterium nucleatum* are the predominant gram-negative anaerobic species from chronic head and neck infections. Anaerobic streptococci (*Peptostreptococcus* spp) are prevalent in all types of URTI and their complications [1]. Although they frequently are recovered in mixed culture with other aerobic or anaerobic organisms, in many instances they are the only pathogens isolated, particularly in blood cultures. Microaerophilic streptococci also are of importance in chronic sinusitis and brain abscesses.

A steadily increasing prevalence rate of penicillin resistance in oral AGNBs has been noted in the last 2 decades. These include pigmented *Prevotella* and *Porphyromonas* spp, *Fusobacterium* spp, and *P oralis*. The main mechanism of resistance is through the production of β-lactamase. Accurate prevalence rates of antibiotic resistance among oral anaerobes are difficult to obtain because these organisms rarely are identified in routine cultures. Studies that evaluated the prevalence of β-lactamase–producing AGNB in URTI have identified them in more than 50% of patients who have chronic otitis media, sinusitis, tonsillitis, and head and neck abscesses [16].

Principles of antimicrobial therapy

Initial selection of antimicrobial choices

Adequate management of mixed aerobic and anaerobic infections necessitates the administration of agents effective against both types of organisms. A number of factors should be considered when choosing appropriate antimicrobial agents. They should be effective against all target organism(s), induce little or no resistance, achieve sufficient concentration in the infected site, have a good safety record, cause minimal toxicity, and have maximum stability.

Table 2
Anaerobic bacteria most frequently encountered in head and neck infections

Organism	Infectious site
Gram-positive cocci	
Peptostreptococcus spp	Respiratory tract, deep neck, and soft tissue infections
Microaerophilic streptococci[a]	Sinusitis, brain abscesses
Non–spore-forming gram-positive bacilli	
Actinomyces spp	Intracranial abscesses, chronic mastoiditis, head and neck infections
P acnes	Infections associated with foreign body
Bifidobacterium spp	Chronic otitis media, cervical lymphadenitis
Spore-forming ram-positive bacilli	
Clostridium spp	
C perfringens	Soft tissue infection
C difficile	Colitis, antibiotic-associated diarrheal disease
C ramosum	Soft tissue infections
Gram-negative bacilli	
B fragilis group	Chronic otitis and sinusitis (rare)
Pigmented *Prevotella* and *Porphyromonas*	Orofacial and deep neck infections, periodontitis
P oralis	Orofacial infections
P oris-buccae	Orofacial infections
Fusobacterium spp	
F nucleatum	Orofacial, deep neck, and respiratory tract infections, brain abscesses, bacteremia
F necrophorum	Bacteremia

[a] Non-obligate anaerobes.

The selection of antimicrobial agents should be guided by their predicted antibacterial spectrum and bioavailability in oral or parenteral forms. Some antimicrobial agents have a narrow spectrum of activity. For example, metronidazole is effective only against most anaerobes and therefore cannot be administered as a single agent for the therapy of mixed infections. Others (eg, the carbapenems) possess a wide spectrum of activity including Enterobacteriaceae. The selection of antimicrobial agents is simplified considerably when reliable culture results are available, but culture results may not always be available because of the difficulty in obtaining appropriate specimens. Many patients therefore are treated empirically on the basis of suspected rather than known pathogen(s). Fortunately, the types of pathogens involved in most mixed or anaerobic infections and their antimicrobial susceptibility patterns tend to be predictable. Some anaerobes, however, have become resistant to selected antimicrobial agents or may become so while a patient is receiving therapy [17]. Controversies exist regarding the need to provide coverage against all resistant isolates. Some studies of the treatment of acute maxillary sinusitis have suggested that narrow-spectrum antimicrobial agents are as effective as antibiotic regimens with a broader spectrum of activity [18]. Other studies, however, have demonstrated the superiority of wider spectrum agents in attaining both clinical and bacteriologic success [19].

The choice of antimicrobial therapy also is influenced by factors other than susceptibility patterns. These include the PK/PD characteristics of the various drugs, their toxicity, effect on the normal flora, and bactericidal activity. The clinical setting and Gram-stain preparation of the specimen may suggest what types of anaerobes are present and the nature of the infectious process.

Duration of therapy

The duration of treatment must be individualized, depending on the clinical response. The duration of therapy for anaerobic infections, which often are chronic, is usually longer than that for infections caused by facultative bacteria. Oral therapy often is substituted for parenteral therapy after an initial period. The number of antimicrobial agents available for oral therapy of anaerobic infections is limited, however; among these agents are amoxicillin-clavulanate, clindamycin, and metronidazole.

Causes of failure of antimicrobial therapy

Antimicrobial therapy may fail for various reasons, including the development of resistance, insufficient tissue concentration of antibiotics, incompatible drug interactions, and the formation of an abscess. The abscess environment is detrimental to many antimicrobial agents. For example, the abscess capsule can interfere with the penetration of antimicrobial agents, and the low pH and high content of binding proteins or inactivating enzymes (ie, β-lactamase) within the abscess may impair their activity [20]. The low pH and the anaerobic environment are especially unfavorable for aminoglycosides and fluoroquinolones [21]. An anaerobic environment with an acidic pH and high osmolarity also can develop at an infection site in the absence of an abscess.

Pharmacokinetic and pharmacodynamic considerations

The ability to predict therapeutic efficacy of antimicrobial agents is based on their PK and PD properties. The PK properties of agents relate to their absorption, distribution, metabolism, and excretion. The PD properties of antibiotics involve the relationship between their tissue concentration and bacterial killing. PD integrates both microbiologic and PK data into clinically relevant relationships and can define the MIC limits at which the PK of a specific antimicrobial agent would not lead to treatment success, can determine the impact of antimicrobial resistance, and can provide the basis for developing dosing strategies that optimize clinical outcomes.

The in vivo bacterial killing of an antimicrobial agent is a function of the duration of its concentration over time relative to its MIC against a specific pathogen. This function is expressed as the area under the curve (AUC). Prediction of therapeutic success in animal models and human studies generally correlates with one of three PK parameters: (1) the time of bacterial exposure to concentrations of the antibiotic above its MIC against the pathogen (T > MIC); (2) the ratio of peak serum concentration of the agent to the MIC of the agent against the pathogen (peak:MIC ratio), and (3) the ratio of the AUC to the MIC of the agent against the pathogen (AUC:MIC ratio) (Fig. 1) [22].

Time-dependent killing of antimicrobial agents

β-Lactam antibiotics exhibit time-dependent killing, and the best predictor of clinical outcome is the duration of T > MIC for the bacteria. Relevant data from in vitro PK simulations, animal models, and human clinical studies suggest that the T > MIC required to achieve bacterial eradication should generally be higher than 40% to 50% of the dosing interval for time-dependent antibiotics [23,24]. Variations in that relation exist, however, because the optimal T > MIC for carbapenems (15%–25%) is lower than that for penicillins (30%–40%) and cephalosporins (40%–50%).

The macrolides (eg, erythromycin and clarithromycin) and azalides (eg, azithromycin) also possess time-dependent killing capabilities. Because of their prolonged postantibiotic effect against gram-positive cocci and *H*

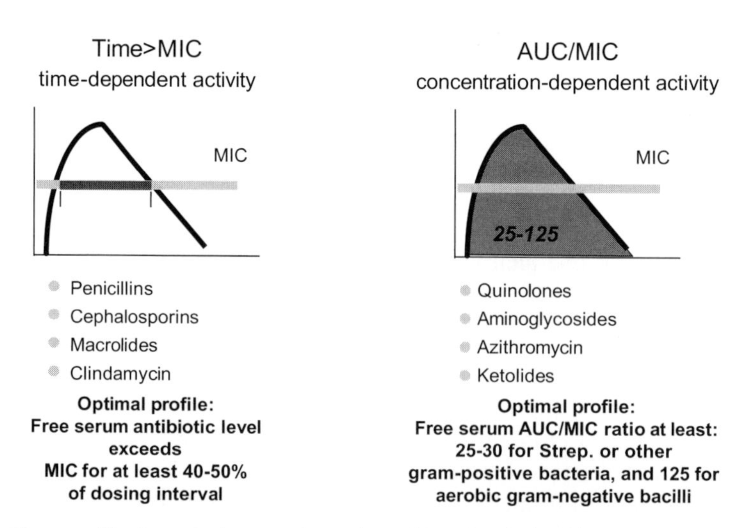

Fig. 1. Pharmacokinetic and pharmacodynamic profiles of antimicrobial agents. AUC, area under the curve; MIC, minimal inhibitory concentration; Strep, streptococcus.

influenzae, however, the parameter that best correlates with efficacy is their AUC:MIC ratio rather than T > MIC. The AUC:MIC ratio leading to maximal efficacy with these agents in animal models is approximately 25 [25]. Azithromycin has the propensity to select for macrolide-resistant bacteria [26]. This propensity may be related to its long serum half-life and prolonged duration of subinhibitory concentrations [27].

Concentration-dependent killing and prolonged persistent effects of antimicrobial agents

The fluoroquinolones, aminoglycosides, and ketolides possess a concentration-dependent mechanism of bacterial killing: they are most effective when their concentrations are significantly above the MIC (see Fig. 1) [24,28]. The AUC:MIC ratio and the peak:MIC ratio are the major parameters that correlate with efficacy. Maximizing the drug concentration at the site of infection is the goal of the dosing regimen. The eradication of organisms by fluoroquinolones is optimal at drug concentrations 10- to 12-fold higher than the MIC for the pathogen; at these concentrations bacterial killing is rapid, and the period of time of drug exposure is minimal [29]. Even though peak:MIC ratios of higher than 10:1 to 12:1 correlate best with optimal bactericidal activity, the AUC:MIC ratio is a better parameter for predicting the efficacy of fluoroquinolones for moderately susceptible bacteria, such as *S pneumoniae*. Based on animal models of sepsis, in vitro pharmacodynamic experiments, and clinical outcome studies, an AUC:MIC ratio of 125 or higher was associated with the highest bacterial eradication rates in the treatment of infections caused by gram-negative enteric pathogens [30]. For gram-positive bacteria such as *S pneumoniae*, the optimal AUC:MIC ratio for therapeutic efficacy is approximately 25 to 30 [31].

Antimicrobial activity according to pharmacokinetic/pharmacodynamic breakpoints

Although the PK/PD breakpoints are the same for all pathogens, the Clinical and Laboratory Standards Institute (CLSI) breakpoints for the same antimicrobial are individualized according to specific pathogens [32]. Whereas the PK/PD breakpoints for *S pneumoniae* are generally similar to the CLSI susceptibility breakpoints, there are significant differences between the PK/PD and CLSI susceptibility breakpoints for several antimicrobial agents against *H influenzae* [6,33]. Because PK/PD breakpoints are based on parameters that resulted in successful outcomes in clinical trials, they are more likely to predict clinical efficacy.

The oral respiratory fluoroquinolones and parenteral ceftriaxone possess the highest in vitro activity against major pathogens in URTIs. Their relative activities against URTI pathogens according to PK/PD breakpoints are

S pneumoniae:
Gatifloxacin/levofloxacin/moxifloxacin (> 99%)
Ceftriaxone/high-dose amoxicillin (± clavulanate) (95%–97%); amoxicillin (± clavulanate)/clindamycin (90%–92%)
Cefpodoxime proxetil/cefuroxime axetil/cefdinir/erythromycin/clarithromycin/azithromycin/telithromycin/cefprozil/TMP/SMX/cefixime (63%–75%)

Loracarbef/cefaclor (< 20%) [6]

H influenzae:
Gatifloxacin/moxifloxacin/ceftriaxone/cefixime/cefpodoxime proxetil/high-dose amoxicillin/clavulanate/amoxicillin/clavulanate (95%–100%)
Cefuroxime axetil/cefdinir/TMP/SMX/amoxicillin (70%–85%)
Cefprozil/cefaclor/loracarbef/doxycycline/erythromycin/clarithromycin/azithromycin/telithromycin (< 25%) [6]
M catarrhalis:
Gatifloxacin/levofloxacin/moxifloxacin/cefixime/high-dose amoxicillin/clavulanate/telithromycin/erythromycin/clarithromycin/azithromycin (100%)
Doxycycline/ceftriaxone/cefpodoxime proxetil/cefdinir (78%–96%)
Cefuroxime axetil (50%)
Cefprozil/amoxicillin/TMP/SMX/cefaclor/loracarbef (< 20%) [6]

Antimicrobial classes useful in head and neck infections

The antimicrobial agents commonly used to treat head and neck infections include the β-lactam antibiotics, macrolides/azalides, lincosamides, metronidazole, fluoroquinolones, tetracyclines, sulfonamides/trimethoprim, rifamycin, and aminoglycosides. Glycopeptides, quinupristin/dalfopristin, linezolid and daptomycin are useful for resistant gram-positive infections, particularly methicillin-resistant *S aureus* (MRSA), penicillin-resistant *S pneumoniae, Streptococcus pyogenes,* and other nosocomial pathogens. The salient features of these antibiotics relevant to the treatment of head and neck infections are summarized here, and their serum half-life, route of administration, and common dosage regimens are shown in Table 3. The FDA recently has reversed its approval of telithromycin (a ketolide) for the treatment of acute bacterial sinusitis and of acute exacerbation of chronic bronchitis, primarily because of serious hepatic toxicities.

β-*Lactam antibiotics*

β-Lactam antibiotics include the penicillins, cephalosporins, carbapenems, and monobactams. Their main mechanism of action is interference of bacterial cell wall biosynthesis. Resistance to β-lactam antibiotics can

Table 3
Selected antibiotic classes useful for the treatment of head and neck infections

Class	Antibiotic	Half-life	Usual adult dose and route of administration	Dosing interval
Natural penicillins	Penicillin G (crystalline)	0.5 h	2 MU IV	q 4 h
	Penicillin G (procaine)	24 h	600,000 U IM	q 12 h
	Penicillin G (benzathine)	10–15 d	1.2 MU IM	weekly
	Penicillin V	0.5–1 h	250–500 mg PO	q 6 h
Aminopenicillins	Ampicillin	1 h	2.0 g IV	q 4 h
	Amoxicillin	1 h	500 mg PO	q 6 h
Amoxicillin	Clavulanate	1.4 h	250/62–500/ 124–875/ 125–2000/125 PO	q 12 h q 6 h
Penicillinase-resistant penicillins	Cloxacillin, oxacillin, or nafcillin	0.5 h	500 mg PO or 2 g IV	q 6 h q 4 h
	Dicloxacillin	0.5–0.9 h	500 mg PO	q 6 h
	Methicillin	0.5 h	2 g IV	q 4 h
Carboxypenicillins	Carbenicillin (indanyl)	1 h	382 mg PO	q 6 h
	Ticarcillin-clavulanate	1–1.5 h	3.1 g IV	q 4 h
Ureidopenicillins	Piperacillin-tazobactam	1 h	3.375 g IV	q 4 h
First-generation cephalosporins	Cefadroxil	1.4 h	500 mg PO	q 6 h
	Cefazolin	1.8 h	1 g IV	q 4 h
	Cephalexin	0.9 h	500 mg PO	q 6 h
	Cephalothin	0.5–0.9 h	1 g IV	q 6 h
	Cephradine	0.7–2 h	500 mg PO or 1 g IV	q 6 h q 4–6 h
Second-generation cephalosporins	Cefaclor	0.75 h	500 mg PO	q 8 h
	Cefamandole	0.5–2.1 h	1 g IV	q 4–8 h
	Cefmetazole	1.2 h	2 g IV	q 6–12 h
	Cefonicid	4–5 h	1 g IV	q 24 h
	Cefotetan	3–4 h	1.5 g IV	q 12 h
	Cefoxitin	0.7 h	1 g IV	q 6 h
	Cefprozil	1.3 h	500 mg PO	q 12 h
	Cefuroxime	1.3–1.7 h	1 g IV	q 8 h
	Cefuroxime-axetil	1.2 h	250 mg PO	q 12 h
Third-generation cephalosporins	Cefdinir-pivoxil	1.7 h	300 mg PO	q 12 h
	Cefixime	3–4 h	200 mg PO	q 12 h
	Cefoperazone	1.9–2.5 h	2 g IV	q 12 h
	Cefotaxime	1.1 h	1.5 g IV	q 8 h
	Cefpodoxime-proxetil	2.4 h	200 mg PO	q 12 h

(*continued on next page*)

Table 3 (*continued*)

Class	Antibiotic	Half-life	Usual adult dose and route of administration	Dosing interval
	Ceftazidime	1.5 h	2 g IV	q 8 h
	Ceftibuten	2.4 h	400 mg PO	q 24 h
	Ceftizoxime	1.4–1.8 h	2 g IV	q 6 h
	Ceftriaxone	6–9 h	1 g IV	q 12 h
Fourth-generation cephalosporin	Cefepime	2 h	2 g IV	q 12 h
Carbapenems	Imipenem-cilastatin	1 h	1 g IV	q 6 h
	Meropenem	1 h	1 g IV	q 8 h
	Ertapenem	4.5 h	1 g IV	q 24 h
Monobactams	Azthreonam	2 h	1-2 g IV	q 6 h
Macrolides	Erythromycin	1.2–1.6 h	250 mg-1 g IV or 500 mg PO	q 6 h
	Clarithromycin	4 h	500 mg PO	q 12 h
	Azithromycin	68 h	250 mg PO	q 24 h
Lincosamide	Clindamycin	2–2.5 h	150–300 mg PO or 600 mg IV	q 8 h
Nitroimidazole	Metronidazole	6–14 h	500 mg PO or 500 mg IV	q 6 h
Fluoroquinolones	Ciprofloxacin	4 h	500–750 mg PO or 400 mg IV	q 12 h
	Levofloxacin	7 h	500–750 mg PO or IV	q 24 h
	Moxifloxacin	12 h	400 mg PO or IV	q 24 h
	Gatifloxacin	7 h	400 mg PO or IV	q 24 h
	Gemifloxacin	7 h	320 mg PO	q 24 h
Tetracyclines	Tetracycline	8 h	250–500 mg PO	q 6 h
	Doxycycline	14–25 h	100 mg PO or IV	q 12 h
	Minocycline	11–26 h	100 mg PO or IV	q 12 h
Sulfonamides and Trimethoprim	Sulfadiazine	8–17 h	1 g PO or 30-50 mg/kg	q 6 h
	Sulfisoxazole	3–7 h	1–2 g PO	q 6 h
	Trimethoprim-sulfamethoxazole	8–15 h (trimethoprim) 7–12 h (sulfamethoxazole)	1–2 DS tablets	q 12 h
Rifamycin	Rifampin	2–5 h	600 mg PO or IV	q 24 h

(*continued on next page*)

Table 3 (*continued*)

Class	Antibiotic	Half-life	Usual adult dose and route of administration	Dosing interval
Aminoglycosides	Gentamicin	2 h	1.5–2 mg/kg IV	q 8 h or 5 mg/kg q 24 h
	Netilmicin	2.5 h	1.5–2.0 mg/kg IV	q 8 h
	Tobramycin	2.5 h	1.5–2.0 mg/kg IV	q 8 h
	Amikacin	2 h	7.5 mg/kg IV	q 12 h
	Streptomycin	2.5 h	15 mg/kg IM or IV	q 12 h
Glycopeptides	Vancomycin	4–6 h	250 mg PO or 15 mg/kg IV	q 12 h
	Teicoplanin	45 h	6–12 mg/kg IV	q 24 h
Miscellaneous	Quinupristin-dalfopristin	1.5 h	7.5 mg/kg IV	q 8 h
	Linezolid	5–7 h	600 mg PO or IV	q 12 h
	Daptomycin	8–9 h	4 mg/kg IV	q 24 h

Abbreviations: BID, twice daily; d, day; h, hour; IM, intramuscularly; IV, intravenously; MU, million units; OD, once daily; PO, by mouth; q, every; QID, four times daily.

be caused by (1) reduced antimicrobial permeability through the bacterial cell wall pores; (2) inactivation by β-lactamases excreted to the extracellular fluid (gram-positive bacteria) or present in the periplasmic space (gram-negative bacteria); or (3) reduced affinity of PBPs for the antibiotic.

Penicillins

Penicillins include the natural penicillins (penicillin G and V), penicillinase-resistant penicillins (methicillin, oxacillin, cloxacillin, nafcillin, dicloxacillin), aminopenicillins (ampicillin, amoxicillin, bacampicillin), carboxypenicillins (carbenicillin, ticarcillin), and ureidopenicillins (piperacillin). They are classified according to antibacterial activity but with considerable overlap among the groups. The combination of a penicillin plus a β-lactamase inhibitor (eg, ampicillin/sulbactam, amoxicillin/clavulanate, ticarcillin/clavulanate, piperacillin/tazobactam) further enhances the antimicrobial spectrum against β-lactamase–producing bacteria, such as *H influenzae, M catarrhalis, Staphylococcus* spp, *Neisseria gonorrhoeae, Escherichia coli, Klebsiella pneumoniae, Proteus* spp, *Bacteroides fragilis* group, *Fusobacterium* spp, *Prevotella* spp, and *Porphyromonas* spp.

Major adverse effects include IgE-mediated immediate hypersensitivity reactions resulting in urticaria, angioneurotic edema, bronchospasm and hypotension, serum sickness, Stevens-Johnson syndrome, vasculitis, interstitial nephritis (frequent with methicillin), and hemolytic anemia. High-dose administration may cause encephalopathy, myoclonus, convulsions, and decreased platelet aggregation resulting in hemorrhagic diathesis (especially with carboxypenicillins).

1. Penicillin G. Procaine and benzathine penicillin are injectable repository forms of aqueous penicillin G. Benzathine penicillin produces prolonged serum levels for 1 or 2 weeks, and procaine penicillin produces serum levels for 12 hours. Penicillin G is active against group A β-hemolytic streptococci (GABHS), alpha-hemolytic streptococcus, meningococci, and *S pneumoniae*. Penicillin-resistant strains of *S pneumoniae* have increased steadily in recent years, but high-dose penicillins are still effective in most oropharyngeal and respiratory infections.
2. Penicillin V is administered orally and resists gastric acidity. Higher serum levels are achieved than with penicillin G. It is less active than penicillin G against gram-negative bacteria, *N gonorrhoeae*, and *H influenzae*. In most other cases it can be used as an oral substitute for penicillin G.
3. Ampicillin usually is administered parenterally and is not penicillinase resistant. It is active against non–β-lactamase–producing *H influenzae*, *Neisseria meningitidis*, pneumococci, and selected gram-negative organisms such as *Salmonella* spp, *Shigella* spp, *Escherichia coli*, and *Proteus mirabilis*.
4. Amoxicillin is better absorbed than ampicillin when administered orally, even with food. Its antibacterial spectrum is similar to that of ampicillin. Intermediate resistance to penicillin by *S pneumoniae* can be overcome by using higher doses of amoxicillin with or without clavulanate. The standard dose of amoxicillin for adults is 1.5 to 1.75 g/d, and the average pediatric dose is 40 to 45 mg/kg/d. When high-dose amoxicillin is prescribed, the dosing is increased to 3.5 to 4.0 g/d or 90 to 100 mg/kg /d. Because of improved PK/PD parameters, high-dose amoxicillin (± clavulanate) has significantly fewer bacteriologic failures against non–β-lactamase–producing ampicillin-resistant *H influenzae*.
5. Methicillin is a semisynthetic compound that is available only in parenteral form and is the least protein-bound among the penicillinase-resistant penicillins. It diffuses well into the brain and joints but is rarely used because of the potential for interstitial nephritis.
6. Oxacillin, cloxacillin, dicloxacillin, and nafcillin are available both orally and parenterally. Only slight differences in absorption and protein binding are observed, and they are considered equivalent clinically. A major concern has been the emergence of resistance among *S aureus* isolates in both hospital- and community-acquired strains.
7. The carboxypenicillins carbenicillin and ticaricillin are active against *Pseudomonas*, *Enterobacter*, and indole-positive *Proteus* spp. Ticarcillin is more active than carbenicillin against *Pseudomonas* spp but is less effective against gram-positive bacteria, especially *Enterococcus* spp.
8. Piperacillin, a ureidopenicillin, is active against *Enterococcus* spp, *Enterobacter*, *Pseudomonas*, *Serratia*, *B fragilis*, and *Acinetobacter* spp.

β-Lactamase–producing strains of *S aureus, N gonorrhoeae, H influenzae*, and Enterobacteriaceae are resistant to piperacillin but are susceptible to the piperacillin-tazobactam combination.

Cephalosporins

More than 20 cephalosporin antibiotics are in use today. These agents are classified based on chemical modifications that enhance their antibacterial spectrum. Similar to the penicillins, they inhibit bacterial cell wall biosyntheses. The main mechanism of resistance is the production of β-lactamases that hydrolyze the β-lactam ring. The different cephalosporins vary greatly in susceptibility to β-lactamases. Whereas the first-generation cephalosporins are the most resistant to hydrolysis by β-lactamases produced by *S aureus*, the second-, third-, and fourth-generation cephalosporins are more resistant to β-lactamases produced by aerobic gram-negative rods. Major adverse effects are similar to those of penicillin, and the incidence of primary allergic reactions is 1% to 3%. Cephalosporins should not be administered to patients who have an immediate hypersensitivy reaction to penicillin (urticaria, anaphylaxis, bronchospasm, and hypotension). Cross-hypersensitivity with the penicillins is about 10%. Granulocytopenia and thrombocytopenia are rare. Ethanol intolerance (disulfiram-like reaction) has been described with cefazolin, cefamandole, cefoperazone, and cefotetan.

Drug interactions are also similar to those of the penicillins. The agents that have a N-methyl-thiotetrazole side chain (cefamandole, cefotetan, cefmetazole, and cefoperazone) are associated with an increased incidence of bleeding when taken concomitantly with oral anticoagulants, heparin, platelet aggregation inhibitors, and thrombolytic agents.

1. First generation: Cephalothin, cefazolin, cephapirin, cephalexin, cephradine, and cefadroxil are active against most gram-positive aerobic cocci (except MRSA, *S epidermidis*, and *Enterococcus* spp). They are not active against aerobic and anaerobic gram-negative bacilli.
2. Second generation: Cefamandole, cefaclor, cefuroxime, cefonicid, cefprozil, cefoxitin, cefotetan, and cefmetazole are slightly less active than the first-generation cephalosporins against gram-positive aerobic cocci . Cefoxitin, cefotetan, and cefmetazole have significant activity against anaerobes, including the *B fragilis* group. As a group, the second-generation cephalosporins are more active against gram-negative aerobic organisms, including Enterobacteriaceae, *Enterobacter* spp, indole-positive *Proteus* spp, and *H influenzae*. Cefaclor and loracarbef have poor overall efficacy against respiratory tract pathogens. Cefprozil and cefuroxime axetil have comparable activity against *S pneumoniae* [34]. Cefuroxime axetil is active against *H influenzae* but has lower efficacy than cefpodoxime proxetil [35]. Cefprozil is markedly less active against *H influenzae* [34].

3. Third generation: Cefotaxime, ceftizoxime, ceftriaxone, cefoperazone, ceftazidime, cefixime, and cefpodoxime-proxetil all possess expanded activity against aerobic gram-negative bacilli but are not very active against anaerobic gram-negative bacilli. They also are less active than the first-generation cephalosporins against gram-positive cocci. Cefdinir and cefpodoxime proxetil are active against both *S pneumoniae* and *H influenzae*. Cefixime is active against *H influenzae* but has limited gram-positive coverage including penicillin-resistant *S pneumoniae* and staphylococci. Cefoperazone and ceftazidime are active against *Pseudomonas aeruginosa*.
4. Fourth generation: Cefepime is effective against *P aeruginosa* as well as gram-positive aerobic cocci.

Carbapenems

The carbapenems, which include imipenem, meropenem, and ertapenem, are the most active penicillins against most aerobic and anaerobic bacteria implicated in head and neck infections. Because their PK/PD profiles exhibit time-dependent killing, their antibacterial effectiveness can be maximized further by increasing the dosing frequency or by prolonged administration of high doses [36,37].

1. Imipenem-cilastatin, a parenteral agent, has a broad spectrum of activity against gram-positive cocci (excluding MRSA and *Enterococcus faecium*), gram-negative bacilli (including *P aeruginosa* but not *Stenotrophomonas maltophilia*), and anaerobic organisms (including β-lactamase–producing gram-negative bacilli). When combined with cilastatin, it is prevented from hydrolysis by renal dehydropeptidase, resulting in an enhanced half-life. Seizures can occur in patients receiving high doses, particularly in those who have renal insufficiency or central nervous system disorders.
2. Meropenem, a parenteral agent, is relatively stable to renal dehydropeptidase and does not require an inhibitor of this enzyme. It has activity similar to that of imipenem but is slightly less active against gram-positive cocci and is more active against gram-negative aerobes (Enterobacteriaceae, *H influenzae*, *Neisseria* spp, and *P aeruginosa*).
3. Ertapenem is a new 1-β-methyl carbapenem and is stable to renal dehydropeptidase. It has a broad antibacterial spectrum for penicillin-susceptible *S pneumoniae*, *S pyogenes*, MRSA, *H influenzae*, *M catarrhalis*, *E coli*, *Citrobacter* spp, Klebsiella spp, *Serratia* spp, *Proteus* spp, *Clostridium perfringens*, *Fusobacterium* spp, *Peptostreptococcus* spp, and anaerobic gram-negative bacilli. In comparison to other available carbapenems, ertapenem has a long half-life of 4.5 hours and is given in a single daily dose, making it suitable for outpatient intravenous antibiotic therapy. It is less effective than the other carbapenems against *P aeruginosa*, *Enterococcus* spp, and *Acinetobacter* spp.

Monobactams

Monobactams (eg, aztreonam) have a monocyclic β-lactam ring and are active only against aerobic gram-negative rods. They can be administered to patients allergic to other β-lactam antibiotics because they have different antigenic characteristics.

Macrolides

Macrolides include erythromycin, clarithromycin, and azithromycin. Their mechanism of action is by inhibition of RNA-dependent protein synthesis by reversibly binding to the 50S ribosome, thus preventing chain elongation. Resistance is mediated by decreased permeability through the bacterial cell wall, by alteration of the 50S and the 23S ribosomal RNA receptor site, or by inactivation by enzymatic hydrolysis. Erythromycin-resistant gram-positive bacteria also are resistant to the other macrolides. Telithromycin, the related ketolide, is no longer approved by the Food and Drug Administration for the treatment of acute sinusitis or acute exacerbation of chronic bronchitis, primarily because of serious hepatic toxicities.

These agents have broad activity against gram-positive and some gram-negative bacteria, as well as treponemes, mycoplasmas, chlamydia, and Rickettsia. All are active against *Corynebacterium diphtheriae*, *Bordetella pertussis*, *Legionella pneumophila*, *Mycoplasma pneumoniae*, *Chlamydia trachomatis,* and *Chlamydophila pneumoniae*. Azithromycin is less active than erythromycin against staphylococci and streptococci but is more active against *H influenzae*. Clarithromycin has good activity against *H influenzae*. The increasing prevalence of macrolide resistance among *S pneumoniae* (about 35% in the United States) and *S pyogenes* (about 12%) is disconcerting because it has been associated with a significant likelihood of clinical failure [38]. Macrolide resistance among these organisms has been correlated with increased clinical usage of macrolides, especially azithromycin [39].

Erythromycin is well absorbed when given orally and also is available for intravenous administration. The base is destroyed by gastric acid, and oral formulations therefore have acid-resistant coatings. Erythromycin is distributed through total body water but does not penetrate well into the cerebrospinal fluid. Clarithromycin and azithromycin have better gastrointestinal absorption. Azithromycin has a very long half-life, resulting in high and prolonged intracellular concentrations. The major adverse effects are gastrointestinal (mostly cramps, nausea, vomiting, and diarrhea with erythromycin), transient hearing loss, allergic reactions (rash, fever, eosinophilia), and cholestatic hepatitis (with estolate). All macrolides prolong the cardiac QT interval. Coadministration with terfenadine (Seldane) or astemizole (Hismanal) is contraindicated because of potential cardiac toxicity. All macrolides except azithromycin increase the serum levels of many drugs such as theophylline, phenytoin, cyclosporine, digoxin, carbamazepine, warfarin, and corticosteroids.

Clindamycin

Clindamycin, a lincosamide antibiotic, binds to the 50S ribosome and inhibits protein synthesis by interfering with chain elongation. It is active against gram-positive cocci such as staphylococci, *S pneumoniae* (including penicillin-resistant strains), *S pyogenes*, and viridans streptococci as well as most anaerobes, including *Peptostreptococcus* spp, *B fragilis, Prevotella, Porphyromonas,* and *Fusobacterium* spp. It also reduces toxin production by *S aureus* and *Clostridium* spp and capsule formation by *S pyogenes* and *S pneumoniae,* and it enhances phagocytosis of susceptible organisms. Development of resistance is increasingly recognized in *B fragilis*. The mechanism of resistance is similar to that of macrolides.

Clindamycin is well absorbed following oral dosing, but gastrointestinal absorption is reduced by the co-administration of kaolin. There is good tissue and bone penetration following oral and parenteral administration, but not in the cerebrospinal fluid. Clindamycin possesses a concentration-dependent mechanism of antimicrobial activity [40].

Major adverse effects include erythema multiforme, anaphylaxis, *Clostridium difficile*–associated diarrhea, and pseudomembranous colitis. Hepatotoxicity, thrombocytopenia, and reversible neutropenia are encountered occasionally.

Metronidazole

Metronidazole is highly active against all anaerobic bacteria with the exception of nonsporulating gram-positive bacilli and some *Capnocytophaga* spp. It has no activity against aerobic and facultative bacteria. Its mechanism of action is by the production of intracellular free radicals that are toxic to bacterial cells by interaction with DNA and other macromolecules. Resistance of anaerobic gram-negative bacilli is rarely encountered. Occasional strains of anaerobic gram-positive cocci and nonsporulating bacilli are highly resistant. Microaerophilic streptococci, *Propionibacterium acnes*, and *Actinomyces* spp are almost uniformly resistant. Metronidazole penetrates well into all tissues and body fluids including the cerebrospinal fluid. Oral and intravenous doses achieve equivalent blood levels.

Major adverse effects include seizures, encephalopathy, disulfiram-like reaction with alcohol (flushing, nausea, tachycardia, vomiting, hypotension, headache), cerebellar dysfunction, ataxia, and peripheral neuropathy.

Fluoroquinolones

The fluoroquinolones are well absorbed from the gastrointestinal tract and are available in oral and intravenous forms. The main mechanism of action is inhibition of DNA topoisomerase (gyrase) in bacterial but not mammalian cells. Resistance may arise during therapy and is caused by mutations in the gene encoding for DNA gyrase or mutations that change the outer porins and efflux pumps. Ciprofloxacin, a second-generation fluoroquinolone, has excellent activity against gram-negative bacteria including *P aeruginosa*. Its AUC:MIC ratio against *S pneumoniae* is only 10 to 20, but it is very active against both *H influenzae* and *M catarrhalis* [24,41]. Levofloxacin has improved activity against *S pneumoniae*. The newer fluoroquinolones (moxifloxacin, gatifloxacin, and gemifloxacin) have excellent activity against *S pneumoniae* (including penicillin-resistant strains), *H influenzae, M catarrhalis*, and respiratory anaerobes [42]. All quinolones show good activity for Rickettsia, Mycoplasma and Legionellae. Their high bioavailability, excellent PK/PD properties, broad spectrum of activity, and generally good overall tolerability have resulted in the extensive clinical use of these agents. Because of toxicities, however, a number of the fluoroquinolones, including temafloxacin, sparfloxacin, grepafloxacin, and trovafloxacin, have been withdrawn from clinical use after initial approval. Another concern is the emergence of cross-resistance among *S pneumoniae* as the result of increased usage of this class of antibiotics.

Major adverse effects include central nervous system manifestations (headache, dizziness, insomnia, agitation, restlessness, abnormal vision, bad dreams, hallucinations, depression, psychotic reactions, grand mal convulsions), anaphylaxis, vasculitis, serum sickness–like reactions, photosensitivity reactions, Achilles tendon rupture and other tendinopathies, increased QT intervals (gatifloxacin, moxifloxacin), rash (gemifloxacin), and hypo- or hyperglycemia (gatifloxacin, levofloxacin). The gastrointestinal absorption of all quinolones is reduced by antacids, dairy products, vitamins, and citric acid.

Tetracyclines

Tetracycline HCP is a short-acting agent (dose interval, 4–8 hours), whereas doxycycline and minocycline are long-acting (dose interval, 12–24 hours). They are well absorbed after oral administration. These agents prevent intracellular protein syntheses at the level of binding of transfer RNA–amino acid complexes to the ribosomes. The main mechanism of resistance is the prevention of penetration of tetracycline into the bacterial cell. All tetracyclines have similar antimicrobial activity. They are active against many gram-positive and gram-negative bacteria. They are also active for *Brucella* spp, *Vibrio cholerae*, *Vibrio vulnificus*, *Mycobacterium marinum*, Chlamydiae, Rickettsia, Mycoplasmas, and *Borrelia burgdorferi*. Many organisms, especially hospital-acquired bacteria, have become resistant, however. Tetracycline, once the drug of choice for anaerobic infections, is presently of limited usefulness because many anaerobic bacteria have developed resistance to tetracycline. The newer tetracycline analogues, doxycycline and minocycline, are more active against anaerobic bacteria than the parent compound. Susceptibility tests should be performed to ensure their efficacy when they are used in severe infections, however. Doxycycline is active against penicillin-susceptible *S pneumoniae*, but resistance to doxycycline by this organism is increasing [6].

Major adverse effects include teeth discoloration and hypoplasia of the enamel in children younger than 8 years, vertigo (minocycline), aggravation of pre-existing renal failure, hepatotoxicity (especially in pregnancy), increase in intracranial pressure, photosensitivity, and superinfection caused by *Candida* spp (thrush, vaginitis). The use of tetracyclines is not recommended before 8 years of age and in pregnancy because of the adverse effect on teeth.

Sulfonamides and trimethoprim

Short-acting sulfonamides include sulfisoxazole, SMX, sulfadiazine, and sulfamethizole. Sulfadoxine is a long-acting agent. Sulfonamides are well absorbed when given orally. They are metabolized by acetylation and glucuronidation in the liver, and their metabolic products are excreted in the urine. The sulfonamides competitively inhibit the incorporation of *p*-aminobenzoic acid into tetrahydropteroic acid that is required for folic acid synthesis. They are active against a broad spectrum of gram-negative and gram-positive bacteria, as well as actinomyces, Chlamydia, Plasmodia, and Toxoplasma. They are inactive against anaerobic bacteria. Resistance is caused by either chromosomal mutations or plasmid exchange and is common, limiting their clinical usefulness.

TMP, which is a dihydrofolate reductase inhibitor, is synergistic with sulfonamides by the sequential inhibition of folic acid synthesis. TMP is active against many gram-positive cocci and most gram-negative rods. It is not active against *P aeruginosa* and *Bacteroides* spp. The combination of TMP/SMX is effective against *S aureus, S pneumoniae, S pyogenes, P mirabilis, Shigella* spp, *E coli, Salmonella* spp, *Pseudomonas cepacia, Pseudomonas pseudomallei, Yersinia enterocolitica,* and *N gonorrhoeae*. It also is effective against *Pneumocystis carinii*. Resistance to TMP generally is caused by plasmid-mediated mutations in dihydrofolate reductase. A high rate of resistance to these drugs is now present in *S pneumoniae* and *H influenzae* (25%–30%) [6]. *M catarrhalis* is intrinsically resistant to TMP. TMP is very well absorbed after oral administration and distributes in most body fluids especially in the prostrate fluid. It is excreted unchanged in the urine.

Major adverse effects of the sulfonamides include hepatic necrosis, serum sickness–like syndrome, acute hemolytic anemia, agranulocytosis, and Stevens-Johnson syndrome. Major adverse effects of TMP include leukopenia, thrombocytopenia, granulocytopenia, and pseudomembranous colitis.

Rifamycin (Rifampin)

Rifampin binds to the β-subunit of RNA polymerase, thus blocking RNA transcription and initiation of chain formation, resulting in a bactericidal effect. Rifamycin is active against a wide range of organisms, including

S aureus, *S epidermidis*, *N meningitidis*, *N gonorrhoeae*, *H influenzae*, *Legionella* spp, *C difficile*, and *Mycobacterium* spp [43]. Resistance develops rapidly, however, because of mutations of the β-subunit of the DNA-dependent RNA polymerase. Rifamycin is available for oral and intravenous administration. Its long half-life allows once-a-day administration. It penetrates well into all tissues and body fluids, including bone. It is used frequently in combination with penicillinase-resistant penicillins, fluoroquinolones, and TMP/SMX for endovascular and orthopedic infections, chronic prostatitis, and infections associated with prosthetic devices.

Because rifampin is an inducer of several cytochrome p450 isoenzymes, it has a high potential for drug interactions. It inhibits the liver uptake of several compounds and shortens the half-life of numerous agents, resulting in decreased levels of ketoconazole, itraconazole, oral contraceptives, methadone, nevirapine, β-adrenergic blockers, delavirdine, digoxin, and disopyramide, among others.

Aminoglycosides

Despite concerns of nephrotoxicity and auditory as well as vestibular dysfunction, aminoglycosides have remained important in clinical practice, particularly for the treatment of antibiotic-resistant gram-negative infections. These agents include gentamicin, netilmicin, tobramycin, and amikacin. Their mechanism of action is inhibition of protein syntheses. Resistance develops through the induction of aminoglycoside-inactivating enzymes or through alterations in intracellular transport, resulting in failure to penetrate the bacterial cells. Gentamicin is active against aerobic gram-negative bacilli and *S aureus* and exhibits excellent synergistic potential with penicillins against aerobic gram-positive bacteria. Netilmicin is similar to gentamicin and tobramycin but has less ototoxicity. Tobramycin is active against many gentamicin-resistant *Pseudomonas* and *Acinetobacter* spp, but not against Enterobacteriaceae resistant to gentamicin. Amikacin is active against many species that are resistant to gentamicin, netilmicin, and tobramycin and is particularly useful for infections caused by resistant *Pseudomonas*, *Serratia*, and *Providencia* spp. Streptomycin is used primarily in combination with isoniazid and rifampin for the treatment of tuberculosis. It has synergistic activity with penicillin against *Enterococcus* spp and is useful for infective endocarditis caused by this organism.

Aminoglycosides are not absorbed orally but are well distributed after intramuscular or intravenous injection. They are poorly protein bound and do not penetrate the central nervous system. They are excreted primarily by glomerular filtration. Peak and trough serum concentrations should be monitored routinely in patients receiving prolonged therapy. Elevated peak concentration correlate with toxicity, and elevated trough concentrations indicate drug accumulation. Once-a-day dosing reduces the nephrotoxic effects of aminoglycosides and is the preferred regimen.

Glycopeptides

Vancomycin and teicoplanin are active against *S aureus* and *S epidermidis* (including strains resistant to methicillin), *S pyogenes, S pneumoniae,* and other *Streptococcus* spp, Enterococci, *Corynebacterium JK*, and *C difficile.* They inhibit the assembly and synthesis of the second stage of cell wall peptidoglycan polymers of susceptible bacteria. Resistance is acquired by mutation and/or alterations in cell wall biosynthesis resulting in a thickened cell wall caused by accumulation of excess amounts of peptidoglycan, thus preventing intracellular penetration to reach their target sites. They are used primarily to treat systemic infections caused by *E faecium*, penicillin-resistant *S pyogenes* or *S pneumoniae,* and methicillin-susceptible or –resistant *S aureus* or *S epidermidis*. The glycopeptides are not absorbed when administered orally but are effective against *C difficile*–associated colitis. Intravenous administration is required for systemic infections. Peak serum levels of 20 to 30 μg/mLand trough levels of 5 to 10 μg/mL are desirable. Teicoplanin has a longer half-life than vancomycin, allowing once-daily dosing, but requires an initial loading dose.

Major adverse effects include rash, "red man syndrome" (caused by rapid intravenous administration and release of histamines), leukopenia, and tinnitus and hearing loss (serum concentration > 40 μg/mL).

Quinupristin/dalfopristin

The combination quinupristin/dalfopristin is used primarily for serious or life-threatening infections associated with vancomycin-resistant *E faecium* bacteremia or complicated skin and soft tissue infections caused by penicillin-resistant *S pyogenes* and methicillin-susceptible or -resistant *S aureus*. In this drug combination, dalfopristin inhibits the early phase, and quinupristin inhibits the late stage of bacterial protein synthesis. Resistance occurs through efflux, target modification, and enzymatic inactivation. It is available for intravenous administration and has a wide tissue distribution. It is metabolized in the liver and is eliminated either by hepatic (75%) or renal (25%) routes.

The major adverse effects are severe and incapacitating muscular inflammation and pain, allergic reactions, phlebitis, pancreatitis, and pseudomembranous colitis.

Linezolid

Linezolid, an oxazolidinone antibiotic, acts by inhibiting the initiation of bacterial protein syntheses. It possesses a wide spectrum of activity against aerobic gram-positive organisms including methicillin-resistant staphylococci, penicillin-resistant pneumococci, and vancomycin-resistant *Enterococcus faecalis* and *E faecium*. Anaerobes such as *Clostridium* spp, *Peptostreptococcus* spp, and *Prevotella* spp also are susceptible. Linezolid is bacteriostatic against most susceptible organisms but displays bactericidal activity against some strains of pneumococci, *B fragilis*, and *C perfringens*. Resistance by clinical isolates of *E faecium* has been reported.

Major adverse effects include thrombocytopenia and leucopenia that emerge after 2 to 3 weeks of therapy.

Daptomycin

Daptomycin, a cyclic lipopeptide antibiotic, is used primarily for the treatment of complicated skin and soft tissue infections caused by susceptible aerobic gram-positive bacteria including methicillin-susceptible and -resistant *S aureus*, vancomycin-resistant enterococci, and penicillin-resistant *S pyogenes* or *S pneumoniae*. Daptomycin binds to components of the cell membrane of susceptible bacteria, causing rapid depolarization and inhibition of intracellular DNA, RNA, and protein synthesis. It is bactericidal in a concentration-dependent manner. It is highly protein bound (92%) and is excreted unchanged in the urine (78%) and the feces (6%).

Major adverse effects include severe myopathy with markedly elevated serum creatinine phosphokinase (10-fold higher than baseline), peripheral neuropathy, anaphylaxis, thrombocytopenia, and respiratory failure.

Antimicrobial management of selected head and neck infections

Although the management of various head and neck infections is discussed in detail in other articles in this issue, the microbiology and antimicrobial therapy of selected head and neck infections are briefly reviewed here and are summarized in Table 4.

Dental infections

Gingivitis

The development of gingivitis is associated with a significant increase in gram-negative anaerobes (*F nucleatum*, *P intermedia*, and *Bacteroides* spp), spirochetes, and motile rods. Necrotizing ulcerative gingivitis, also known as "acute narcotizing ulcerative gingivitis," "trench mouth," or "Vincent's angina," is caused by a synergistic infection between unusually large spirochetes and fusobacteria [44,45]. The unique organisms associated with this infection are fairly constant and include oral treponemes, *Selenomonas* spp, *P intermedia*, and *Fusobacterium* spp. This condition responds dramatically to systemic metronidazole [46]. Other regimens, including penicillin G, clindamycin, and amoxicillin-clavulanate, are also effective [47].

Periodontitis

Periodontal disease develops in the presence of two events in the oral cavity: a quantitative increase in bacterial counts of anaerobic gram-negative

Table 4
Initial empiric antibiotic treatment for selected head and neck infections

Infection	Common pathogens	Recommended regimens
Dental		
Acute necrosing ulcerative gingivitis	Treponemes, *Selenomonas* spp, *P intermedia*, *Fusobacterium* spp	Metronidazole ± penicillin IV
Periodontal abscess	*A actinomycetemcomitans* and *P gingivalis*	Metronidazole PO; amoxicillin-clavulanate PO
Otologic		
Otitis media, acute	*S pneumoniae*, *H influenzae*, *M catarrhalis*	Amoxicillin (high dose) PO
Otitis media, chronic	*P aeruginosa* and *S aureus*; AGNB and *Peptostreptococcus* spp	Amoxicillin-clavulanate PO; ciprofloxacin + clindamycin PO; imipenem or piperacillin-tazobactam IV
Mastoiditis, acute and chronic	*S pneumoniae, S pyogenes, S aureus, H influenzae, P* a*eruginosa, Enterobacteriaceae,* AGNB and *Peptostreptococcus* spp	Amoxicillin-clavulanate PO; ticarcillin-clavulanate IV; imipenem or piperacillin-tazobactam IV
Rhinologic		
Sinusitis, acute	*S pneumoniae, H influenzae, M catarrhalis, S pyogenes* and *S aureus*	Amoxicillin-clavulanate PO; levofloxacin, moxalactam, gatifloxacin or gemifloxacin PO
Sinusitis, chronic	*S aureus, S pneumoniae, H influenzae,* AGNB, *Peptostreptococcus* spp	Amoxicillin-clavulanate PO; ticarcillin-clavulanate IV; gemifloxacin PO; moxalactam, or gatifloxacin IV or PO
Oropharyngeal		
Pharyngotonsillitis	Groups A, B, C and G streptococci, *N gonorrhoeae, N meningitidis, C diphtheriae, A hemolyticum*	Penicillin PO; amoxicillin PO; clindamycin or macrolides PO
Peritonsillar, retropharyngeal, and odontogenic deep neck infections	*Prevotella, Porphyromonas, Fusobacterium, Peptostreptococcus* spp, GABHS, *S aureus, H influenzae.*	Ticarcillin-clavulanate IV; piperacillin-tazobactam IV; imipenem or meropenem IV
Parotitis & Sialoadenitis	*S aureus,* AGNB, *Peptostreptococcus* spp *Streptococcus* spp (including *S pneumoniae*), gram-negative bacilli (including *E coli*)	Nafcillin or cloxacillin plus clindamycin IV; cefazolin IV; amoxicillin-clavulanate PO; ticarcillin-clavulanate IV

(*continued on next page*)

Table 4 (*continued*)

Infection	Common pathogens	Recommended regimens
Suppurative thyroiditis	*S aureus*, GABHS, *S pneumoniae*, AGNB, *Peptostreptococcus* spp, *Actinomyces* spp	Dicloxacillin or moxicillin-clavulanate PO; macrolides or clindamycin IV or PO; ticarcillin-clavulanate IV
Cervical lymphadenitis	Viral causes most common if bilateral, but bacterial causes associated with an oropharyngeal infection (*S aureus* and GABHS, oral anaerobes, *Mycobacterium* spp) should be suspected if unilateral	Dicloxacillin or amoxicillin-clavulanate PO; macrolides or clindamycin IV or PO
Infected thyroglossal duct or branchial cleft cysts	*S aureus*, *S pyogenes*, other *Streptococcus* spp, oral anaerobes	Cefoxitin or clindamycin IV; ticarcillin-clavulanate IV
Wound infection complicating head & neck surgery	*S aureus*, enteric gram-negative rods, AGNB, *Peptostreptococcus* spp	Cefoxitin or clindamycin IV; ampicillin-sulbactam PO; clindamycin or metronidazole plus a fluoroquinolone PO or IV

Abbreviations: AGNB, anaerobic gram-negative bacilli, including pigmented *Prevotella* and *Porphyromonas* spp, *Bacteroides* spp, and *Fusobacterium* spp; GABHS, group A β-hemolytic streptococci; IV, intravenous; PO, by mouth.

bacteria and a change in the balance of bacterial types from harmless to disease-causing bacteria. Among the bacteria most often implicated in periodontal disease and bone loss are *Actinobacillus actinomycetemcomitans* and *Porphyromonas gingivalis*. Other bacteria associated with periodontal disease are *Bacteroides forsythus*, *Treponema denticola*, *Treponema sokranskii*, and *P intermedia* [48]. Aggressive periodontitis is now recognized as a contagious infection that can be passed between family members. *A actinomycetemcomitans* and *P gingivalis* are believed to have a major role in this infection. Therapy should include the combination of antimicrobial agents and drainage of the infected root and resection of inflamed periodontal tissues [49]. Although penicillin has been effective, its use has been associated with the increasing recovery of BLPB [50]. Other agents that are resistant to β-lactamase may be superior in such a setting, but controlled clinical trials are not available. Systemic therapy with tetracyclines has been effective in the past, but the rapid emergence of tetracycline-resistant aerobic and anaerobic bacteria limits their usefulness. Furthermore, tetracyclines are contraindicated in children younger than 8 years of age because of tooth staining. Metronidazole has been shown to be superior or comparable to penicillin in the treatment of periodontal infection [51].

Otitis and mastoiditis

Acute otitis media

S pneumoniae, *H influenzae*, and *M catarrhalis* are the principal etiologic agents in bacterial acute otitis media (AOM), accounting for about 80% of the bacterial isolates [52]. Of special concern is the increased rate of penicillin-resistant strains of *S pneumoniae* [53] and amoxicillin-resistant *H influenzae* isolated from infected ears [53]. The incidence of such strains reached 50% in some geographic areas. Whereas the rate of *S pneumoniae* has decreased following the introduction of the pneumococcal conjugate vaccine in 2000, the frequency of isolation of nontypeable *H influenzae* has increased [54]. Viruses were recovered in the middle ear fluid in 14.3% of children [55]. Anaerobes are infrequently studied in AOM but were recovered from 5% to 15% of acutely infected ears [56] and from 42% of culture-positive aspirates of serous otitis media [57,58]. *Peptostreptococcus* spp and *Propionibacterium acnes* were the predominant isolates, and AGNB were also recovered.

Antimicrobial therapy should be directed at eradication of the primary pathogen(s) and prevention of recurrences and other complications. Although spontaneous resolution is common and may occur in 75% of patients, it is impossible to predict which patient will require antimicrobial agents to hasten improvement. The new guidelines for the treatment of AOM from the American Academies of Pediatrics and Family Practice offer an option of initial observation rather than antibacterial treatment in children between the ages of 6 months and 12 years who have an uncertain diagnosis and nonsevere illness [59]. If empiric antibacterial treatment is contemplated, increasing the dose of amoxicillin to 90 mg/kg/d to overcome β-lactamase–producing *S pneumoniae* and *H influenzae* is recommended, although controlled trials demonstrating superiority of this approach are lacking. The combination of amoxicillin plus clavulanic acid is effective against penicillinase-producing *H influenzae* and *M catarrhalis*. The newer second- or third-generation cephalosporins (cefuroxime, cefdinir, and cefpodoxime) also have been effective. The growing resistance of *S pneumoniae* to macrolides (about 35%) and the poor pharmacokinetics of azithromycin for *H influenzae* render the initial selection of macrolides less attractive. Anaerobes recovered in AOM are susceptible to aminopenicillins and other antibiotics commonly used to treat AOM. TMP/SMX, however, is active against only 50% of *Peptostreptococcus* spp, the major anaerobe isolated in AOM.

Chronic otitis media

Bacterial isolates from chronic suppurative otitis media usually are polymicrobial, with recovery of mixed aerobes and anaerobes ranging between two and six isolates per specimen. Many of these organisms produce β-lactamase that may have contributed to the high failure rate of β-lactam antibiotics. The most common aerobic isolates are *P aeruginosa* and

S aureus. Anaerobes are isolated from approximately 50% of patients, predominantly AGNB and *Peptostreptococcus* spp [1,60].

Antimicrobial treatment includes clindamycin, cefoxitin, a combination of metronidazole plus either clindamycin or a macrolide, or a penicillin (ie, amoxicillin, ticarcillin) plus a β-lactamase inhibitor (ie, clavulanic acid, sulbactam) [61]. In instances in which *P aeruginosa* is considered a true pathogen, parenteral therapy with a fluoroquinolone (ciprofloxacin), an anti-pseudomonal β-lactam (piperacillin-tazobactam, imipenem-cilastatin), or an aminoglycoside should be added. Parenteral therapy with a carbapenem or a ureidopenicillin provides adequate coverage for all potential pathogens, including anaerobic as well as aerobic bacteria.

Acute and chronic mastoiditis

S pneumoniae, S pyogenes, *S aureus,* and *H influenzae* are the most common aerobes recovered in acute mastoiditis [62]. *P* aer*uginosa,* Enterobacteriaceae, *S aureus,* AGNB, and *Peptostreptococcus* spp are the predominant isolates in chronic mastoiditis. *S pneumoniae* and *H influenzae* are rarely recovered [63]. Treatment should be guided by culture and susceptibility testing. Parenteral agents with the combination of a penicillin plus a β-lactamase inhibitor (ie, ticarcillin-clavulanate) are appropriate. Treatment should be continued for 7 to 10 days.

Sinusitis

Acute sinusitis

Bacteria commonly recovered from pediatric and adult patients who have community-acquired acute purulent sinusitis include *S pneumoniae, H influenzae, M catarrhalis*, *S pyogenes*, and *S aureus* [64–66]. *S aureus* is a common pathogen in sphenoid sinusitis [67]. The infection is polymicrobial in about one third of the cases. Enteric bacteria are recovered less commonly. Approximately 8% of isolates recovered from acute maxillary sinusitis have an odontogenic origin, mostly as an extension of the infection from the roots of the premolar or molar teeth [68]. *P aeruginosa* and other gram-negative rods are common in sinusitis of nosocomial origin (especially in patients who have nasal tubes or catheters), the immunocompromised, and patients who have cystic fibrosis or HIV infection [69]. Anaerobic also bacteria can be recovered in these patients, however.

The choice of antimicrobial therapy is similar to that for AOM. The recommendations of the Sinus and Allergy Partnership guidelines for the optimal treatment of acute bacterial sinusitis are based on predicted microbiologic data and PK/PD parameters of antimicrobial agents with expected clinical efficacy rates [61]. For adults, the best antibacterial efficacy rates are predicted for amoxicillin-clavulanate and the respiratory fluoroquinolones (> 90% efficacy). They are followed by high-dose amoxicillin, cefpodoxime proxetil, cefuroxime axetil, and TMP/SMX (80%–90% efficacy), clindamycin, doxycycline, cefprozil, and macrolides (70%–80% efficacy), and cefaclor or loracarbef (50%–60% efficacy). These predictions have not been subjected to randomized clinical trials for direct comparison. Fluoroquinolones are not advocated in children. Macrolides or TMP-SMX is recommended in patients who have hypersensitivity to β—lactams.

In patients who do not show significant improvement within 48 hours or who show signs of deterioration, antral puncture for surgical drainage is recommended, and aspirate cultures and susceptibility testing should be performed to guide further antimicrobial therapy [70,71].

Chronic sinusitis

Although the etiology of chronic sinusitis is uncertain, bacteria are frequently isolated in the sinus cavity of these patients [67]. The clinical significance of some of the low-virulence organisms, such as *S epidermidis*, is questionable because they regularly colonize the nasal cavity [72–76]. When adequate anaerobic culture techniques were employed, however, strict anaerobes were recovered from more than half of the patients [67]. Chronic sinusitis caused by anaerobes is a particular concern because many of the complications (eg, mucocele formation, osteomyelitis, intracranial abscess) are associated with recovery of these organisms [1].

Antimicrobial therapy for chronic sinusitis should be directed against both aerobic and anaerobic bacteria, including BLPB. Choices include clindamycin, metronidazole plus a penicillin or a macrolide, or a penicillin–β-lactamase inhibitor combination (eg, amoxicillin-clavulanate or ticarcillin-clavulanate). The newer fluoroquinolones that provide antianaerobic coverage (eg, moxifloxacin, gatifloxacin, gemifloxacin) are suitable alternatives and are available in both oral and parenteral forms. Treatment for chronic sinusitis should be extended to at least 21 days. Fungal sinusitis can be treated with surgical débridement and antifungal agents.

Pharyngotonsillitis

The pathogens implicated in acute pharyngotonsillitis include groups A, B, C, and G streptococci, *N gonorrhoeae, N meningitidis, Corynebacterium diphtheriae,* and *Arcanobacterium hemolyticum.* Indirect evidence supports the involvement of obligate anaerobes (*Fusobacterium* spp, pigmented *Prevotella* and *Porphyromonas* spp, and *Peptostreptococcus* spp) in both acute and chronic tonsillitis [77]. For example, obligate anaerobes frequently are recovered from tonsillar, peritonsillar, or retropharyngeal abscesses, in many cases without any aerobic bacteria [78]. Obligate anaerobes are isolated from 25% of suppurative cervical lymph nodes associated with dental or tonsillar infections [79], and encapsulated pigmented *Prevotella* and *Porphyromonas* spp are found frequently within acutely inflamed tonsils [1], often directly from the core of recurrently inflamed tonsils that fail to yield GABHS [80,81]. Furthermore, an immune response against *P intermedia* can be detected in patients who have non-GABHS tonsillitis [82] and against *P intermedia* and *F nucleatum* in patients who recovered from peritonsillar cellulitis or abscesses [83].

The growing inability of penicillin to eradicate GABHS from the oropharynx leading to clinical and bacteriologic failure is an important clinical dilemma. Recent studies have shown that treatment with oral penicillin failed to eradicate GABHS in 35% of patients who had acute-onset pharyngitis treated with oral penicillin V and in 37% of those who received intramuscular penicillin [84]. Various theories have been proposed to explain this failure of penicillin therapy (Box 1) [20,85,86]. The success rate in the treatment of acute GABHS tonsillitis was found to be consistently higher with cephalosporins than with penicillin. The greater efficacy of cephalosporins may result from their activity against aerobic BLPB such as *S aureus, Haemophilus* spp, and *M catarrhalis*. Another possibility is that the normal resident oropharyngeal flora, which may compete with GABHS, is less susceptible to cephalosporins than to penicillin [85]. Nevertheless, penicillin still is recommended as the antibiotic of choice in recent treatment guidelines because of its proven efficacy, safety, narrow spectrum, and low cost [87]. More importantly, penicillin is effective in preventing the nonsuppurative sequelae of acute rheumatic fever, an important goal for antimicrobial therapy of GABHS pharyngotonsillitis. This advantage has not been established for other available therapeutic regimens. The macrolides are an alternative choice. Compliance with the newer macrolides (clarithromycin and azithromycin) is better than with erythromycin, because of improved gastrointestinal tolerance. The

Box 1. Possible causes for antibiotic failure or relapse in therapy of GABHS tonsillitis

Bacterial interactions
- The presence of BLPB that "protect" GABHS from penicillins
- Co-aggregation between GABHS and *M catarrhalis*
- Absence of members of the oral bacterial flora capable of interfering with the growth of GABHS (through production of bacteriocins and/or competition for nutrients)

Internalization of GABHS (survives within epithelial cells, escaping eradication by penicillins)
Resistance (ie, erythromycin) or tolerance (ie, penicillin) to the antibiotic used
Inappropriate dose, duration of therapy, or choice of antibiotic
Poor compliance
Reacquisition of GABHS from a contact or an object (ie, toothbrush or dental braces)
Carrier state, not disease

increased use of macrolides for the treatment of various respiratory tract infections has resulted in a significant increase in resistance by GABHS to these agents, however [88–92]. When *C diphtheriae* is suspected, erythromycin is the drug of choice, with penicillin or rifampin as alternatives.

Peritonsillar, retropharyngeal, and odontogenic deep neck infections

Deep neck infections commonly originate from an odontogenic or oropharyngeal infection and generally are polymicrobial, involving both aerobic and anaerobic bacteria from the primary source. Predominant anaerobic organisms include *Prevotella, Porphyromonas, Fusobacterium*, and *Peptostreptococcus* spp; aerobic organisms include GABHS, *S aureus*, and *H influenzae*. More than two thirds of deep neck abscesses contain BLPB [78,93]. Retropharyngeal cellulitis and abscess in young children is more likely to involve aerobic isolates alone, such as *S pyogenes* and *S aureus* [94]. *Fusobacterium necrophorum* is especially common in deep neck infections associated with septic thrombophlebitis of the internal jugular vein resulting in bacteremia and metastatic abscesses (Lemierre disease) [95]. Accurate localization of the primary source of infection as well as the anatomic route of spread by appropriate imaging techniques is critical to a successful outcome. Surgical drainage of loculated pus and protection of the airway are essential. Because these infections are life threatening, initial empiric antimicrobial therapy should include broad coverage for BLPB including *S aureus*, *S pyogenes*, AGNB, and *Peptostreptococcus* spp. A penicillin–β-lactamase inhibitor combination (ticarcillin-clavulanate or piperacillin-tazobactam) or a carbapenem (imipenem or meropenem) is appropriate in view of the severity of these infections. If MRSA is suspected, the addition of vancomycin or linezolid is warranted.

Parotitis and sialadenitis

The parotid gland is the salivary gland most commonly affected by inflammation. The pathogens most commonly associated with acute bacterial parotitis and sialadenitis are *S aureus* and anaerobic bacteria. The predominant anaerobes include AGNB and *Peptostreptococcus* spp. Isolation of *Streptococcus* spp (including *S pneumoniae*) and gram-negative bacilli (including *E coli*) also has been reported [96,97]. Gram-negative organisms often are seen in hospitalized patients. Organisms less frequently found are Arachnia, *H influenzae, K pneumoniae, Salmonella* spp, *P aeruginosa, Treponema pallidum*, cat-scratch bacillus, and *Eikenella corrodens*. *M tuberculosis* and atypical mycobacteria are rare causes of parotitis. Broad-spectrum antimicrobial therapy is indicated to cover all possible aerobic and anaerobic pathogens, including *S aureus*, GABHS, and anaerobic bacteria. A penicillinase-resistant penicillin or a first-generation cephalosporin generally is adequate. Clindamycin plus a fluoroquinolone is an alternative. Vancomycin for MRSA and ceftazidime for broader coverage of gram-negative organisms may be required in seriously ill patients.

Suppurative thyroiditis

S aureus, GABHS, *S epidermidis,* and *S pneumoniae* are the predominant aerobic isolates in suppurative thyroiditis. The most common anaerobic bacteria are AGNB, *Peptostreptococcus* spp, and *Actinomyces* spp [98,99]. Agents that are rarely recovered include *Klebsiella* spp, *H influenzae, Streptococcus viridans, Salmonella* spp, Enterobacteriaceae, *M tuberculosis*, atypical mycobacteria, *Aspergillus* spp, *Coccidioides immitis*, *Candida* spp, *Treponema pallidum*, and *Echinococcus* spp. Viruses associated with subacute thyroiditis include measles, mumps, influenza, enterovirus, Epstein-Barr virus, adenovirus, echovirus, and St. Louis encephalitis virus. Treatment with broad-spectrum antibiotics is indicated at least until culture results are available. Empiric therapy should cover *S aureus* and GABHS. A penicillinase-resistant penicillin (ie, dicloxacillin) or a penicillin–β-lactamase inhibitor combination (ie, amoxicillin-clavulanate) is suitable for oral therapy. Patients allergic to penicillin can be treated with a macrolide or clindamycin. Antibiotic treatment should be administered for at least 14 days.

Cervical lymphadenitis

The cervical lymphatic system is a first line of defense against various infections of the head and neck, including the upper respiratory tract, oropharynx, and soft tissues of the face and scalp. Viruses, including Epstein-Barr virus, cytomegalovirus, herpes simplex virus, adenovirus, enterovirus, roseola, rubella, and HIV, are the most common cause of bilateral cervical lymphadenitis in children [100]. Other pathogens include *M pneumoniae* and *C diphtheriae*. The most common bacterial organisms causing acute unilateral infection associated with facial trauma or impetigo are *S aureus* and GABHS [79,100,101]. Anaerobic bacteria are associated with a dental or periodontal source of infection; the predominate isolates include AGNB and *Peptostreptococcus* spp [79,101]. Other causes include *Bartonella henselae, H influenzae, Francisella tularensis, Pasteurella multocida, Yersinia pestis, Y enterocolitica, Listeria monocytogenes, A actinomycetemcomitans, Burkholderia gladioli, Spirillum minor, Nocardia brasiliensis, Mycobacterium tuberculosis,* and non-TB *mycobacterium* [102]. Cervical adenitis in the newborn often is associated with group B streptococci. The most common fungi involved in cervical lymphadenitis are *Histoplasma capsulatum, C immitis,* and *Paracoccidioides* spp.

Most patients who have cervical lymphadenitis do not require specific antibiotic therapy because these infections are commonly associated with a viral pharyngitis or stomatitis. Empiric antimicrobial therapy should provide adequate coverage for *S aureus* and GABHS with a penicillinase-resistant penicillin such as cloxacillin and dicloxacillin, or a penicillin–β-lactamase inhibitor combination (ie, amoxicillin-clavulanate). Patients allergic to penicillin can be treated with a macrolide or clindamycin. Treatment should be administered for at least 14 days. When mycobacterial or cat-scratch disease is suspected, incision and drainage should be avoided because chronically draining cutaneous fistulae may develop. Therapy with rifampin, TMP/SMX, or gentamicin, directed at *B henselae*, should be considered in cat-scratch disease. Total surgical removal is the most effective therapy for nontuberculous mycobacterial infection. Empiric antituberculous therapy with rifampin and isoniazid usually is initiated until the organisms are identified positively as atypical mycobacteria.

Infected thyroglossal duct and branchial cleft cysts

The organisms causing infections of the thyroglossal duct and brachial cleft cysts usually originate from the skin or the oropharynx and include *S aureus, S pyogenes,* other *Streptococcus* spp, and oral anaerobes [103,104]. Surgical drainage of an abscess is the therapy of choice, but administration of antimicrobial agents is required also. Because aerobic and anaerobic BLPB are isolated from the majority of these infections, antimicrobial therapy effective against these organisms is recommended. Effective agents include cefoxitin or clindamycin, a penicillin–β-lactamase inhibitor combination (eg, ticarcillin-clavulanate), or a carbapenem (ie, imipenem or meropenem) for seriously ill patients. A penicillinase-resistant penicillin (ie, nafcillin) or first-generation cephalosporin generally is adequate when the infection is caused by staphylococci. If MRSA is suspected, the addition of vancomycin or linezolid may be warranted.

Wound infection complicating head and neck surgery

Wound infections result from disruption of the oral mucosa at the surgical site and exposure to oropharyngeal flora. They generally are polymicrobial; the most frequently recovered isolates include *S aureus*, enteric gram-negative rods, AGNB, and *Peptostreptococcus* spp [105]. Cefoxitin, ampicillin-sulbactam, or a combination of clindamycin or metronidazole with a fluoroquinolone is suitable for initial empiric therapy [106]. Antimicrobial prophylaxis with cefoxitin or clindamycin is effective in preventing postsurgical wound infections of the head and neck and should be administered for only 24 hours.

References

[1] Finegold SM. Anaerobic infections in humans: an overview. Anaerobe 1995;1:3–9.
[2] Brook I. The role of beta-lactamase-producing bacteria in the persistence of streptococcal tonsillar infection. Rev Infect Dis 1984;6:601–7.
[3] Butler JC. Epidemiology of pneumococcal serotypes and conjugate vaccine formulations. Microb Drug Resist 1997;3:125–9.

[4] Joloba ML, Windau A, Bajaksouzian S, et al. Pneumococcal conjugate vaccine serotypes of *Streptococcus pneumoniae* isolates and the antimicrobial susceptibility of such isolates in children with otitis media. Clin Infect Dis 2001;33:1489–94.

[5] Nagai K, Davies TA, Ednie LM, et al. Activities of a new fluoroketolide, HMR 3787, and its (des)-fluor derivative RU 64399 compared to those of telithromycin, erythromycin A, azithromycin, clarithromycin, and clindamycin against macrolide-susceptible or -resistant *Streptococcus pneumoniae* and S. *pyogenes*. Antimicrob Agents Chemother 2001;45:3242–5.

[6] Jacobs MR, Felmingham D, Appelbaum PC, et al. The Alexander Project 1998–2000: susceptibility of pathogens isolated from community-acquired respiratory tract infection to commonly used antimicrobial agents. J Antimicrob Chemother 2003;52:229–46.

[7] Mera RM, Miller LA, Daniels JJ, et al. Increasing prevalence of multidrug-resistant *Streptococcus pneumoniae* in the United States over a 10-year period: Alexander Project. Diagn Microbiol Infect Dis 2005;51:195–200.

[8] Fedler KA, Biedenbach DJ, Jones RN. Assessment of pathogen frequency and resistance patterns among pediatric patient isolates: report from the 2004 SENTRY Antimicrobial Surveillance Program on 3 continents. Diagn Microbiol Infect Dis 2000;56:427–36.

[9] Fasola E, Bajaksouzian S, Appelbaum P, et al. Variation in erythromycin and clindamycin susceptibilities of *Streptococcus pneumoniae* in four test methods. Antimicrob Agents Chemother 1997;41:129–34.

[10] Tait-Kamradt A, Davies T, Cronan M, et al. Mutations in 23S rRNA and ribosomal protein L4 account for resistance in pneumococcal strains selected in vitro by macrolide passage. Antimicrob Agents Chemother 2000;44:2118–25.

[11] Gill MJ, Brenwald NP, Wise R. Identification of an efflux pump gene, pmrA, associated with fluoroquinolone resistance in *Streptococcus pneumoniae*. Antimicrob Agents Chemother 1999;43:187–9.

[12] Felmingham D, Washington J. Trends in the antimicrobial susceptibility of bacterial respiratory tract pathogens—findings of the Alexander Project 1992–1996. J Chemother 1999;11: 5–21.

[13] Ubukata K, Shibasaki Y, Yamamoto K, et al. Association of amino acid substitutions in penicillin-binding protein 3 with beta-lactam resistance in beta-lactamase-negative ampicillin-resistant *Haemophilus influenzae*. Antimicrob Agents Chemother 2001;45:1693–9.

[14] Jacobs MR, Bajaksouzian S, Zilles A, et al. Susceptibilities of *Streptococcus pneumoniae* and *Haemophilus influenzae* to 10 oral antimicrobial agents based on pharmacodynamic parameters: 1997 U.S. Surveillance study. Antimicrob Agents Chemother 1999;43:1901–8.

[15] Peric M, Bozdogan B, Jacobs MR, et al. Effects of an efflux mechanism and ribosomal mutations on macrolide susceptibility of *Haemophilus influenzae* clinical isolates. Antimicrob Agents Chemother 2003;47:1017–22.

[16] Brook I. Antibiotic resistance of oral anaerobic bacteria and their effect on the management of upper respiratory tract and head and neck infections. Semin Respir Infect 2002;17: 195–203.

[17] Hecht DW. Antibiotic resistance, clinical significance, and the role of susceptibility testing. Anaerobe 2006;12:115–21.

[18] Lindbaek M. Acute sinusitis: guide to selection of antibacterial therapy. Drugs 2004;64: 805–19.

[19] Brook I, Foote PA, Hausfeld JN. Eradication of pathogens from the nasopharynx after therapy of acute maxillary sinusitis with low- or high-dose amoxicillin/clavulanic acid. Int J Antimicrob Agents 2005;26:416–9.

[20] Brook I. The role of beta-lactamase producing bacteria and bacterial interference in streptococcal tonsillitis. Int J Antimicrob Agents 2001;17:439–42.

[21] Verklin RM, Mandell GL. Alteration of antibiotics by anaerobiosis. J Lab Clin Med 1977; 89:65–72.

[22] Craig WA, Andes D. Pharmacokinetics and pharmacodynamics of antibiotics in otitis media. Pediatr Infect Dis J 1996;15:255–9.

[23] Vogelman B, Gudmundsson S, Leggett J, et al. Correlation of antimicrobial pharmacokinetic parameters with therapeutic efficacy in an animal model. J Infect Dis 1988;158: 831–47.
[24] Craig W. Pharmacokinetic/pharmacodynamic parameters: rationale for antibacterial dosing of mice and men. Clin Infect Dis 1998;26:1–10.
[25] Maglio D, Nicolau DP. The integration of pharmacokinetics and pathogen susceptibility data in the design of rational dosing regimens. Methods Find Exp Clin Pharmacol 2004; 26:781–8.
[26] Leach A, Shelby-James T, Mayo M, et al. A prospective study of the impact of community-based arithromycin treatment of trachoma on carriage and resistance of *Streptococcus pneumoniae*. Clin Infect Dis 1997;24:356–62.
[27] Doern GV. Macrolide and ketolide resistance with *Streptococcus pneumoniae*. Med Clin North Am 2006;90:1109–24.
[28] Moore RD, Lietman PS, Smith CR. Clinical response to aminoglycoside therapy: importance of the ratio of peak concentration to minimal inhibitory concentration. J Infect Dis 1987;155:93–9.
[29] Lister PD, Sanders CC. Pharmacodynamics of moxifloxacin, levofloxacin, and sparfloxacin against *Streptococcus pneumoniae*. J Antimicrob Chemother 2001;47:811–8.
[30] Forrest A, Nix D, Ballow C. Pharmacodynamics of intravenous ciprofloxacin in seriously ill patients. Antimicrob Agents Chemother 1993;37:1073–81.
[31] Lacy MK, Lu W, Xu X, et al. Pharmacodynamic comparisons of levofloxacin, ciprofloxacin, and ampicillin *against Streptococcus pneumoniae* in an in vitro model of infection. Antimicrob Agents Chemother 1999;43:672–7.
[32] Stass H, Dalhoff A. The integrated use of pharmacokinetic and pharmacodynamic models for the definition of breakpoints. Infection 2005;33(Suppl 2):29–35.
[33] Jacobs MR, Bajaksouzian S, Windau A, et al. Effects of various test media on the activities of 21 antimicrobial agents against *Haemophilus influenzae*. J Clin Microbiol 2002;40: 2369–76.
[34] Doern GV. Activity of oral β-lactam antimicrobial agents versus respiratory tract isolates of *Streptococcus pneumoniae*, *Haemophilus influenzae*, and *Moraxella catarrhalis* in the era of antibiotic resistance. Otolaryngol Head Neck Surg 2002;127:S17–23.
[35] Steele RW, Thomas MP, Begue RE. Compliance issues related to the selection of antibiotic suspensions for children. Pediatr Infect Dis J 2001;20:1–5.
[36] Mattoes HM, Kuti JL, Drusano GL, et al. Optimizing antimicrobial pharmacodynamics: dosage strategies for meropenem. Clin Ther 2004;26:1187–98.
[37] Kuti JL, Nightingale CH, Nicolau DP. Optimizing pharmacodynamic target attainment using the MYSTIC antibiogram: data collected in North America in 2002. Antimicrob Agents Chemother 2004;48:2464–70.
[38] Dagan R, Leibovitz E, Fliss DM, et al. Bacteriologic efficacies of oral azithromycin and oral cefaclor in treatment of acute otitis media in infants and young children. Antimicrob Agents Chemother 2000;44:43–50.
[39] Doern GV. Antimicrobial use and emergence of antimicrobial resistance with *Streptococcus pneumoniae* in the United States. Clin Infect Dis 2001;33(Suppl 3):S187–92.
[40] Christianson J, Andes DR, Craig WA. Pharmacodynamic characteristics of clindamycin against *Streptococcus pneumoniae* in a murine thigh-infection model [abstract A-1100]. Presented at the 41st Interscience Conference on Antimicrobial Agents and Chemotherapy. Chicago (IL), December 16–19, 2001.
[41] Craig WA. Does the dose matter? Clin Infect Dis 2001;33(Suppl 3):S233–7.
[42] Ambrose P, Owens R. New antibiotics in pulmonary critical care medicine; focus on advanced generation quinolones and cephalosporins. Semin Respir Crit Care Med 2002;21: 19–32.
[43] Doern GV, Heilmann KP, Huynh HK, et al. Antimicrobial resistance among clinical isolates of *Streptococcus pneumoniae* in the United States during 1999–2000, including

a comparison of resistance rates since 1994–1995. Antimicrob Agents Chemother 2001;45: 1721–9.

[44] Loesche WJ, Syed SA, Laughon BE, et al. The bacteriology of acute necrotizing ulcerative gingivitis. J Periodontol 1982;53:223–30.

[45] Socransky SS, Haffajee AD. Evidence of bacterial etiology: a historical perspective. Periodontol 2000, 1994;5:7–25.

[46] Shinn DL. Vincent's disease and its treatment. In: Finegold SM, editor. Metronidazole. Bridgewater (NJ): Excerpta Medica; 1977. p. 307–8.

[47] Brook I, Douma M. Antimicrobial therapy guide for the dentist. Newton (PA): Handbooks in Healthcare Co.; 2004.

[48] Darby I, Curtis M. Microbiology of periodontal disease in children and young adults. Periodontol 2000, 2001;26:33–53.

[49] Loesche WJ. Rationale for the use of antimicrobial agents in periodontal disease. Int J Technol Assess Health Care 1990;6:403–17.

[50] Heimdahl A, Von-Konow L, Nord CE. Isolation of beta-lactamase producing *Bacteroides* strains associated with clinical failures with penicillin treatment of human orofacial infections. Arch Oral Biol 1980;25:689–92.

[51] Loesche WJ, Giordano JR. Treatment paradigms in periodontal disease. Compend Contin Educ Dent 1997;18:221–32.

[52] Pichichero ME, Pichichero CL. Persistent otitis media: causative pathogen. Pediatr Infect Dis J 1995;14:178–83.

[53] Leibovitz E, Raiz S, Piglansky L, et al. Resistance pattern of middle ear fluid isolates in acute otitis media recently treated with antibiotics. Pediatr Infect Dis J 1998;17:463–9.

[54] Casey JR, Pichichero ME. Changes in frequency and pathogens causing acute otitis media in 1995-2003. Pediatr Infect Dis J 2004;23:824–8.

[55] Heikkinen T, Thint M, Chonmaitree T. Prevalence of various respiratory viruses in the middle ear during acute otitis media. N Engl J Med 1999;340:260–4.

[56] Brook I, Anthony BV, Finegold SM. Aerobic and anaerobic bacteriology of acute otitis media in children. J Pediatr 1978;92:13–5.

[57] Brook I, Yocum P, Shah K, et al. The aerobic and anaerobic bacteriology of serous otitis media. Am J Otolaryngol 1983;4:389–92.

[58] Brook I, Frazier EH. Microbial dynamics of persistent purulent otitis media in children. J Pediatr 1996;128:237–40.

[59] American Academy of Pediatrics Subcommittee on Management of Acute Otitis Media. Diagnosis and management of acute otitis media. Pediatrics 2004;113:1451–65.

[60] Brook I. Prevalence of beta-lactamase-producing bacteria in chronic suppurative otitis media. Am J Dis Child 1985;139:280–4.

[61] Clinical practice guidelines: management of sinusitis. Pediatrics 2001;108:798–807.

[62] Niv A, Nash M, Peiser J, et al. Outpatient management of acute mastoiditis with periosteitis in children. International Journal of Pediatric Otorhinolaryngology 1998;46:9–13.

[63] Brook I. Aerobic and anaerobic bacteriology of chronic mastoiditis in children. Am J Dis Child 1981;135:478–9.

[64] Gwaltney JM Jr, Scheld WM, Sande MA, et al. The microbial etiology and antimicrobial therapy of adults with acute community-acquired sinusitis: a fifteen-year experience at the University of Virginia and review of other selected studies. J Allergy Clin Immunol 1992;90: 457–62.

[65] Wald ER, Milmore GJ, Bowen AD, et al. Acute maxillary sinusitis in children. N Engl J Med 1981;304:749–54.

[66] Brook I, Foote PA, Hausfeld JN. Frequency of recovery of pathogens causing acute maxillary sinusitis in adults before and after introduction of vaccination of children with the 7-valent pneumococcal vaccine. J Med Microbiol 2006;55:943–6.

[67] Nord CE. The role of anaerobic bacteria in recurrent episodes of sinusitis and tonsillitis. Clin Infect Dis 1995;20:1512–24.

[68] Brook I. Microbiology of acute and chronic maxillary sinusitis associated with an odontogenic origin. Laryngoscope 2005;115:823–5.
[69] Decker CF. Sinusitis in the immunocompromised host. Curr Infect Dis Rep 1999;1:27–32.
[70] Brook I. Management of chronic suppurative otitis media: superiority of therapy effective against anaerobic bacteria. Pediatr Infect Dis J 1994;13:188–93.
[71] Sinus and Allergy Health Partnership. Antimicrobial treatment guidelines for acute bacterial rhinosinusitis. Otolaryngol Head and Neck Surg 2004;130(Suppl 1):1S–45S.
[72] Gordts F, Halewyck S, Pierard D, et al. Microbiology of the middle meatus: a comparison between normal adults and children. J Laryngol Otol 2000;14:184–8.
[73] Brook I. Bacteriology of acute and chronic ethmoid sinusitis. J Clin Microbiol 2005;43: 3479–80.
[74] Brook I. Bacteriology of acute and chronic frontal sinusitis. Arch Otolaryngol Head Neck Surg 2002;128:583–5.
[75] Brook I, Foote PA, Frazier EH. Microbiology of acute exacerbation of chronic sinusitis. Ann Otol Rhinol Laryngol 2005;114:573–6.
[76] Brook I, Frazier EH, Foote PA. Microbiology of the transition from acute to chronic maxillary sinusitis. J Med Microbiol 1996;45:372–5.
[77] Brook I. The role of anaerobic bacteria in tonsillitis. Int J Pediatr Otorhinolaryngol 2005; 69:9–19.
[78] Brook I. Aerobic and anaerobic microbiology of peritonsillar abscess in children. Acta Paediatr Scand 1981;70:831–5.
[79] Brook I. Aerobic and anaerobic bacteriology of cervical adenitis in children. Clin Pediatr 1980;19:693–6.
[80] Brook I, Yocum P. Comparison of the microbiology of group A streptococcal and non-group A streptococcal tonsillitis. Ann Otol Rhinol Laryngol 1988;97:243–6.
[81] Brook I, Gober AE. Treatment of non-streptococcal tonsillitis with metronidazole. Int J Pediatr Otorhinolaryngol 2005;69:65–8.
[82] Brook I, Foote PA Jr, Slots J, et al. Immune response to *Prevotella intermedia* in patients with recurrent non-streptococcal tonsillitis. Ann Otol Rhinol Laryngol 1993;102:113–6.
[83] Brook I, Foote PA, Slots J. Immune response to *Fusobacterium nucleatum* and *Prevotella intermedia* in patients with peritonsillar cellulitis and abscess. Clin Infect Dis 1995;20:S220–1.
[84] Kaplan EL, Johnson DR. Unexplained reduced microbiological efficacy of intramuscular benzathine penicillin G and of oral penicillin V in eradication of group A streptococci from children with acute pharyngitis. Pediatrics 2001;108:1180–6.
[85] Brook I. The role of bacterial interference in otitis, sinusitis and tonsillitis. Otolaryngol Head Neck Surg 2005;133:139–46.
[86] Brook I, Gober AE. Increased recovery of *Moraxella catarrhalis* and *Haemophilus influenzae* in association with group A beta-haemolytic streptococci in healthy children and those with pharyngo-tonsillitis. J Med Microbiol 2006;55:989–92.
[87] Bisno AL, Gerber MA, Gwaltney JM Jr, et al. Practice guidelines for the diagnosis and management of group A streptococcal pharyngitis. Infectious Disease Scoeity of America. Clin Infect Dis 2002;35:113–25.
[88] Colakoglu S, Alacam R, Hascelik G. Prevalence and mechanisms of macrolide resistance in Streptococcus pyogenes in Ankara, Turkey. Scand J Infect Dis 2006;38:456–9.
[89] Richter SS, Heilmann KP, Beekmann SE, et al. Macrolide-resistant *Streptococcus pyogenes* in the United States, 2002-2003. Clin Infect Dis 2005;41:599–608.
[90] Casey JR, Pichichero ME. Meta-analysis of cephalosporins versus penicillin for treatment of group A strepharyngo-tonsillitisococcal tonsillopharyngitis in adults. Clin Infect Dis 2004;38:1526–34.
[91] Brook I. Antibacterial therapy for acute group a streptococcal pharyngotonsillitis: short-course versus traditional 10-day oral regimens. Paediatr Drugs 2002;4:747–54.
[92] Khayr W, Taepke J. Management of peritonsillar abscess: needle aspiration versus incision and drainage versus tonsillectomy. Am J Ther 2005;12:344–50.

[93] Brook I. Microbiology of abscesses of the head and neck in children. Ann Otol Rhinol Laryngol 1987;96:429–33.
[94] Asmar BI. Bacteriology of retropharyngeal abscess in children. Pediatr Infect Dis J 1990;9: 595–6.
[95] Hughes CE, Spear RK, Shinabarger CE, et al. Septic pulmonary emboli complicating mastoiditis: Lemierre's syndrome. Clin Infect Dis 1994;18:633–5.
[96] Brook I. Aerobic and anaerobic microbiology of suppurative sialadenitis. J Med Microbiol 2002;51:526–9.
[97] Brook I. Acute bacterial suppurative parotitis: microbiology and management. J Craniofac Surg 2003;14:37–40.
[98] Shah SS, Baum SB. Infectious thyroiditis: diagnosis and management. Curr Infect Dis Rep 2000;2:147–53.
[99] Jeng LB, Lin JD, Chen MF. Acute suppurative thyroiditis: a ten year review in a Taiwanese hospital. Scand J Infect Dis 1994;26:297–300.
[100] Peters TR, Edwards KM. Cervical lymphadenopathy and adenitis. Pediatr Rev 2000;21: 399–405.
[101] Brook I, Frazier EH. Microbiology of cervical lymphadenitis in adults. Acta Otolaryngol 1998;118:443–6.
[102] Hazra R, Robson CD, Perez-Atayde AR, et al. Lymphadenitis due to nontuberculous mycobacteria in children: presentation and response to therapy. Clin Infect Dis 1999;28:123–9.
[103] Brook I. Microbiology of infected epidermal cysts. Arch Dermatol 1989;125:1658–61.
[104] Lemierre A. On certain septicemias due to anaerobic organisms. Lancet 1936;2:701–3.
[105] Brook I, Hirokawa R. Post surgical wound infection after head and neck cancer surgery. Ann Otol Rhinol Laryngol 1989;98:322–5.
[106] Fraioli R, Johnson JT. Prevention and treatment of postsurgical head and neck infections. Curr Infect Dis Rep 2004;6:172–80.

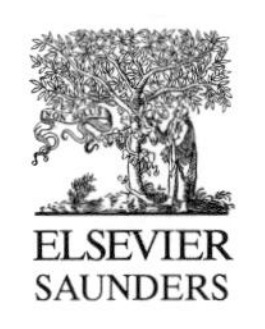

INFECTIOUS
DISEASE CLINICS
OF NORTH AMERICA

Infect Dis Clin N Am 21 (2007) 393–408

Periorbital and Orbital Infections

Ellen R. Wald, MD

Department of Pediatrics, University of Wisconsin School of Medicine and Public Health, Box 4108, 600 Highland Avenue, Madison, WI 53792, USA

Infections of the eye can be preseptal or orbital in origin (Box 1). They must be distinguished from noninfectious causes of swelling in or around the eye, including (1) blunt trauma (leading to the proverbial "black" eye), (2) tumor, (3) local edema, and (4) allergy. In cases of blunt trauma, history provides the key to the diagnosis. Eyelid swelling continues to increase for 48 hours and then resolves over several days. Tumors that characteristically involve the eye include hemangioma of the lid, ocular tumors such as retinoblastoma [1] and choroidal melanoma, and orbital neoplasms such as neuroblastoma and rhabdomyosarcoma [2]. Tumors usually cause gradual onset of proptosis in the absence of inflammation. Orbital pseudotumor, an autoimmune inflammation of the orbital tissues, presents with eyelid swelling, red eye, pain, and decreased ocular motility [3,4]. Hypoproteinemia and congestive heart failure cause eyelid swelling because of local edema. Characteristic findings are bilateral, boggy, nontender, nondiscolored soft tissue swelling. Allergic inflammation includes angioneurotic edema or contact hypersensitivity [5]. Superficially, these problems can resemble the findings in acute infection. The presence of pruritus and the absence of tenderness are helpful distinguishing characteristics of allergic inflammation.

Pathogenesis

Knowledge of the anatomy of the eye is important for understanding its susceptibility to spread of infection from contiguous structures. Veins that drain the orbit, the ethmoid and maxillary sinuses, and the skin of the eye and periorbital tissues (Fig. 1) constitute an anastomosing and valveless network [2]. This venous system provides opportunities for spread of infection from one anatomic site to another and predisposes to involvement of the

E-mail address: erwald@wisc.edu

doi:10.1016/j.idc.2007.03.008

Box 1. Infectious causes of preseptal and orbital cellulitis

Preseptal cellulitis

Localized infection of the eyelid or adjacent structure
- Conjunctivitis
- Hordeolum
- Dacryoadenitis
- Dacryocystitis
- Bacterial cellulitis (trauma)

Hematogenous dissemination
- Bacteremic periorbital cellulitis

Acute sinusitis
- Inflammatory edema

Orbital cellulitis

Acute sinusitis
- Subperiosteal abscess
- Orbital abscess
- Orbital cellulitis
- Cavernous sinus thrombosis

Hematogenous dissemination
- Endophthalmitis

Traumatic inoculation
- Endophthalmitis

cavernous sinus. Bacterial cellulitis of the soft tissue of the facial structures can cause contiguous phlebitis that may progress to involve distant sites.

Fig. 2 demonstrates the relationship between the eye and the paranasal sinuses. The roof of the orbit is the floor of the frontal sinus, and the floor of the orbit is the roof of the maxillary sinus. The medial wall of the orbit is formed by the frontal maxillary process, the lacrimal bone, the lamina papyracea of the ethmoid bone, and a small part of the sphenoid bone [6]. Infection originating in the mucosa of the paranasal sinuses can spread to involve the bone (osteitis with or without subperiosteal abscess) and the intraorbital contents. Orbital infection can occur through natural bony dehiscences in the lamina papyracea of the ethmoid or frontal bones or through foramina through which the ethmoidal arteries pass [5].

Fig. 3 shows the position of the orbital septum. This structure is a connective-tissue extension of the periosteum (or periorbita) that is reflected into the upper and lower eyelids. Infection of tissues anterior to the orbital septum is described as "periorbital" or "preseptal" [7]. The septum provides a nearly impervious barrier to spread of infection to the orbit. Although preseptal cellulitis or periorbital cellulitis (the terms can be used

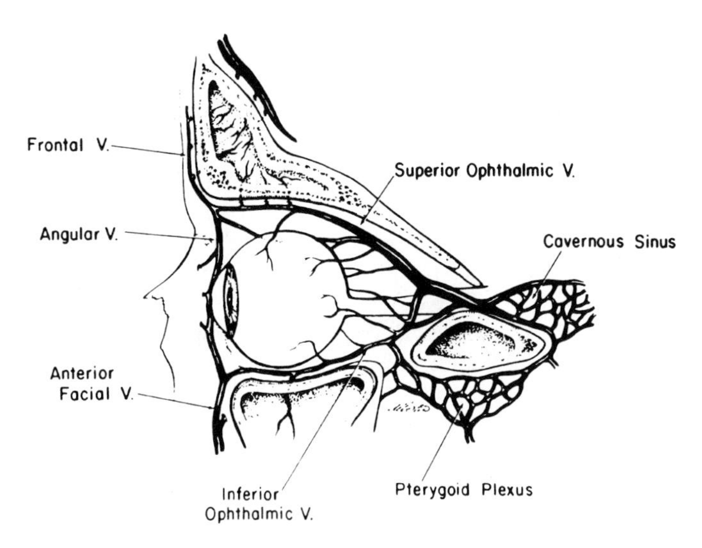

Fig. 1. The valveless venous system of the orbit and its many anastomoses. V, vein. (*From* Harris GJ. Subperiosteal abscess of the orbit. Arch Ophthalmol 1983;101:753–4; with permission.)

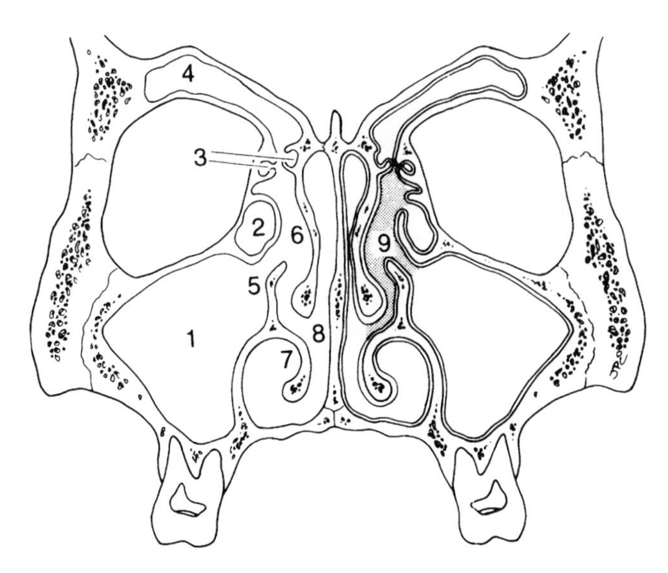

Fig. 2. The relationship between the eye and the paranasal sinuses is shown schematically. The roof of the orbit, the medial wall, and the floor are shared by the frontal, ethmoid, and maxillary sinuses, respectively. 1, maxillary sinus; 2, ethmoidal bulla; 3, ethmoidal cells; 4, frontal sinus; 5, uncinate process; 6, middle turbinate; 7, inferior turbinate; 8, nasal septum; 9, osteomeatal complex. (*From* Shapiro ED, Wald ER, Brozanski BA. Periorbital cellulitis and paranasal sinusitis: a reappraisal. Pediatr Infect Dis J 1982;1:91–4; with permission.)

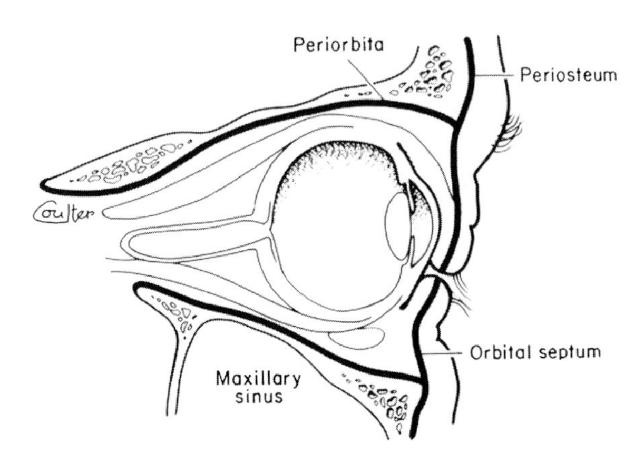

Fig. 3. The orbital septum is a connective tissue extension of the periosteum that is reflected into the upper and lower lid. (*From* Shapiro ED, Wald ER, Brozanski BA. Periorbital cellulitis and paranasal sinusitis: a reappraisal. Pediatr Infect Dis J 1982;1:91–4; with permission.)

interchangeably) often is considered a "diagnosis," the term is an inadequate diagnostic label unless accompanied by a modifier that indicates likely pathogenesis.

Infectious causes of preseptal cellulitis occur in the following three settings: (1) secondary to a localized infection or inflammation of the conjunctiva, eyelids, or adjacent structures (eg, conjunctivitis, hordeolum, acute chalazion, dacryocystitis, dacryoadenitis, impetigo, traumatic bacterial cellulitis); (2) secondary to hematogenous dissemination of nasopharyngeal pathogens to the periorbital tissue; and (3) as a manifestation of inflammatory edema in patients who have acute sinusitis (see Box 1) [7].

Infections behind the septum that cause eye swelling include subperiosteal abscess, orbital abscess, orbital cellulitis, cavernous sinus thrombosis, panophthalmitis, and endophthalmitis. Although all these entities can be labeled "orbital cellulitis," a systematic approach allows a more specific diagnosis, thereby directing management.

Preseptal infections

Conjunctivitis

Conjunctivitis is the most common disorder of the eye for which children are brought for medical care. In most cases, the lids are crusted and thickened with hyperemic conjunctiva. The usual causes of conjunctivitis in children older than neonates but less than 6 years old are *Haemophilus influenzae* (nontypeable) and *Streptococcus pneumoniae* [8–10]. Acute otitis media is a complicating feature in approximately 20% to 25% of children who have conjunctivitis caused by *H influenzae* [11]. In this case, systemic antibiotics are preferable to topical ophthalmic preparations for treatment. Several large outbreaks of conjunctivitis caused by an unencapsulated strain of *S pneumoniae* have been reported recently among college students [12]. These organisms also may cause sporadic cases of conjunctivitis [13]. In cases of bacterial conjunctivitis without acute otitis media, topical therapy with polymyxin-bacitracin [14], ciprofloxacin [15], norfloxacin [16], and chloramphenicol [17] hastens resolution [18].

Adenovirus is the most common cause of viral conjunctivitis in children older than 6 years [19]. Occasionally, individuals who have adenovirus infection have diffuse swelling of the lids that can be mistaken for a more serious problem (Fig. 4) [20]. To establish the microbiologic diagnosis in patients who have conjunctivitis, a swab of the conjunctival surface should be obtained for bacterial and viral pathogens.

Hordeolum and chalazion

An external hordeolum, or stye, is a bacterial infection of the glands of Zeis or Moll (sebaceous gland or sweat gland, respectively) associated with a hair follicle on the eyelid. In most cases, infection is localized and points to the lid margin as a pustule or inflammatory papule. The lid can be slightly swollen and erythematous around the area of involvement. An external hordeolum usually lasts a few days to a week and resolves spontaneously.

An internal hordeolum is a bacterial infection of a meibomian gland, a long sebaceous gland whose orifice is at the lid margin [21]. The infection usually causes inflammation and edema of the neck of the gland, which can result in obstruction. If there is no obstruction, infection points to the lid margin. If obstruction is present, infection points to the conjunctival surface of the eye [21]. Sometimes the swelling caused by an acute internal hordeolum is diffuse rather than localized, and a pustule is not obvious on the lid margin. To clarify the cause, it is necessary to evert the eyelid and examine the tarsal conjunctiva. A tiny, delicate pustule is diagnostic of an internal hordeolum.

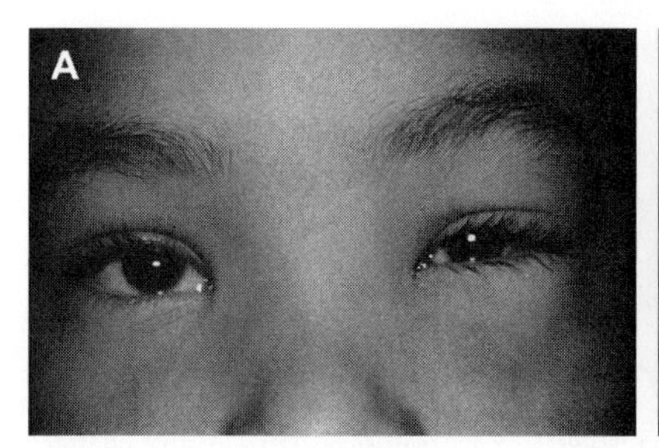

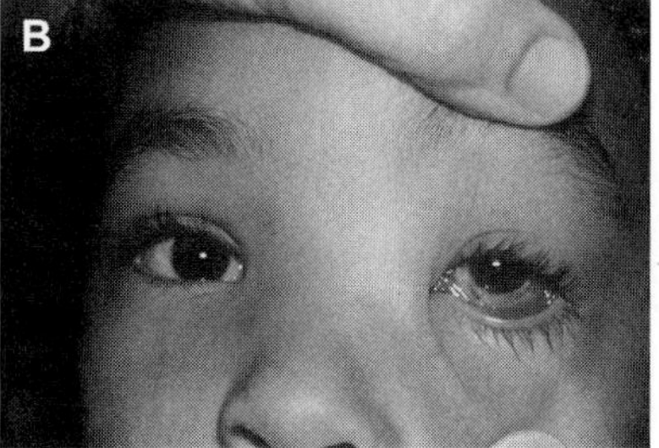

Fig. 4. (*A* and *B*) A child who has hemorrhagic conjunctivitis caused by adenovirus.

The usual cause of acute internal or external hordeola is *Staphylococcus aureus* [22]. An antibiotic ophthalmic ointment containing bacitracin can be applied to the site of infection. The main purpose of the topical therapy is to prevent spread of infection to adjacent hair follicles. Warm compresses may facilitate spontaneous drainage.

In contrast to the internal hordeolum, a chalazion manifests as a persistent (more than 2 weeks in duration), nontender, localized bulge or nodule (3–10 mm) in the lid; the overlying skin is completely normal. It is a sterile lipogranulomatous reaction. When a chalazion is large and causes local irritation, incision may be required.

Dacryoadenitis

Dacryoadenitis is an infection of the lacrimal gland. Sudden onset of soft tissue swelling that is maximal over the outer portion of the upper lid margin is typical. Occasionally, the eyeball is erythematous, the eyelid swollen, and the patient can have remarkable constitutional symptoms. The location of the swelling is a distinguishing characteristic (Fig. 5). When dacryoadenitis is caused by viral infection (mumps virus, Epstein-Barr virus [23], cytomegalovirus, coxsackievirus, echoviruses, or varicella-zoster virus), the area is only modestly tender. By contrast, when the infection is caused by bacterial agents, discomfort is prominent. In addition to *S aureus,* which is the most common cause of bacterial dacryoadenitis, causative agents include streptococci, *Chlamydia trachomatis, Brucella melitensis,* and, occasionally, *Neisseria gonorrhoeae* [24]. Fungal and rare parasitic infections of the lacrimal gland have been reported, including *Cysticercus cellulosae* and *Schistosoma haematobium* [25].

If parenteral therapy is required for suspected bacterial dacryoadenitis caused by *S aureus*, nafcillin, 150 mg/kg/d divided into doses every 6 hours,

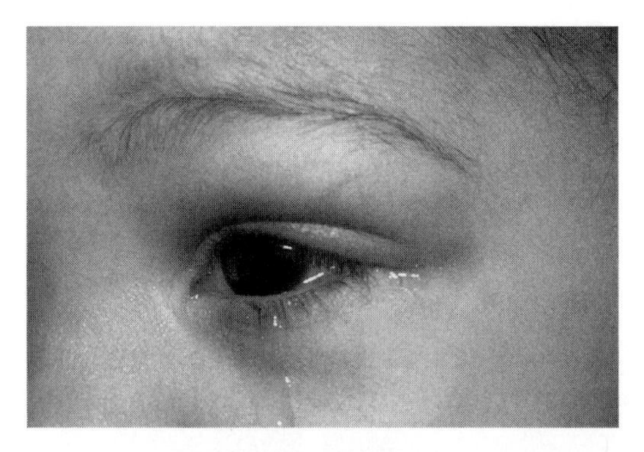

Fig. 5. A patient who has dacryoadenitis caused by an unspecified viral infection. The nontender swelling over the lateral portion of the left upper lid evolved while an antibiotic was being administered for acute otitis media. Swelling resolved in several days without any change in medical treatment.

is appropriate. In circumstances in which methicillin-resistant *S aureus* (MRSA) is a concern, vancomycin, 40 mg/kg in three to four divided doses, is recommended. Oral treatment of acute dacryoadenitis is undertaken with a semisynthetic penicillin such as dicloxacillin (100 mg/kg/d divided into four doses), cephalexin, or cefadroxil (100 or 50 mg/kg/d, respectively, divided into doses every 6 or 12 hours, respectively). If MRSA is suspected, alternatives include sulfamethoxazole-trimethoprim (based on 40 mg/kg/d of trimethoprim in two doses), clindamycin (40 mg/kg/d divided into doses every 6 hours), or linezolid (20 mg/kg/d divided into doses every 12 hours). Treatment is continued until all signs and symptoms have disappeared.

The differential diagnosis of swelling of the upper outer aspect of the eyelid includes inflammatory noninfectious problems such as Sjögren's syndrome and sarcoidosis as well as benign and malignant tumors [25].

Dacryocystitis

Dacryocystitis is a bacterial infection of the lacrimal sac. Although it is uncommon, it can occur at any age as a bacterial complication of a viral upper respiratory tract infection (URI). Because of the course traversed by the lacrimal duct, which drains to the inferior meatus within the nose, it is surprising that the duct and sac are not infected more often. Delayed opening, inspissated secretions, and anatomic abnormalities lead to disproportionate representation of infants younger than 3 months among children who have dacryocystitis [26].

Patients who have dacryocystitis often have had a viral URI for several days. They then experience fever and impressive erythema and swelling in addition to exquisite tenderness, which is most prominent in the triangular area just below the medial canthus (Fig. 6). Pressure over the lacrimal sac causes considerable discomfort but can result in expression of purulent material from the lacrimal puncta. Common causative organisms are gram-positive cocci. *S pneumoniae* is most common in neonates, although *S aureus, H influenzae,* and *Streptococcus agalactiae* also have been reported

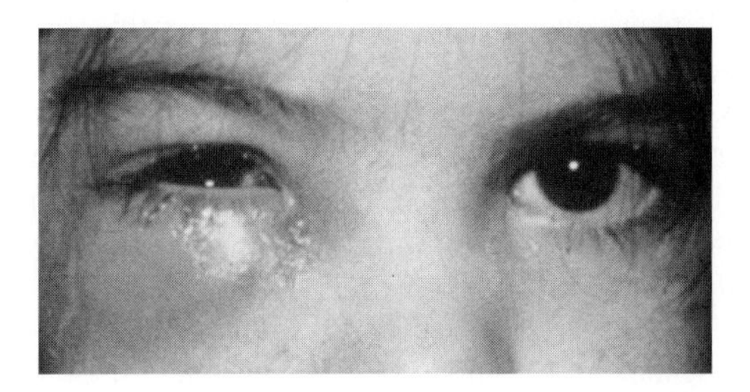

Fig. 6. A 6-year-old girl who has dacryocystitis. The area beneath the medial canthus is erythematous, indurated, and exquisitely tender.

[26,27]. *S aureus* and *Staphylococcus epidermidis* are most commonly implicated in acquired dacryocystitis in the older patient [28]. It is important to obtain material from the punctum, because other organisms (including enteric gram-negative bacilli, anaerobic bacteria, and yeast) have been observed occasionally [29]. Unusual pathogens, such as *Pasteurella multocida* and *Aeromonas hydrophila,* have been reported rarely [30].

Most patients who have dacryocystitis require admission to the hospital. Often they appear ill or toxic [29]. Because of the potential for any case of bacterial facial cellulitis to result in cavernous sinus thrombosis, therapy with parenteral antibiotics is indicated until the infection begins to subside. Nafcillin (at a dose of 150 mg/kg/d divided into doses every 6 hours) or cefazolin (at a dose of 100 mg/kg/d divided into doses every 8 hours) is appropriate except when infection caused by MRSA is suspected. In the latter case, vancomycin (40 mg/kg/d divided into doses every 6 hours) is best initiated. In penicillin-allergic patients, vancomycin or clindamycin (40 mg/kg/d divided into doses every 6 hours) suffices. After substantial improvement is observed in local findings, an oral agent can be substituted to complete a 10- to 14-day course of therapy.

The role of nonmedical management of dacryocystitis is controversial. Although surgical manipulation of the lacrimal duct is not necessary for most patients, both probing of the duct and incision and drainage have been reported to be successful in neonates [27]. Incision and drainage and direct application of antibiotics inside the sac have been promoted by some practitioners who care for adults [31].

Preseptal cellulitis after trauma

Occasionally, preseptal cellulitis results from secondary bacterial infection of sites of local skin trauma (including insect bites) or with spread of infection from a focus of impetigo. The traumatic injury may be extremely modest or completely unapparent. Loosely bound periorbital soft tissues permit impressive swelling to accompany minor infection. The overlying skin can be bright red with subtle textural changes, or intense swelling can lead to shininess (Fig. 7). Some patients have fever, but many are afebrile despite dramatic local findings. The peripheral white blood cell count is variable. In these cases, cellulitis, similar to that on any other cutaneous area, is caused by *S aureus* (including MRSA) or group A streptococcus [32,33].

Several less common causes of lid cellulitis have been reported. Periocular cellulitis and abscess formation have resulted from infection with *P multocida* in a healthy child who sustained a cat bite and cat scratch to the eyelid [34]. Ringworm (caused by *Trichophyton* species) also has been recognized as a cause of lid infection (leading to preseptal cellulitis) characterized by redness, swelling, ulceration, and vesicle formation [35,36]. Palpebral myiasis involving the eyelid of a 6-year-old child was reported from the Massachusetts Eye and Ear Infirmary [37]. A small draining fistula through which

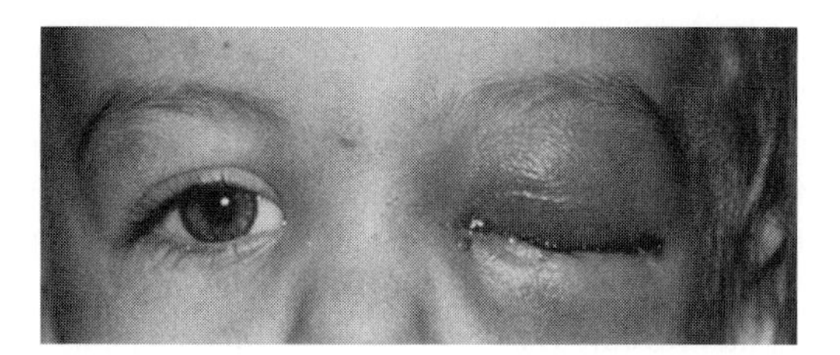

Fig. 7. A 3-year-old boy had rapid onset of left-eyelid swelling and erythema after he incurred a small laceration at the lateral margin of the left eye. He had had an upper respiratory tract infection for 10 days. Group A streptococcus was recovered from the wound.

the larvae were extracted was noted at the site of the erythematous and edematous lid. Several cases of cellulitis of the eyelid caused by *Bacillus anthracis* have been reported from Turkey [38]. The diagnosis was suspected when the erythematous and swollen lid developed an eschar. Scrapings showed the presence of gram-positive rods that were confirmed by culture. A primary case of lymphocutaneous *Nocardia brasiliensis* of the eyelid has been reported in an adult who was hunting in England 2 weeks before presentation following a small abrasion on this lower eyelid [39]. In countries where *Mycobacterium tuberculosis* is endemic, this cause also should be considered in patients who present with a swollen lid. Raina and colleagues [40] reported seven children who had tuberculous lesions of their eyelids. In most cases the presentation was relatively indolent (2 days to 2 months), and fistulas occurred during the course of conventional antibiotic treatment for more typical bacterial disease. Diagnosis was confirmed by a positive tuberculin skin test, the identification of a primary focus of tuberculosis in lung or bone, and response to antituberculous therapy.

Patients who have bacterial cellulitis of traumatized areas rarely have bacteremia. Precise bacteriologic diagnosis is made through culture of exudate from the wound. If there is no drainage, a careful attempt at tissue aspiration is undertaken if it can be done safely (ie, far enough from the orbit that there can be no potential damage to the eye). A tuberculin syringe with a 25-gauge needle can be used for aspiration of "tissue juice." Usually, only a minuscule amount of infected material can be aspirated. A small volume of nonbacteriostatic saline (0.2 mL) is drawn into the syringe before the procedure. The saline is not injected into the skin; instead, it is used to expel the small volume of tissue fluid onto chocolate agar for culture [41]. In patients who have bacterial cellulitis, parenteral treatment similar to that advised for dacryocystitis is recommended to hasten resolution and avoid spread of infection to the cavernous sinus.

Bacteremic periorbital cellulitis

Bacteremic periorbital cellulitis, most often seen in infants younger than 18 months of age, is preceded by a viral URI for several days. There is a sudden increase in temperature (to $>39°C$) accompanied by the acute onset and rapid progression of eyelid swelling. Swelling usually begins in the inner canthus of the upper and lower eyelid and can obscure the eyeball within 12 hours. Periorbital tissues are markedly discolored and usually are erythematous, although the area may have a violaceous discoloration if the swelling has been rapidly progressive [42,43]. The child's resistance to examination commonly leads to the erroneous impression of tenderness. Retraction or separation of the lids reveals that the globe is normally placed and extraocular eye movements are intact. If retraction of the lids is not possible, orbital CT scan may be necessary [44]. The young age, high fever, and rapid progression of findings differentiate bacteremic preseptal cellulitis from other causes of swelling around the eye.

In the era before universal *H influenzae* type b (Hib) immunization, this organism was the most common cause of bacteremic periorbital cellulitis in approximately 80% of cases [45]; *S pneumoniae* accounted for the remaining 20%. The substantial decline that has been observed in the total number of cases of bacteremic periorbital cellulitis is attributable to the widespread use of the Hib vaccine since 1991 and the introduction of pneumococcal conjugate vaccine in 2000 [45,46]. A precise bacteriologic diagnosis is made by recovery of the organism from blood culture. If a careful tissue aspiration is performed, culture of the specimen may have a positive result.

The pathogenesis of most of these infections, which usually occur during the course of a viral URI, is hematogenous dissemination from a portal of entry in the nasopharynx. This process is akin to the mechanism of most infections caused by Hib and some infections caused by *S pneumoniae*. In the current era, with routine immunization for *H influenzae* and *S pneumoniae,* these infections are rare [47].

In patients who have bacteremic periorbital cellulitis, radiographs of the paranasal sinuses often are abnormal. The abnormalities, however, almost certainly reflect the viral respiratory syndrome that precedes and probably predisposes to the bacteremic event, rather than a clinically significant sinusitis [7]. Bacteremic cellulitis rarely arises from the paranasal sinus cavities, as evidenced by the finding that typeable *H influenzae* organisms almost never are recovered from maxillary sinus aspirates and likewise rarely are recovered from abscess material in patients who have serious local complications of paranasal sinus disease, such as subperiosteal abscess. Although *S pneumoniae* can cause subperiosteal abscess in patients who have acute sinusitis, such patients usually are not bacteremic.

Treatment for suspected bacteremic periorbital cellulitis requires parenteral therapy. A nonvaccine strain of *S pneumoniae* or *Streptococcus pyogenes* is the most likely cause in a child who has received both the Hib and heptavalent pneumococcal conjugate vaccine [48]. Because this infection is usually bacteremic in the age group in whom the meninges are susceptible to inoculation, it may be prudent to use an advanced-generation cephalosporin such as cefotaxime or ceftriaxone (150 or 100 mg/kg/d, respectively, divided into 8- or 12-hour doses, respectively). Lumbar puncture should be performed unless the clinical picture precludes meningitis. Addition of vancomycin (60 mg/kg/d divided into doses every 6 hours) or rifampin (20 mg/kg once daily, not to exceed 600 mg/d) is appropriate if cerebrospinal fluid pleocytosis is present. When evidence of local infection has resolved and there is no meningitis, oral antimicrobial therapy is prescribed to complete a 10-day course.

Preseptal (periorbital) cellulitis caused by inflammatory edema of sinusitis

Several complications of paranasal sinusitis can result in the development of swelling around the eye. The most common and least serious complication often is referred to as "inflammatory edema" or a "sympathetic effusion" [6]. This complication is a form of preseptal cellulitis, although infection is confined to the sinuses [49].

Typically, a child at least 2 years old has had a viral URI for several days when swelling is noted. Often, there is a history of intermittent early morning periorbital swelling that resolves after a few hours. On the day of presentation, the eyelid swelling does not resolve typically but progresses gradually. Surprisingly, striking degrees of erythema can also be present. Eye pain and tenderness are variable. Eyelids can be very swollen and difficult to evert, requiring the assistance of an ophthalmologist. There is no displacement of the globe or impairment of extraocular eye movements, however. Fever, if present, is usually low grade.

The peripheral white blood cell count is unremarkable. Blood culture results are always negative. If a tissue aspiration is performed, culture of the specimen has a negative result. Sinus radiographs show ipsilateral ethmoiditis or pansinusitis. The age of the child, gradual evolution of lid swelling, and modest temperature elevation differentiate inflammatory edema from bacteremic periorbital cellulitis.

The pathogenesis of sympathetic effusion or inflammatory edema is attributable to the venous drainage of the eyelid and surrounding structures. The inferior and superior ophthalmic veins, which drain the lower lid and upper lid, respectively, pass through or just next to the ethmoid sinus. When the ethmoid sinuses are completely congested, physical impedance of venous drainage occurs, resulting in soft tissue swelling of the eyelids, maximal at the medial aspect of the lids. In this instance, infection is confined within the paranasal sinuses. The globe is not displaced, and there is no impairment of the extraocular muscle movements. Inflammatory edema, however, is part of a continuum with more serious complications resulting from the spread of infection outside the paranasal sinuses into the orbit [50]. Rarely, infection progresses despite initial optimal management of sympathetic effusions [49].

The infecting organisms in cases of inflammatory edema are the same as those that cause uncomplicated acute sinusitis (ie, *S pneumoniae,* nontypeable *H influenzae,* and *Moraxella catarrhalis*). Antibiotic therapy can be given orally if, at the time of the first examination, the eyelid swelling is modest, the child does not appear toxic, and the parents will adhere to management. Otherwise, admission to the hospital and parenteral treatment should be undertaken.

The only potential source of bacteriologic information is that which may be obtained by maxillary sinus aspiration; however, this procedure is rarely performed if infection is confined to the sinuses. Outpatient treatment should be considered only if the eyelid is at least 50% open and very close follow-up can be assured. Appropriate agents for outpatient therapy have activity against beta-lactamase–producing organisms (eg, amoxicillin–potassium clavulanate, cefuroxime axetil, and cefpodoxime proxetil). Parenteral agents include cefuroxime (150 mg/kg/d divided into doses every 8 hours) and ampicillin-sulbactam (200 mg/kg/d divided into doses every 6 hours). The latter combination, although not approved for children younger than 12 years, is an attractive choice. Although the use of topically applied intranasal decongestants such as oxymetazoline has not been evaluated systematically, such agents may be helpful during the first 48 hours. After several days, once the affected eye has returned to near normal, an oral antimicrobial agent is substituted to complete a 14-day course of therapy.

Orbital infections

The child or adolescent who has true orbital disease secondary to sinusitis usually has sudden onset of erythema and swelling about the eye after several days of a viral URI (Fig. 8). Eye pain can precede swelling and often is dramatic. The presence of fever, systemic signs, and toxicity is variable. At least 30% of patients in one series were afebrile at presentation [51]. Orbital infection is suggested by proptosis (with the globe displaced, usually anteriorly and downward), impairment of extraocular eye movements (most often upward gaze), or loss of visual acuity or chemosis (edema of the bulbar conjunctiva). Fortunately, orbital infection is the least common cause of the "swollen eye."

Nearly all orbital infections involve the formation of a subperiosteal abscess. In young children, subperiosteal abscess results from ethmoiditis and

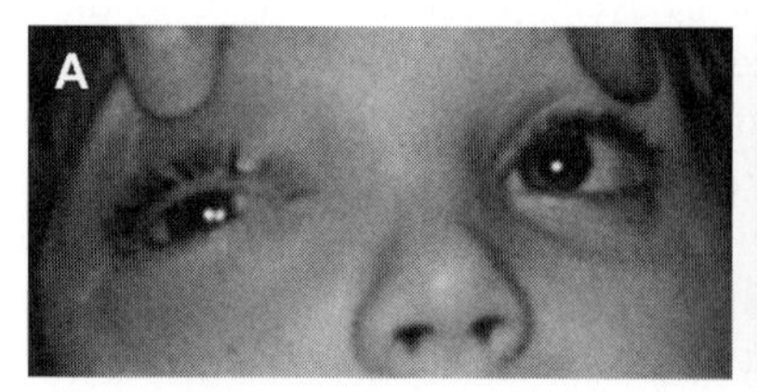

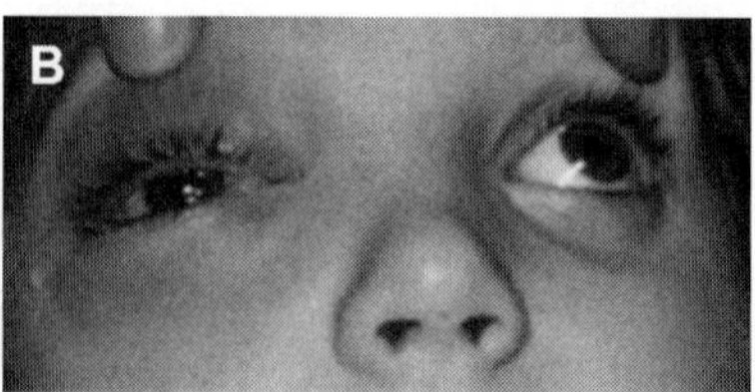

Fig. 8. (*A* and *B*) A 7-year-old boy who has orbital cellulitis. He had a 5-day history of eye pain and progressive swelling of the eyelids, which were markedly erythematous. When his eyelids were retracted, anterior and lateral displacement of the globe and impairment of upward gaze were noted.

ethmoid osteitis. For the adolescent, subperiosteal abscess can be a complication of frontal sinusitis and osteitis. True orbital abscesses are very uncommon [52]. Rarely, orbital cellulitis evolves, without formation of subperiosteal abscess, by direct spread from the ethmoid sinus to the orbit through natural bony dehiscences in the bones that form the medial wall of the orbit [49].

Imaging studies usually are performed if orbital disease is suspected. They help determine whether subperiosteal abscess, orbital abscess, or orbital cellulitis is the cause of the clinical findings (Fig. 9). In the presence of a large, well-defined abscess, complete ophthalmoplegia, or impairment of vision, prompt operative drainage of the paranasal sinuses and the abscess is commonly performed [53–55]. Several studies, however, have reported on the successful drainage of a subperiosteal abscess by endoscopy. This method, performed through an intranasal approach, has avoided an external incision [56,57]. Small abscesses may be managed with intravenous antibiotics alone [58–62]. In many cases, a well-defined abscess is not seen. Instead, inflammatory tissue (a so-called "phlegmon") is observed interposed between the lateral border of the ethmoid sinus and the swollen medial rectus muscle. Usually, patients who have these findings also are managed successfully with antimicrobial therapy alone [53,58,59,63]. On occasion, the CT scan can be misleading, suggesting abscess when inflammatory edema is present [50]; accordingly, the clinical course is the ultimate guide to management.

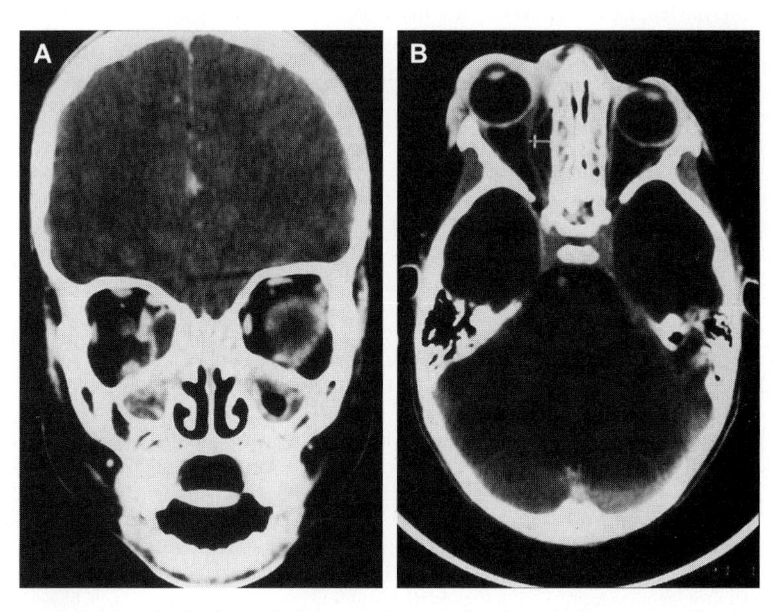

Fig. 9. (*A*) Axial and (*B*). Coronal CT scans show a subperiosteal abscess extending from the left ethmoid sinus.

Empiric antimicrobial therapy should be chosen to provide activity against *S aureus, S pyogenes,* and anaerobic bacteria of the upper respiratory tract (anaerobic cocci, *Bacteroides* spp, *Prevotella* spp, *Fusobacterium* spp, and *Veillonella* spp) in addition to the usual pathogens associated with acute sinusitis (ie, *S pneumoniae, H influenzae,* and *M catarrhalis*) [63,64]. Appropriate selections include cefuroxime (150 mg/kg/d divided into doses every 8 hours) or ampicillin-sulbactam (200 mg/kg/d divided into doses every 6 hours). Clindamycin (40 mg/kg/d divided into doses every 6 hours) or metronidazole (30 to 35 mg/kg/d divided into doses every 8 to 12 hours) can be added if cefuroxime is used and anaerobic infection is likely. If a patient presents with life- or vision-threatening disease, vancomycin may be added to ampicillin/sulbactam for coverage of community-acquired MRSA or penicillin-resistant *S pneumoniae* [51]. If surgery is performed, Gram stain of material drained from the sinuses or the abscess guides consideration of additional drugs or an altered regimen. When final results of culture are available, antibiotic therapy may be changed, if appropriate. Intravenous therapy is maintained until the infected eye appears nearly normal. At that time, oral antibiotic therapy can be substituted to complete a 3-week course of treatment.

References

[1] Abramson DH, Frank CM, Susman M, et al. Presenting signs of retinoblastoma. J Pediatr 1998;132:505–8.

[2] VanDyke RB, Desky AB, Daum RS. Infections of the eye and periorbital structures. Adv Pediatr Infect Dis 1988;3:125–80.

[3] Sirbaugh PE. A case of orbital pseudotumor masquerading as orbital cellulitis in a patient with proptosis and fever. Pediatr Emerg Care 1997;13:337–9.

[4] Greenberg MF, Pollard ZF. The red eye in childhood. Pediatr Clin North Am 2003;50: 105–24.

[5] Lessner A, Stern GA. Preseptal and orbital cellulitis. Infect Dis Clin North Am 1992;6: 933–52.

[6] Chandler JR, Langenbrunner DJ, Stevens ER. The pathogenesis of orbital complications in acute sinusitis. Laryngoscope 1970;80:1414–28.

[7] Shapiro ED, Wald ER, Brozanski BA. Periorbital cellulitis and paranasal sinusitis: a reappraisal. Pediatr Infect Dis 1982;1:91–4.

[8] Block SL, Hedrick J, Tyler R, et al. Increasing bacterial resistance in pediatric acute conjunctivitis (1997–1998). Antimicrob Ag Chemo 2000;44:1650–4.

[9] Bingen E, Cohen R, Jourenkova N, et al. Epidemiologic study of conjunctivitis-otitis syndrome. Pediatr Infect Dis J 2005;24:731–2.

[10] Buznach N, Dagan R, Greenberg D. Clinical and bacterial characteristics of acute bacterial conjunctivitis in children in the antibiotic resistance era. Pediatr Infect Dis J 2005;24:823–8.

[11] Bodor FF. Conjunctivitis-otitis syndrome. Pediatr 1982;69:695–8.

[12] Martin M, Turco JH, Zegans ME, et al. An outbreak of conjunctivitis due to atypical Streptococcus pneumoniae. N Engl J Med 2003;348:1112–21.

[13] Porat N, Greenberg D, Gvon-Lavi N, et al. The important role of nontypeable Streptococcus pneumoniae international clones in acute conjunctivitis. J Infect Dis 2006;194:689–96.

[14] Gigliotti F, Hendley JO, Morgan J, et al. Efficacy of topical antibiotic therapy in acute conjunctivitis in children. J Pediatr 1984;104:623–6.

[15] Leibowitz HM. Antibacterial effectiveness of ciprofloxacin 0.3% ophthalmic solution in the treatment of bacterial conjunctivitis. Am J Ophthalmol 1991;112:29S–33S.
[16] Miller IM, Wittreich J, Vogel R, et al. The safety and efficacy of topical norfloxacin compared with placebo in the treatment of acute, bacterial conjunctivitis. The Norfloxacin placebo ocular study group. Eur J Ophthalmol 1992;2:58–66.
[17] Rose PW, Hamden A, Brueggermann AB, et al. Chloramphenicol treatment for infective conjunctivitis in children in primary care: a randomized double-blind placebo-controlled trial. Lancet 2005;366:37–43.
[18] Sheikh A, Hurwitz B. Topical antibiotics for acute bacterial conjunctivitis: Cochrane systematic review and meta-analysis update. Br J Gen Pract 2005;55:962–4.
[19] Wald ER. Conjunctivitis in infants and children. Pediatr Infect Dis J 1997;16:S7–20.
[20] Ruttum MS, Ogawa G. Adenovirus conjunctivitis mimics preseptal and orbital cellulitis in young children. Pediatr Infect Dis J 1996;15:266–7.
[21] Sullivan JH. Lids and lacrimal apparatus. In: Vaughn D, Asbury T, Riordan-Eva P, editors. General ophthalmology. 13th edition. Norwalk (CT): Appleton & Lange; 1992. p. 28–80.
[22] Lederman C, Miller M. Hordeola and chalazia. Pediatr Rev 1999;20:283–4.
[23] Rhem MN, Wilhelmus KR, Jones DB. Epstein-Barr virus dacryoadenitis. Am J Ophthalmol 2000;129:372–5.
[24] Gungor K, Bekir NA, Namiduru M. Ocular complications associated with brucellosis in an endemic area. Eur J Ophthalmol 2002;12:232–7.
[25] Boruchoff SA, Boruchoff SE. Infections of the lacrimal system. Infect Dis Clin North Am 1992;6:925–32.
[26] Campolattaro BN, Lueder GT, Tychsen L. Spectrum of pediatric dacryocystitis: medical and surgical management of 54 cases. J Pediatr Ophthalmol Strabismus 1997;34:143–53.
[27] Pollard ZF. Treatment of acute dacryocystitis in neonates. J Pediatr Ophthalmol Strabismus 1991;28:341–3.
[28] Hurwitz JJ, Rodgers KJ. Management of acquired dacryocystitis. Can J Ophthalmol 1983; 18:213–6.
[29] Faden HS. Dacryocystitis in children. Clin Pediatr 2006;45:567–9.
[30] Meyer DR, Wobig JL. Acute dacryocystitis caused by *Pasteurella multocida*. Am J Ophthalmol 1990;110:444–5.
[31] Cahill KV, Burns JA. Management of acute dacryocystitis in adults. Ophthal Plast Reconstr Surg 1993;9:38–41.
[32] Powell K. Orbital and periorbital cellulites. Pediatr Rev 1995;16:163–7.
[33] Vayalumkal JV, Jadavji T. Children hospitalized with skin and soft tissue infections. Paediatr Drugs 2006;8:99–111.
[34] Hutcheson KA, Magbalon M. Periocular abscess and cellulitis from Pasteurella multocida in a healthy child. Am J Ophthal 1999;128:514–5.
[35] Velazquez AJ, Goldstein MH, Driebe WT. Preseptal cellulitis caused by Trichophyton (Ringworm). Cornea 2002;21:312–4.
[36] Rajalekshmi PS, Evans SL, Morton CE, et al. Ringworm causing childhood preseptal cellulitis. Ophthal Plast Reconstr Surg 2003;19:244–6.
[37] Jun BK, Shin JC, Woog JJ. Palpebral myiasis. Korean J Ophthalmol 1999;13:138–40.
[38] Caca I, Cakmak SS, Unlu K, et al. Cutaneous anthrax on eyelids. Jpn J Ophthalmol 2004;48: 268–71.
[39] Brannan PA, Kersten RC, Hudak DT, et al. Primary Nocardia brasiliensis of the eyelid. Am J Ophthalmol 2004;138:498–9.
[40] Raina UK, Jain S, Monga S, et al. Tubercular preseptal cellulitis in children—a presenting feature of underlying systemic tuberculosis. Ophthalmology 2004;111:291–6.
[41] Todd JK. Office laboratory diagnosis of skin and soft tissue infections. Pediatr Infect Dis J 1985;4:84–7.
[42] Smith TF, O'Day D, Wright PF. Clinical implication of preseptal (periorbital) cellulitis. Pediatrics 1978;62:1006–9.

[43] Thirumoorthi MB, Asmar BI, Dajani AS. Violaceous discoloration in pneumococcal cellulitis. Pediatrics 1978;62:492–3.
[44] Goldberg F, Berne AS, Oski FA. Differentiation of orbital cellulitis from preseptal cellulitis by computed tomography. Pediatrics 1978;62:1000–5.
[45] Barone SR, Aiuto LT. Periorbital and orbital cellulitius in *Haemophilus influenzae* vaccine era. J Pediatr Ophthalmol Strabismus 1997;34:293–6.
[46] Donahue SP, Schwartz G. Preseptal and orbital cellulitis in childhood—a changing microbiologic spectrum. Ophthalmology 1998;105:1902–6.
[47] Givner LB, Mason EO Jr, Barson WJ, et al. Pneumococcal facial cellulitis in children. Available at: http://www.pediatrics.org/cgi/content/full/106/5/e61. Accessed January 2007.
[48] Schwartz GR, Wright SW. Changing bacteriology of periorbital cellulitis. Ann Emerg Med 1996;28:617–20.
[49] Wald ER. Periorbital and orbital infections. Pediatr Rev 2004;25:312–20.
[50] Skedros DG, Haddad J Jr, Bluestone CD, et al. Subperiosteal orbital abscess in children: diagnosis, microbiology and management. Laryngoscope 1993;103:28–32.
[51] Nageswaran S, Woods CR, Benjamin DK, et al. Orbital cellulitis in children. Pediatr Infect Dis J 2006;25:695–9.
[52] Jain A, Rubin PAD. Orbital cellulitis in childen. Int Ophthalmol Clin 2001;41:71–86.
[53] Sobol SE, Marchand J, Tewfik TL, et al. Orbital complications of sinusitis in children. J Otolaryngol 2002;31:131–6.
[54] Eustis HS, Armstrong DC, Buncie JK, et al. Staging of orbital cellulitis in children: computerized tomography characteristics and treatment guidelines. J Pediatr Ophthalmol Strabismus 1986;23:246–51.
[55] Wong VYM, Duncan NO, Edwards MS. Medical management of orbital infection. Pediatr Infect Dis J 1994;13:1012–3.
[56] Pereira KD, Mitchell RB, Younis RT, et al. Management of medial subperiosteal abscess of the orbit in children—a five year experience. Int J Pediatr Otorhinolaryngol 1997;38:247–54.
[57] Deutsch E, Eilon A, Herron I, et al. Functional endoscopic sinus surgery of orbital subperiosteal abscess in children. Int J Pediatr Otorhinolaryngol 1996;34:181–90.
[58] Rubin SE, Rubin LG, Zito J, et al. Medical management of orbital subperiosteal abscess in children. J Pediatr Ophthalmol Strabismus 1989;26:21–7.
[59] Souliere CR Jr, Antoine GA, Martin M, et al. Selective non-surgical management of subperiosteal abscess of the orbit: computerized tomography and clinical course as indication for surgical drainage. Int J Pediatr Otorhinolaryngol 1990;19:109–19.
[60] Ferguson MP, McNab AA. Current treatment and outcome in orbital cellulitis. Aust N Z J Ophthalmol 1999;27:375–9.
[61] Starkey CR, Steele RW. Medical management of orbital cellulitis. Pediatr Infect Dis J 2001; 20:1002–5.
[62] Greenberg MF, Pollard ZF. Medical treatment of pediatric subperiosteal orbital abscess secondary to sinusitis. J AAPOS 1998;2:351–5.
[63] Harris GJ. Subperiosteal abscess of the orbit age as a factor in the bacteriology and response to treatment. Ophthalmology 1994;101:585–95.
[64] Harris GJ. Subperiosteal abscess of the orbit. Arch Ophthalmol 1983;101:753–4.

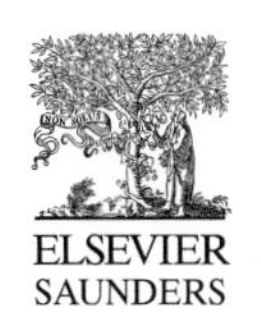

ELSEVIER
SAUNDERS

INFECTIOUS
DISEASE CLINICS
OF NORTH AMERICA

Infect Dis Clin N Am 21 (2007) 409–426

Diagnosis and Treatment of Acute Otitis Media: Evaluating the Evidence

John H. Powers, MD, FACP, FIDSA[a,b,c,*]

[a]*Scientific Applications International Corporation in support of the Collaborative Clinical Research Branch, National Institute of Allergy and Infectious Diseases, National Institutes of Health, USA*
[b]*George Washington University School of Medicine, Washington, DC, USA*
[c]*University of Maryland School of Medicine, Baltimore, MD, USA*

Acute otitis media (AOM) is inflammation of the middle ear that occurs primarily in children, presenting with a rapid onset of local and/or systemic symptoms. The issues surrounding the diagnosis and treatment of AOM are some of the most common and challenging for clinicians. AOM is diagnosed more than 5 million times per year in the United States [1]. Data compiled by the Centers for Disease Control and Prevention (CDC) from 1975 to 1990 showed that the disease is responsible for an estimated 24.5 million office visits per year [2]. Some data suggest that the incidence of the disease might be increasing, but challenges in the diagnosis of this disease make it difficult to interpret these analyses. For instance, the CDC data include International Classification of Disease(ICD-9) codes of suppurative otitis media, nonsuppurative otitis media, and unspecified otitis media. Many of these patients may not truly have AOM. What is clear, however, is over the 15-year span of the CDC evaluation, office visits for AOM increased 150%. Visits for boys under the age of 2 years rose from 32.0 to 111.3 visits per 100 persons per year. In girls in this age group, the increase was from 31.1 to 92.7 visits per 100 persons per year. An increase of lesser magnitude occurred in children between the ages of 2 and 5 years [2]. A diagnosis of AOM also is the most common reason for prescribing an antimicrobial agent to children and is one of the most common reasons overall for anyone in the United States to receive an antimicrobial agent [3,4]. It is estimated

The author has served as a consultant for Astra_Zeneca Cerexa, Forrest, Merck Methylgene, Theravance Wyeth, and Takeda.

* 6700B Rockledge Drive, Room 1123, Bethesda, MD 20892.
E-mail address: powersjohn@mail.nih.gov.

0891-5520/07/$ - see front matter
doi:10.1016/j.idc.2007.03.013 ***id.theclinics.com***

that the cost of AOM in the United States is approximately $3.8 billion per year, most of which comes from the cost of antimicrobial drugs [5,6].

Given the commonness of this condition, one would assume there should be an adequate evidence base for clinicians supporting the diagnosis and treatment of AOM. Unfortunately, the opposite seems to be true. A recent review by the Agency for Healthcare Research and Quality (AHRQ) called the present evidence base for AOM "woeful" and outlined the need for quality research in this area [7]. Of the six recommendations in the 2004 guidelines published by the American Academy of Pediatrics (AAP) and the American Academy of Family Physicians, only one, the assessment and treatment of ear pain with analgesics, was based on "strong recommendation." Review articles on the topic of AOM often reference other review articles. One wonders if this practice perpetuates beliefs and biases in the absence of new data on which to base new recommendations.

The reasons for the suboptimal evidence in this field are open to speculation. The possibilities include the general neglect of studies in pediatrics for years and clinicians' reluctance, once practice patterns (even those based on admittedly less than optimal evidence) become entrenched, to address questions that were inadequately answered by previous research. Unfortunately, these discussions sometimes revolve around misperceptions regarding the ethics of conducting trials, but it is not unethical to perform studies when the evidence is unclear. When a practice pattern becomes commonplace, clinicians sometimes ask for data that "prove" that the intervention is not effective. However, this mindset starts with the presumption that an invervention is effective and then attempts to prove it is not. This is near impossible, as clinical trials usually ask one question at a time, and one can always find a clinical situation that a given trial does not address. Therefore, clinical trials traditionally use proof by contradiction: they start with a null hypothesis that an intervention is not effective and gather evidence to determine if this hypothesis is unlikely to be true. It sometimes is unfortunate that treatment guidelines based on the evidence as it exists today become a blockade to performing future trials because the recommendations are termed "standard of care" in the guidelines. This mindset—that the answers have already been determined even when evidence is suboptimal—can stall future therapeutic advances forever. A final reason for the absence of substantial evidence may be the focus on organisms instead of patient outcomes. A mindset that the goal of administering an antimicrobial is merely to attempt to sterilize the middle ear cavity, and that clinical outcomes regarding how patients feel or function are "confounded," misrepresents the definition of confounding and provides little impetus for study of patient-related outcomes. Patients or their parents do not present to the office complaining that their *Streptococcus pneumoniae* hurts; the goal of antimicrobial therapy is to improve how patients feel, function, or survive. The effect on an organism by an antimicrobial is a mechanism of action, not an outcome.

A more important question is why clinicians should care about the evidence base in AOM. First, clinicians need to recognize the gaps in the evidence so they know when it is logical and ethical to deviate from treatment guidelines. The art of medicine comes in applying the data from groups of patients studied in clinical trials to individual patients, and clinicians must know these data to know when and when not to apply them. Second, it is in the best interest of patient care that clinicians continue to fill in gaps in their knowledge to ascertain whether they are doing their patients more good than harm. Hippocrates' dictum of "first, do no harm" still applies today. Evidence is needed to ascertain the balance of risks and benefits to patients. Discussions of use of antimicrobial agents often focus on their benefits, with little discussion of the harms. Even if antimicrobial agents prevent rare complications in AOM, a quantitative assessment of risks compared with benefits is still needed to determine if the number of children who experience serious adverse consequences of antimicrobial therapy is greater than those whose complications of the disease might be prevented by such therapy. Inappropriate use of antimicrobial agents can result in spread of resistance, so the use of drugs for self-resolving illnesses may negate the use of those same or related drugs for serious and life-threatening diseases. The population effects of inappropriate prescribing on resistance seems to move clinicians little when faced with a sick patient [8]. An issue of more immediate concern to clinicians, however, should be the unwarranted adverse effects of drugs directly experienced by patients who receive no benefit. Even if these adverse events are relatively uncommon, anaphylaxis, liver failure, and Stevens-Johnson syndrome are a high price to pay in children who do not have AOM or who do not benefit from antimicrobial agents. In addition, some studies point to the potential for long-term consequences related to the administration of antimicrobial agents. These studies show associations between receipt of antimicrobial agents and such adverse events as development of allergic diseases and loss of enamel on teeth [9–12]. These associations are not direct evidence of causality, and further evidence is needed to draw firm conclusions, but these studies are suggestive and remind us that prescribing of antimicrobial agents comes at a price. Third, an issue that receives little attention is that once clinicians prescribe an antimicrobial agent, they tend to discontinue the search for other causes of the patient's illness while "awaiting a response." Although there is much discussion about the consequences of delaying antimicrobial therapy with "watchful waiting" as a strategy for decreasing antimicrobial use, there is little discussion of the consequences of delaying the true diagnosis in children who received an inaccurate diagnosis of AOM. Finally, it is important to evaluate the evidence so that those interested in clinical research know where to focus future study.

With these considerations in mind, rather than discussing treatment options that are ably described elsewhere [13], this article outlines the issues with the evidence regarding diagnosis and treatment of AOM. There are four possible conclusions one may draw about any clinical research study: the results represent true findings, the results are the product of random error (chance), the results are the product of systemic biases, or the results are the product of confounding (that is, they reflect some factor[s] other than the intervention tested when there is a difference in the proportion of subjects between groups with that factor). One should attempt to rule out the last three forms of error to decide whether results are likely to represent true findings. This article discusses issues concerning the quality of the evidence and points out areas where further research is needed to help clinicians make more informed decisions.

Diagnosis

Definitions

Otitis media is inflammation of the middle ear. Clinicians need to differentiate AOM from other forms of middle ear inflammation. The syndrome of AOM is characterized by the rapid onset of local and/or systemic signs and symptoms accompanying middle ear inflammation as evidenced by the presence of middle ear effusion (MEE). On the other hand, otitis media with effusion, also called "glue ear" or serous otitis media, presents with serous or mucoid fluid in the middle ear cavity without acute symptoms of ear pain. Chronic suppurative otitis media is persistent inflammation of the middle ear cavity or mastoid air cells. This discussion concentrates on the syndrome of AOM.

Making an appropriate diagnosis of AOM is challenging. The criterion standard for bacterial AOM is the presence of signs and symptoms in association with a tympanocentesis to ascertain both the presence of MEE and the presence of bacteria. The presence of bacteria alone does not diagnose the disease, and it is unclear what investigators mean when they refer to "asymptomatic" AOM, because it is symptoms that bring the patient to the clinician's care. It seems logical that the patients who have bacterial otitis would be the most likely to benefit from antibacterial drugs. There is, however, surprisingly little evidence comparing various signs and symptoms against this criterion standard. Six studies have evaluated the diagnostic accuracy of various signs and symptoms of AOM [14–19]. Two of these studies compared signs and symptoms with tympanocentesis [16,18]. One performed evaluations for pathogens in MEE [18], and the other evaluated only for the presence of fluid [16]. The remaining four studies compared clinical signs and symptoms with clinical criteria rather than with a separate criterion standard. In none of the studies were assessors blinded, and many of the studies suffer from spectrum bias: that is, the characteristics of children enrolled (ie, those seen at specialty clinics) may not reflect the average child seen in clinical practice [20]. A more recent systematic review evaluated most of these studies and converted the analyses of their results into positive and negative likelihood ratios (LR)

[21]. The LR is the probability of a given test result among people who have a disease divided by the probability of that test result among people who do not have the disease. LRs are more useful than sensitivity, specificity, or positive and negative predictive values for several reasons: they are less likely to change with the prevalence of the disease; one can calculate LRs for several levels of the symptom/sign or test; one can combine the results of multiple diagnostic tests; and one can use them to calculate posttest probability for a disease. A positive test or presence of a finding in association with a positive LR greater than one increases the likelihood of the disease. A negative test or absence of a finding in association with a negative LR less than one decreases the likelihood of the disease.

Symptoms

The symptoms of AOM can include ear pain, ear tugging or rubbing, fever (which can be a symptom when described as "feverishness" or obtained by history or a sign when body temperature is measured directly), excessive crying, restless sleep, and/or poor appetite. In evaluating symptoms, the presence of ear pain had the highest positive LR across various studies, ranging from 3.0 (95% confidence interval [CI], 2.1–4.3) [19,21] to 7.3 (95% CI, 4.4–12.1) [14,21]. The absence of ear pain decreased the likelihood of disease somewhat with negative LRs of 0.6 (95% CI, 0.5–0.7) to 0.4 (95% CI, 0.4–0.5) [14,19,21]. Despite some opinion that fever is helpful in making the diagnosis, the presence or absence of fever is of variable utility. One study showed a positive LR of 2.6 (95% CI, 1.9–3.6) but two other studies showed fever did not contribute to the diagnosis, with positive LRs of 0.8 (95% CI, 0.6–1.0) and 0.9 (95% CI, 0.8–1.0). The absence of fever in ruling out the disease is also inconsistent, with negative LRs of 1.2 (95% CI, 1.0 CI, 1.5) and 1.4 (95% CI, 0.9–2.0) in two studies but 0.3 (95% CI, 0.2–0.5) in another [14,19,21]. Other findings, such as excessive crying (with a positive LR of 1.8 [95% CI, 1.4–2.3]), poor appetite (with an LR of 1.1 [95% CI, 0.8–1.4]), and restless sleep (with LR of 1.3 [95% CI, 1.1–1.6]) were less helpful. The one study that compared symptoms with a positive culture by tympanocentesis combined various symptoms into an overall symptom score, so it was not possible to evaluate the impact of individual symptoms on the diagnosis [18]. It is common teaching that ear rubbing or tugging is not helpful in making a diagnosis, but in one study it had a positive LR of 3.3 (95% CI, 2.1–5.1), and a negative LR of 0.7 (95% CI, 0.6–0.8) [19,21]. This finding is in contrast to an older study that found ear tugging of little utility, but this study did not specify the criteria used to define AOM [22].

Signs

The signs of AOM on ear examination can include changes in the position of the tympanic membrane (TM) (bulging), changes in TM color (redness), and alterations in TM mobility indicative of MEE as measured by pneumatic otoscopy or tympanometry. Two studies compared TM signs to results of tympanocentesis. One of the studies evaluated only the presence of MEE by tympanocentesis, not the presence of bacteria, so these data are not helpful in evaluating the usefulness of various signs in predicting a bacterial cause of AOM [16,18]. The interpretation of these trials also is hindered by verification bias, because the investigators selectively chose which patients would undergo tympanocentesis [23]. A recent study attempted to adjust the results of a previous study for verification bias [21]. This study found that TM bulging had a positive LR of 51 (95% CI, 36–73), TM cloudiness had an LR of 34 (95% CI, 28—42), and TM immobility was associated with a LR of 31 (95% CI, 27–37) when compared with the presence of MEE by tympanocentesis. Despite teaching that redness of the TM is not helpful, this study showed that distinct redness of the TM was associated with a LR of 8.4 (95% CI, 6.7–11.0). A slightly red TM was less helpful, with a LR of 1.4 (95% CI, 1.1–1.8). Normal color or normal mobility of the TM decreases the likelihood of AOM substantially, with negative LRs of 0.2 for both variables. Assuming baseline prevalence of true AOM of 20%, normal color or mobility of the TM decreases the probability of AOM to less than 5%. The independence of the signs of color, mobility, and position could not be assessed from these data. Another, more recent study comparing positive cultures from tympanocentesis with TM signs found no difference overall in a scoring system devised for that study that combined various TM abnormalities in patients who had positive viral/culture negative taps compared with those positive for bacteria. When evaluated alone, however, TM bulging was associated with the presence of bacteria in MEE. The positive predictive value of TM bulging in this study was 74%, with a negative predictive value of 45%. Thus more than 25% of patients who had bulging TMs did not have positive bacterial cultures of MEE, and more than half of children who do not have bulging TMs still have positive cultures [18].

Impact of lack of clarity of diagnosis

Given the lack of data on making a definitive diagnosis, it is not surprising that clinicians and clinical trials vary widely in their specific definitions of the disease. The lack of uniform criteria for diagnosis complicates clinical practice and makes it challenging to compare or pool the results of various trials. A study from 1981 showed a wide variety of definitions of the disease used in clinical studies. This study reviewed clinical trials in AOM published in six journals between 1955 and 1979 [24]. The study included 43 trials, among which 17 (40%) did not describe the criteria used by the investigators to define the disease. Of the 26 trials that did define the disease, investigators used 18 different sets of criteria. This article also contained a survey of 165 clinicians, who used 147 different criteria to define the illness in their practices. Eleven criteria were used by more than one respondent, and no single set was used by more than six respondents to the survey. The AHRQ group developed a definition of AOM based on group consensus that included three components: rapid onset of symptoms within 48 hours, the presence of middle ear effusion, and one or more of the signs and symptoms of otalgia, otorrhea, irritability, or fever [7]. This group evaluated 80 studies and found that none of the studies used all three components, 22.5% (18) used two criteria, and 42.5% (34) used one criterion. Twenty-eight (35%) of the studies used none of the components. Middle ear effusion was included most often, in 52.5% of the studies, followed by signs and symptoms of inflammation in 32.5%, and rapid onset in 2.5% of the studies. A more recent study of more current trials showed the situation has not improved. This study compared trials published between 1994 and 2005 to the definition of AOM proposed by the AAP to evaluate the consistency of diagnostic criteria [25]. The AAP definitions also had three components: (1) a history of acute onset of signs and symptoms (timing not defined); (2) the presence of middle ear effusion indicated by bulging, absent mobility, or air–fluid level behind the TM or otorrhea; and (3) signs and symptoms of middle ear inflammation as evidenced by erythema of the tympanic membrane or otalgia [13]. Note that various combinations of signs and symptoms proposed in this defintion are either poorly defined for purposes of clinical trials or predict AOM with differing or unknown frequency. The authors also compared their findings with another, similar definition that included bulging of the TM as evidence of inflammation [26]. The authors found that 20% of 88 studies used all three components of the AAP criteria.

The uncertainty in clinical trial results is reflected in the practice patterns of clinicians. The evidence suggests clinicians overdiagnose AOM, resulting in potentially unnecessary antimicrobial prescribing. One study suggested that clinicians expressed certainty in the diagnosis of AOM in 90% of cases, but 70% of those cases met the AHRQ criteria, with 29% of prescriptions deemed unnecessary [27]. In another study, clinicians prescribed antimicrobial agents in three of four cases when the odds of a correct diagnosis of AOM were less than 50%. One in four clinicians prescribed antimicrobial agents when the odds of AOM were less than 25%.

There seems to be substantial interobserver variability in evaluating TM signs. One study compared TM findings of pediatric residents with those of pediatric otolaryngologists and evaluated the kappa correlation between the two observer groups. A kappa correlation of 1 represents a perfect correlation, and zero indicates that the correlation is no greater than chance. The correlation between residents and attending physicians was 0.3, interpreted as "fair." Based on the data presented previously, TM bulging seems to be the most helpful sign in making a diagnosis of AOM. Bulging, however, seems to be in the eye of the beholder, because the investigators in this study found the poorest interobserver correlation in evaluating TM position, with a kappa coefficient of 0.16. The correlation of TM mobility between observer groups was 0.21 [28].

In summary, the presence of acute onset of less than 48 hours of ear pain in association with a bulging, cloudy, or distinctly red, immobile TM may provide the highest likelihood of selecting patients who have bacterial AOM, although data are incomplete. Even under these conditions, however, as many as 25% of patients may not have bacterial disease, and there is substantial interobserver variability in detecting these findings. Therefore, in clinical trials evaluating new therapies, where high specificity of diagnosis is critical, investigators should use tympanocentesis in all patients who enter clinical trials to assure they have the correct diagnosis of disease under study. Investigators can use the signs and symptoms noted previously to select the patients most likely to have bacterial disease to undergo tympanocentesis. Assuring patients have the disease is part of the definition of substantial evidence from adequate and well-controlled trials used by the US Food and Drug Administration (FDA) in evaluating new drugs [29]. Indeed, at an FDA Advisory Committee meeting in 2002, the majority of participants voted that AOM trials should include baseline tympanocentesis [28,30]. In addition, clinical trials are evaluating new interventions of unknown effectiveness, and one should not expose research subjects to the potential for harm when there is no potential for benefit in patients who do not have AOM or bacterial disease. Clinical trials are distinct from clinical practice, and the fact that clinicians often do not use tympanocentesis in clinical practice is a different consideration than in the setting of clinical trials. Perhaps the use of tympanocentesis in clinical practice should be readdressed also, given the lack of diagnostic accuracy of clinical criteria alone. In any case, the lack of ability in clinical practice to diagnose the disease specifically based on signs and symptoms alone points to an urgent need for rapid diagnostics to help evaluate which patients have an infection, which infections are bacterial, and the susceptibility patterns of those bacteria. Better diagnostics would help clinicians better select patients who might benefit from antimicrobial therapy while minimizing unwarranted adverse effects and deterring the emergence of resistance. This information could aid both in clinical practice and in clinical trials. Such tests probably will include some evaluation of host response in combination with microbiologic testing.

Treatment

There are several possible treatments for AOM, including antimicrobial therapy, analgesics, myringotomy, and tympanostomy tubes. This section concentrates on the use of antimicrobial agents to treat acute symptoms. Discussions of the effect of analgesics and prevention of future episodes by either prolonged antimicrobial therapy or vaccination are presented elsewhere [28,30–35].

Goals of antimicrobial therapy

The overall goal of administering therapy in AOM is to improve patients' health in terms of how they feel, function, or survive. The mortality rate in untreated AOM is very low, so one could not expect therapies in AOM to demonstrate a decrease in mortality. Suppurative complications in AOM also are low, about 0.12% in untreated cases [28,30,36]. There is little evidence that antimicrobial agents decrease the incidence of suppurative complications, other than the historical evaluation that complications such as mastoiditis are less common today than in years past. This historical assessment is confounded by other changes in medical care over time [37]. There also is an absence of evidence that treating AOM has long-term benefits in preventing hearing loss or learning deficits. Therefore, the most clinically relevant goal of treating AOM is cure of patient's symptoms. Previous analyses combining data from various studies show that the spontaneous rate of clinical resolution of symptoms in AOM is relatively high, with approximately 60% of children recovering within 24 hours and approximately 80% cured in 3 days [36]. These values are highly variable, however, given random variation from trial to trial, differing definitions of disease, and differing definitions and timing of outcomes. Therefore, there is no universally applicable "placebo rate" that investigators can use in designing clinical trials. Some have advocated measuring a surrogate end point of microbiologic outcomes in AOM clinical trials, but microbiologic assessments are not a direct measure of clinical benefit to patients. Because investigators rarely perform a second tympanocentesis in clinical trials, and clinicians do so even more rarely in their practice, this outcome is not routinely measurable. In addition, there seems to be a poor correlation between overall microbiologic outcomes and clinical outcomes, because symptoms resolve in two thirds of children who still have a pathogen in MEE on day 2 to 4 of therapy [38]. Therefore, assumptions about "presumed eradication" of pathogens used in previous clinical trials of AOM are not justifiable. A persistently positive culture may be associated with a more prolonged course of the disease, but this prolongation may result from inherent characteristics of the patient population rather than the effect of specific drugs [37]. Antimicrobial agents in AOM can decrease the burden of organisms in the middle ear, but this is a mechanism of action, not a goal of therapy. The questions of interest are whether lowering the burden of organisms results in faster cure for patients compared with no therapy or whether the host immune system cures the patient just as quickly with no treatment.

Benefits versus harm

The evaluation of the evidence of benefits and harms of potential therapies in AOM is complicated by various issues in the design and analysis of the clinical trials in this area. As noted previously, the definitions of AOM used in clinical trials vary widely, making comparisons and pooling of data difficult. In addition, the populations in placebo-controlled trials also vary, from patients who have routine otitis media to recurrent cases. It is not clear if the natural history of an individual episode of recurrent AOM differs from that of a single episode of AOM. There are no validated severity scores in AOM. In this setting,"severity" means baseline factors that may predict a more prolonged course or worse outcome of the disease. For instance, the Pneumonia Severity Index uses baseline factors in patients who have community-acquired pneumonia to attempt to predict 30-day all-cause mortality [39]. Unfortunately, investigators have not compared currently published "severity" instruments with the clinical course of the illness in AOM. Many of these scales contain fever as part of a severity index, but, as noted previously, fever is poorly associated with AOM. Some studies have claimed that higher fever at baseline may be associated with *Streptococcus pneumoniae* as the causative pathogen, but it is not clear if higher fever overall portends a worse outcome on average. Some of the trials in AOM were not blinded [40]. On average, unblinded trials exaggerate the size of treatment effect by about 19% [41]. Many clinical trials in AOM do not standardize concomitant medications such as analgesics that may act as confounders when assessing outcomes. The outcome measurements in many clinical trials of AOM also vary widely in both their definitions and their timing. Many of the clinical trials in AOM do not use a true intention-to-treat analysis, because they exclude patients from analysis based on postrandomization events, such as not taking a specified percentage of medication. This may affect the integrity of randomization, thereby creating the possibility of selection bias. Many of these trials also evaluate multiple end points at multiple time points with multiple subgroup analyses, all of which increase the chance of false-positive findings [42]. Finally, some of the trials contain little information on adverse events of the interventions against which to balance any potential benefits against potential harms.

Interpreting meta-analyses of clinical trials

Several authors have attempted to pool the results of various placebo-controlled trials in AOM in the form of meta-analyses. Various authors have published at least five systematic reviews or meta-analyses on the effect of antimicrobial agents in treating AOM [43–47]. These meta-analyses combine different studies in different ways, and therefore each presents different conclusions. At least two of these meta-analyses contain no information on adverse events. Meta-analyses pool data in an attempt to control for one type of error in trials, namely random error that may result from chance. The increased sample sizes in meta-analyses allow calculation of more precise results. Meta-analyses, however, do not control for other types of error in trials, namely bias and confounding. Increasing the sample size actually may increase the effects of bias and confounding on measured outcomes. For instance, two of the six trials included in a recent meta-analysis [47] were not blinded, because they were designed primarily to address parental acceptability of delayed initiation of antimicrobials [40,63]. The potential bias of unblinded trials is not decreased by the pooling of data. Various authors recognized and discussed issues with the evidence in individual trials in AOM, and these issues do not disappear when the results are pooled [48], even when data from individual patients in previous trials are analyzed [47]. These meta-analyses may not pool like with like [49]. Indeed, one study found that subsequent large, randomized, controlled trials failed to support the conclusions of previous meta-analyses in 35% of studies [50]. The more precise answer obtained by a meta-analysis may be more precisely wrong, and this possibility is of most concern when the trials included in the meta-analysis have known biases and confounders, as is the case with AOM studies. Meta-analyses can be useful in forming hypotheses for testing in future trials, but one should exercise care when forming definitive conclusions [51].

Placebo-controlled trials

Given the issues with pooling of trials in AOM, it may be more instructive to evaluate individual placebo-controlled trials. There is insufficient space here to discuss each trial in detail, but there are several main themes. Over an almost 40-year time span between 1968 and 2005, various authors have published 11 randomized trials comparing groups of subjects receiving various antimicrobial agents at various doses and durations with concurrent placebo groups in the treatment of AOM [52–62]. In addition, three other randomized trials (and one nonrandomized trial) evaluated immediately compared to delayed initiation of antimicrobials [40,63–65]. Investigators designed these four trials primarily to evaluate a management strategy, not specifically to address the question of the magnitude of the benefit of antimicrobials compared to placebos. The continued publication of placebo-controlled trials during this period provides evidence that uncertainty still exists in evaluating the treatment effect of antimicrobial agents. Five of these trials have been published since 2000, and two of them were published in 2005, showing that investigators can and are performing placebo-controlled trials in AOM. These trials compared penicillin, amoxicillin, amoxicillin-clavulanate, erythromycin, and sulfa drugs with placebo. No placebo-controlled trials have evaluated cephalosporins or fluoroquinolones. Most of the trials were in children who had routine otitis. In one trial, subjects had what the investigators defined as recurrent otitis [52]. One of the trials evaluated microbiologic outcomes only, and the other 10 evaluate clinical outcomes using various definitions and timing of end points. The timing of outcome evaluations in these trials varied from 2 to 56 days after initiation of study drugs. The placebo success rate in these trials varied from 66% to 93%, showing the variability in the natural history of the illness from trial to trial and the impact of differing enrollment and outcome definitions. Sample sizes ranged from 106 to more than 500 patients. Five of the 10 trials with clinical endpoints failed to provide evidence of a benefit of antimicrobial agents compared with placebo, demonstrating that the effect of antimicrobial agents is inconsistent from trial to trial. In the trials that did show an effect of antimicrobial agents, the point estimates of the difference between the antibiotics and placebo groups ranged from 2.1% to 16%, with 95% confidence intervals ranging from a lower bound of 0.6% to an upper bound of approximately 25%. This finding means the number of children needed to treat for one child to benefit may range from 4 to 166. The largest treatment effects were seen in the trials that were not blinded [40,58]. For instance, the primary end point in two trials was the evaluation of parental acceptability of withholding of antimicrobial agents for 3 days, which required parental knowledge of treatment assignment [40,64]. A secondary end point in one trial was the difference in effectiveness between amoxicillin and placebo in the watchful-waiting group compared with immediate use of antimicrobial agents, but this assessment obviously could not be blinded based on the primary purpose of the trial [40]. Trials for which there were multiple comparisons at multiple time points and those that used vague end points (eg, undefined scoring systems) were more likely to show larger effects [60]. The assessments that children under the age of 2 years may be more likely to benefit from antimicrobial agents is based on subgroup analyses from the these clinical trials. Subgroup analyses can form hypotheses for future trials, but it is challenging to form firm conclusions based on them, given the increased probability of false-positive findings [66].

The reporting of the potential harms of therapy in many of the placebo-controlled trials generally has been incomplete. An adequate evaluation of the harms of therapy is needed to assess the balance of risks and benefits. One systematic review of 689 children aged 6 months to 15 years found that antimicrobial agents increased the risk of vomiting, diarrhea, and rashes by 7% [44]. This finding translates into one child with an adverse events for every 17 children treated. Given the variability in the assessment of benefits from placebo-controlled trials, it is unclear how to compare this number with the number of children needed to treat to benefit. In addition, this assessment will differ for different antimicrobial agents, given their differing adverse-event profiles.

The lack of validity of noninferiority trials

The uncertainty in the evidence from placebo-controlled trials has raised another issue related to the evaluation of new antimicrobial agents in AOM. These trials compare a new antimicrobial agent with an older antimicrobial agent with the goal of ruling out a margin of inferiority of the new drug compared with the old drug. These noninferiority trials are not designed to show that two drugs are "equivalent" or "as good as each other" but only to show how much less effective a new drug might be than an old drug [66]. The efficacy of all cephalosporins and fluoroquinolones for AOM has been studied in the setting of noninferiority trials. It seems logical that one could not allow the new drug to be more inferior to the old drug by an amount that is larger than the benefit of the old drug compared with placebo. For instance, if an old drug is reliably and reproducibly shown to be 2% more effective than placebo, a new drug that is as much as 10% less effective than the old drug may be as much as 8% less effective than placebo. Most recent noninferiority trials in AOM are designed to rule out margins of inferiority of 10% to 15% for new drugs compared with an old drug. The analysis of previous placebo-controlled trials shows that antimicrobial agents are not reliably and reproducibly 10% to 15% more effective than placebo from trial to trial. Therefore, a trial designed to show that a new drug may be as much as 10% to 15% worse than an older drug may not ensure that the new drug is more effective than a placebo. The issues with noninferiority trials are not just about statistics, which addresses only the issue of random error. If one changes the conditions of the trial (eg, by changing the definition of the disease or the definition or timing of outcomes) the constancy of the effect of the control drug compared to the placebo is not certain in the current trial. Therefore, it will not be clear whether either the old drug or the new drug is more effective than placebo under the conditions of that trial. Trials that do not ensure that subjects enrolled actually have bacterial otitis but instead enroll children with self-resolving viral upper respiratory tract illnesses will be more likely to show similarity of two drugs but not ensure that either drug is effective in bacterial disease in the setting of that trial. For this reason, Pocock [67] points out that previous approval by a regulatory agency or widely held beliefs that a drug is effective does not necessarily mean that a drug can be used as a control drug in a noninferiority trial. The FDA has approved 19 drugs for AOM, all based on the use of noninferiority trials. The problem with serial testing of drugs in noninferiority trials is exemplified by recent studies in recurrent otitis. Appelman [52] studied amoxicillin-clavulanate in a placebo-controlled trial in children who had recurrent otitis. This trial had many of the problems described previously, and it did not provide evidence of a benefit of the drug compared with placebo. The FDA, however, approved high-dose amoxicillin-clavulanate in recurrent otitis based on one noncomparative trial and another trial comparing high-dose and standard-dose amoxicillin-clavulanate that did not show superiority of the high dose to the lower dose [68]. Because the benefit of amoxicillin clavulanate compared with placebo was not clear, the benefit of the higher dose also is unclear. The potential for a slippery slope becomes apparent when one sees that investigators subsequently compared gatifloxacin to amoxicillin-clavulanate in children who had recurrent otitis in a noninferiority trial [69]. The benefit of gatifloxacin compared to a placebo is unclear, because it is based on a series of previous trials in which the benefit of the control drug was uncertain.

Need for placebo-controlled trials

It has become clear that noninferiority trials do not provide evidence that a new drug is any more effective than a placebo in AOM, and investigators should perform future trials as placebo-controlled trials. It is not unethical to perform placebo-controlled trials when the effect of the control drug is unclear, as stated in the note to paragraph 29 in the Declaration of Helsinki [70]. International guidance on study design outlines these issues in detail [71,72]. Investigators can perform trials with an early escape for patients who are not well at 72 hours. Several recent trials in watchful waiting have used this design of withholding antimicrobial agents for only a few days, but they were not designed primarily to address the question of treatment benefit, and these trials were not blinded [40,70–73]. In addition, the lack of clarity regarding the effect of antimicrobial agents compared with placebo also raises issues about the clinical impact of in vitro resistance on clinical outcomes in AOM. If the benefit of antimicrobial agents compared with placebo in disease caused by susceptible pathogens is unclear, then the impact of in vitro resistance on clinical outcomes with "resistant" pathogens also is unclear. None of the newer antimicrobial agents has demonstrated superiority to older drugs despite differences in activity in vitro [7]. If older drugs are hypothesized to be no longer effective in treating disease because of resistant pathogens, it makes little sense to design trials to show how much inferior a new drug may be to a drug that is no longer effective. The AAP guidelines rightly point out that the recommendations as to which antimicrobial to choose and at which dose are based on pharmacokinetic principles and expert opinion, not data from clinical trials [13].

Summary

Research is an iterative process. With more knowledge, more new questions become apparent. Expert consensus has deemed that the potential benefit of antimicrobial therapy in AOM seems to outweigh the risks in selected situations in clinical practice. In other situations watchful waiting is appropriate. The evidence on which these assessments are based is less than optimal, however, and better evidence is needed for the basis of future treatment recommendations. Investigators can use placebo-controlled superiority trials or trials comparing a new drug with an older drug and with placebo to determine accurately the effect of new drugs and to allow a better assessment of risks to benefits. Future research in defining severity scales that would allow enrollment of more homogenous patients in trials and might allow more accurate prescribing would be extremely helpful. The development of rapid diagnostics to aid in the diagnosis of AOM would revolutionize both clinical practice and trials. Finally, the use of novel end points in superiority trials, such as time to resolution of symptoms using validated patient-reported outcome instruments, would allow more accurate assessments of outcomes and might yield valuable information regarding duration of therapy.

References

[1] Hendley JO. Clinical practice. Otitis media. N Engl J Med 2002;347:1169–74.
[2] Anderson JR, Madans JH, Feldman JJ, et al. Vital and health statistics: advance data from vital and health statistics numbers 211-220. Centers for Disease Control and Prevention 1995; Available at: http://www.cdc.gov/nchs/data/series/sr_16/sr16_022.pdf. Accessed May 16, 2007.
[3] Froom J, Culpepper L, Jacobs M, et al. Antimicrobials for acute otitis media? A review from the International Primary Care Network. BMJ 1997;315:98–102.
[4] McCaig LF, Besser RE, Hughes JM. Trends in antimicrobial prescribing rates for children and adolescents. JAMA 2002;287:3096–102.
[5] Boccazzi A, Careddu P. Acute otitis media in pediatrics: are there rational issues for empiric therapy? Pediatr Infect Dis J 1997;16:S65–9.
[6] Gates GA. Cost-effectiveness considerations in otitis media treatment. Otolaryngol Head Neck Surg 1996;114:525–30.
[7] Chan LS, Takata GS, Shekelle P, et al. Evidence assessment of management of acute otitis media: II. Research gaps and priorities for future research. Pediatrics 2001;108:248–54.
[8] Metlay JP, Shea JA, Crossette LB, et al. Tensions in antibiotic prescribing: pitting social concerns against the interests of individual patients. J Gen Intern Med 2002;17:87–94.
[9] Cohet C, Cheng S, MacDonald C, et al. Infections, medication use, and the prevalence of symptoms of asthma, rhinitis, and eczema in childhood. J Epidemiol Community Health 2004;58:852–7.
[10] Hong L, Levy SM, Warren JJ, et al. Association of amoxicillin use during early childhood with developmental tooth enamel defects. Arch Pediatr Adolesc Med 2005;159:943–8.
[11] Noverr MC, Noggle RM, Toews GB, et al. Role of antibiotics and fungal microbiota in driving pulmonary allergic responses. Infect Immun 2004;72:4996–5003.
[12] Wickens K, Pearce N, Crane J, et al. Antibiotic use in early childhood and the development of asthma. Clin Exp Allergy 1999;29:766–71.
[13] American Academy of Pediatrics Subcommittee on Management of Acute Otitis Media. Diagnosis and management of acute otitis media. Pediatrics 2004;113:1451–65.
[14] Heikkinen T, Ruuskanen O. Signs and symptoms predicting acute otitis media. Arch Pediatr Adolesc Med 1995;149:26–9.
[15] Ingvarsson L. Acute otalgia in children—findings and diagnosis. Acta Paediatr Scand 1982; 71:705–10.
[16] Karma PH, Penttila MA, Sipila MM, et al. Otoscopic diagnosis of middle ear effusion in acute and non-acute otitis media. I. The value of different otoscopic findings. Int J Pediatr Otorhinolaryngol 1989;17:37–49.
[17] Kontiokari T, Koivunen P, Niemela M, et al. Symptoms of acute otitis media. Pediatr Infect Dis J 1998;17:676–9.
[18] McCormick DP, Lim-Melia E, Saeed K, et al. Otitis media: can clinical findings predict bacterial or viral etiology? Pediatr Infect Dis J 2000;19:256–8.
[19] Niemela M, Uhari M, Jounio-Ervasti K, et al. Lack of specific symptomatology in children with acute otitis media. Pediatr Infect Dis J 1994;13:765–8.
[20] Sackett DL. Bias in analytic research. J Chronic Dis 1979;32:51–63.
[21] Rothman R, Owens T, Simel DL. Does this child have acute otitis media? JAMA 2003;290: 1633–40.
[22] Baker SG, Kramer BS. A perfect correlate does not a surrogate make. BMC Med Res Methodol 2003;3:16.
[23] Bates AS, Margolis PA, Evans AT. Verification bias in pediatric studies evaluating diagnostic tests. J Pediatr 1993;122:585–90.
[24] Hayden GF. Acute suppurative otitis media in children. Diversity of clinical diagnostic criteria. Clin Pediatr (Phila) 1981;20:99–104.
[25] Chandler SM, Garcia SM, McCormick DP. Consistency of diagnostic criteria for acute otitis media: a review of the recent literature. Clin Pediatr (Phila) 2007;46:99–108.

[26] Hoberman A, Marchant CD, Kaplan SL, et al. Treatment of acute otitis media consensus recommendations. Clin Pediatr (Phila) 2002;41:373–90.
[27] Rosenfeld RM. Diagnostic certainty for acute otitis media. Int J Pediatr Otorhinolaryngol 2002;64:89–95.
[28] Steinbach WJ, Sectish TC, Benjamin DK Jr, et al. Pediatric residents' clinical diagnostic accuracy of otitis media. Pediatrics 2002;109:993–8.
[29] U.S.Government Printing Office. U.S. Code of Federal Regulations, Title 21, Part 314.126. Available at: http://a257.g.akamaitech.net/7/257/2422/10apr20061500/edocket.access.gpo.gov/cfr_2006/aprqtr/21cfr314.126.htm. Accessed May 16, 2007.
[30] US Food and Drug Administration. Transcripts of the Anti-infective Drugs Advisory Committee: clinical trial design in studies of acute bacterial otitis media. Available at: http://www.fda.gov/ohrms/dockets/ac/02/transcripts/3875T2.PDF. Accessed July 11, 2002.
[31] Roark R, Berman S. Continuous twice daily or once daily amoxicillin prophylaxis compared with placebo for children with recurrent acute otitis media. Pediatr Infect Dis J 1997;16: 376–81.
[32] Straetemans M, Sanders EA, Veenhoven RH, et al. Pneumococcal vaccines for preventing otitis media. Cochrane Database Syst Rev 2004;1:CD001480.
[33] Teele DW, Klein JO, Word BM, et al. Antimicrobial prophylaxis for infants at risk for recurrent acute otitis media. Vaccine 2000;19(Suppl 1):S140–3.
[34] Williams RL, Chalmers TC, Stange KC, et al. Use of antibiotics in preventing recurrent acute otitis media and in treating otitis media with effusion. A meta-analytic attempt to resolve the brouhaha. JAMA 1993;270:1344–51.
[35] Bertin L, Pons G, d'Athis P, et al. A randomized, double-blind, multicentre controlled trial of ibuprofen versus acetaminophen and placebo for symptoms of acute otitis media in children. Fundam Clin Pharmacol 1996;10:387–92.
[36] Rosenfeld RM, Kay D. Natural history of untreated otitis media. Laryngoscope 2003;113: 1645–57.
[37] Powers JH. Microbiologic surrogate end points in clinical trials of infectious diseases: example of acute otitis media trials. Pharmacotherapy 2005;25:109S–23S.
[38] Johann-Liang R, Zalkikar J, Powers JH. Correlation between bacteriologic and clinical endpoints in trials of acute otitis media. Pediatr Infect Dis J 2003;22:936–7.
[39] Fine MJ, Auble TE, Yealy DM, et al. A prediction rule to identify low-risk patients with community-acquired pneumonia. N Engl J Med 1997;336:243–50.
[40] McCormick DP, Chonmaitree T, Pittman C, et al. Nonsevere acute otitis media: a clinical trial comparing outcomes of watchful waiting versus immediate antibiotic treatment. Pediatrics 2005;115:1455–65.
[41] Juni P, Altman DG, Egger M. Systematic reviews in health care: assessing the quality of controlled clinical trials. BMJ 2001;323:42–6.
[42] Bender R, Lange S. Adjusting for multiple testing—when and how? J Clin Epidemiol 2001; 54:343–9.
[43] Damoiseaux RA, van Balen FA, Hoes AW, et al. Antibiotic treatment of acute otitis media in children under two years of age: evidence based? Br J Gen Pract 1998;48:1861–4.
[44] Delmar MC, Glasziou P, Hayem M. Are antibiotics indicated as initial treatment for children with acute otitis media? A meta-analysis. BMJ 1997;314:1526–9.
[45] Marcy M, Takata G, Chan LS, et al. Management of acute otitis media. Evid Rep Technol Assess (Summ) 2000;15:1–4.
[46] Rosenfeld RM, Vertrees JE, Carr J, et al. Clinical efficacy of antimicrobial drugs for acute otitis media: metaanalysis of 5400 children from thirty-three randomized trials. J Pediatr 1994;124:355–67.
[47] Rovers MM, Glasziou P, Appelman CL, et al. Antibiotics for acute otitis media: a meta-analysis with individual patient data. Lancet 2006;368:1429–35.
[48] Wald ER. Acute otitis media: more trouble with the evidence. Pediatr Infect Dis J 2003;22: 103–4.

[49] Bailar JC III. The promise and problems of meta-analysis. N Engl J Med 1997;337:559–61.
[50] LeLorier J, Gregoire G, Benhaddad A, et al. Discrepancies between meta-analyses and subsequent large randomized, controlled trials. N Engl J Med 1997;337:536–42.
[51] Anello C, Fleiss JL. Exploratory or analytic meta-analysis: should we distinguish between them? J Clin Epidemiol 1995;48:109–16.
[52] Appelman CL, Claessen JQ, Touw-Otten FW, et al. Co-amoxiclav in recurrent acute otitis media: placebo controlled study. BMJ 1991;303:1450–2.
[53] Burke P, Bain J, Robinson D, et al. Acute red ear in children: controlled trial of non-antibiotic treatment in general practice. BMJ 1991;303:558–62.
[54] Damoiseaux RA, van Balen FA, Hoes AW, et al. Primary care based randomised, double blind trial of amoxicillin versus placebo for acute otitis media in children aged under 2 years. BMJ 2000;320:350–4.
[55] Halsted C, Lepow ML, Balassanian N, et al. Otitis media. Clinical observations, microbiology, and evaluation of therapy. Am J Dis Child 1968;115:542–51.
[56] Howie VM, Ploussard JH. Efficacy of fixed combination antibiotics versus separate components in otitis media. Effectiveness of erythromycin estrolate, triple sulfonamide, ampicillin, erythromycin estolate- triple sulfonamide, and placebo in 280 patients with acute otitis media under two and one-half years of age. Clin Pediatr (Phila) 1972;11: 205–14.
[57] Kaleida PH, Casselbrant ML, Rockette HE, et al. Amoxicillin or myringotomy or both for acute otitis media: results of a randomized clinical trial. Pediatrics 1991;87:466–74.
[58] Laxdal OE, Merida J, Jones RH. Treatment of acute otitis media: a controlled study of 142 children. Can Med Assoc J 1970;102:263–8.
[59] LeSaux SN, Gaboury I, Baird M, et al. A randomized, double-blind, placebo-controlled noninferiority trial of amoxicillin for clinically diagnosed acute otitis media in children 6 months to 5 years of age. CMAJ 2005;172:335–41.
[60] Mygind N, Meistrup-Larsen KI, Thomsen J, et al. Penicillin in acute otitis media: a double-blind placebo-controlled trial. Clin Otolaryngol Allied Sci 1981;6:5–13.
[61] Thalin A, Densert O, Larsson A, Is penicillin necessary in the treatment of acute otitis media? Proceedings of the international conference on acute and secretory otitis media Part 1, 441–446. 1986.
[62] van Buchem FL, Dunk JH, van't Hof MA. Therapy of acute otitis media: myringotomy, antibiotics, or neither? A double-blind study in children. Lancet 1981;2:883–7.
[63] Little P, Gould G, Williamson I, et al. Pragmatic randomised controlled trial of two prescribing strategies for childhood otitis media. BMJ 2001;322:336–42.
[64] Siegel RM, Kiely M, Bien JP, et al. Treatment of otitis media with observation and safety-net antibiotic prescription. Pediatrics 2003;112:527–31.
[65] Cates C. An evidence based approach to reducing antibiotic prescribing use in children with acute otitis media: controlled before and after study. BMJ 1999;318:715–6.
[66] Powers JH. Interpreting the results of clinical trials on antimicrobial agents. In: Mandell GL, Bennett JE, Dolin R, editors. Principles and practice of infectious diseases. 6th edition. Philadelphia: Elsevier Churchill Livingstone; 2005. p. 619–28.
[67] Pocock SJ. The pros and cons of noninferiority trials. Fundam Clin Pharmacol 2003;17: 483–90.
[68] Augmentin ES-600 prescription drug labeling. In: Physicians desk reference. Monvale (NJ): Thomson Scientific; 2007.
[69] Saez-Llorens X, Rodriguez A, Arguedas A, et al. Randomized, investigator-blinded, multicenter study of gatifloxacin versus amoxicillin/clavulanate treatment of recurrent and nonresponsive otitis media in children. Pediatr Infect Dis J 2005;24:293–300.
[70] World Medical Association. Declaration of Helsinki. Available at: http://www.wma.net/e/policy/b3.htm. Accessed May 16, 2007.
[71] International Conference on Harmonisation. Choice of control group and related issues in clinical trials (ICH E-10). 2006.

[72] International Conference on Harmonisation. Statistical principles for clinical trials (ICH E-9). Available at: http://www.ich.org/MediaServer.jser?@_ID=485&@_MODE=GLB. 2006. Accessed May 16, 2007.
[73] Siegel RM, Bien J, Lichtenstein P, et al. A safety-net antibiotic prescription for otitis media: the effects of a PBRN study on patients and practitioners. Clin Pediatr (Phila) 2006;45: 518–24.

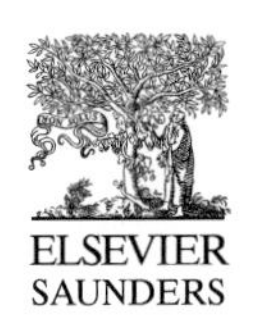

ELSEVIER
SAUNDERS

INFECTIOUS DISEASE CLINICS OF NORTH AMERICA

Infect Dis Clin N Am 21 (2007) 427–448

Acute and Chronic Bacterial Sinusitis

Itzhak Brook, MD, MSc

Department of Pediatrics and Medicine, Georgetown University School of Medicine, 4431 Albemarle St. NW, Washington, DC 20016, USA

Sinusitis is defined as inflammation of the mucous membrane lining the paranasal sinuses. Sinusitis can be classified chronologically into five categories [1]:

Acute sinusitis: a new infection that may last up to 4 weeks and can be subdivided symptomatically into severe and nonsevere
Recurrent acute sinusitis: four or more separate episodes of acute sinusitis that occur within 1 year
Subacute sinusitis: an infection that lasts between 4 to 12 weeks, representing a transition between acute and chronic infection
Chronic sinusitis: signs and symptoms that last for more than 12 weeks
Acute exacerbation of chronic sinusitis: signs and symptoms of chronic sinusitis exacerbate but return to baseline after treatment

In addition to chronicity of infection, sinusitis also can be categorized by mode of transmission and underlying conditions. These classifications include nosocomial sinusitis, sinusitis in severely immunocompromised hosts, and sinusitis of odontogenic origin.

Anatomic considerations and pathogenesis

The paranasal sinuses (maxillary, ethmoid, frontal, and sphenoid) comprise four symmetrical air-filled spaces lined by pseudostratified, ciliated, columnar epithelium. They are interconnected through small tubular openings, the sinus ostia, which drain into various regions of the nasal cavity (Fig. 1). The frontal, anterior ethmoid, and maxillary sinuses open into the middle meatus, whereas the posterior ethmoid and sphenoid sinuses open into the superior meatus. The osteomeatal complex (OMC) is an important anatomic site that represents the confluence of the drainage areas of the

E-mail address: ib6@georgetown.edu

doi:10.1016/j.idc.2007.02.001

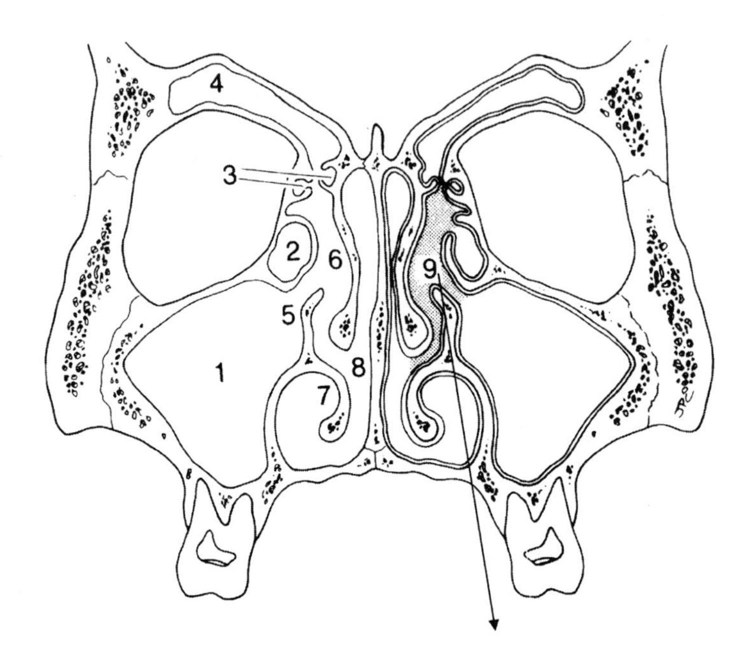

1. **Maxillary sinus**
2. **Ethmoidal bulla**
3. **Ethmoidal cells**
4. **Frontal sinus**
5. **Uncinate process**
6. **Middle turbinate**
7. **Inferior turbinate**
8. **Nasal septum**
9. **Osteomeatal complex**

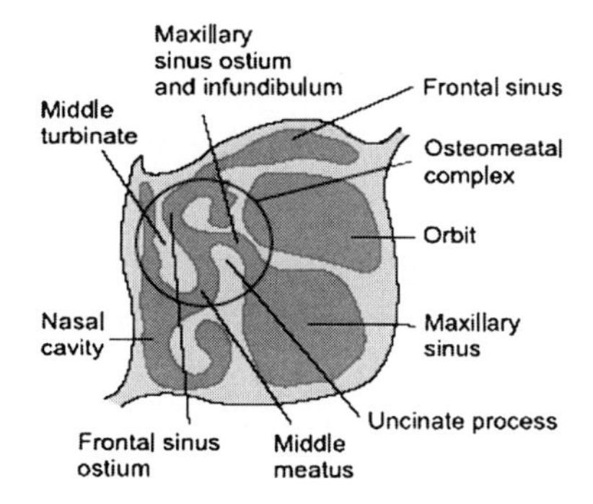

Osteomeatal Complex

Fig. 1. Coronal view of the paranasal sinuses and the osteomeatal complex. (*From* Wald ER. Chronic sinusitis in children. J Pediatr 1995;127:341; with permission)

frontal, ethmoid, and maxillary sinuses (see Fig. 1). It is bound by the middle turbinate medially, the basal lamella posteriorly and superiorly, and the lamina papyracea laterally. It is open for drainage anteriorly and inferiorly. Blockage or inflammation at the OMC is responsible for the development of bacterial sinusitis, because the obstruction interferes with effective mucociliary clearance [2]. Because the mucous membranes lining the nasal chambers and the sinuses are continuous through the natural ostium and are histologically alike, any upper respiratory infection commonly results in an inflammatory sinusitis. Sinus infection, however, usually does not persist after the nasal infection has subsided unless there is continued blockage at the OMC. At this stage, the sealed-off sinus fails to drain freely and is prone to secondary bacterial infection.

The sinuses develop gradually throughout childhood and reach full development during adolescence. Because the infant is born with mainly the maxillary and ethmoid sinuses present, the frontal sinuses rarely become infected before 6 years of age. Occlusion of the sinus ostium is the major predisposing factor causing suppurative infection and most often is the result of a viral or other upper respiratory infection, a common event in early childhood. Other important contributory factors are congenital and genetic factors [3] and acquired immune deficiencies [4,5]. Mechanical obstruction resulting in sinusitis can be related to various causative factors such as septal dislocation resulting from birth trauma, unilateral choanal atresia, foreign bodies placed in the nose, or fractures of the nose following trauma. Up to 30% of patients who have cystic fibrosis may have polyps complicating the already abnormal sinus secretions that predispose them to sinusitis [6]. Allergy, especially asthma, is an important predisposing factor in sinusitis [7]. Cyanotic congenital heart disease frequently is complicated by sinusitis. Dental infections also are a source of sinusitis [8].

Organisms introduced into the sinuses that eventually cause sinusitis originate in the nasal cavity. The normal flora at that site comprises certain bacterial species, which include *Staphylococcus aureus*, *Staphylococcus epidermidis*, alpha- and gamma-streptococci, *Propionibacterium acnes*, and facultative diphtheroids [9–12]. Potential sinus pathogens have been isolated from the healthy nasal cavity, but relatively rarely.

Dynamics of the upper respiratory flora

The pattern of many upper respiratory infections, including sinusitis, evolves through several phases (Fig. 2). The early phase is often a viral infection (mostly rhinovirus, adenovirus, influenza, and parainfluenza viruses) that generally lasts up to 10 days. Complete recovery occurs in 99% of individuals [13]. In a small number of patients, a secondary acute bacterial infection may develop, generally caused by aerobic bacteria (ie, *Streptococcus pneumoniae*, *Haemophilus influenzae*, and *Moraxella catarrhalis*). If resolution does not take place, anaerobic bacteria from the oropharyngeal flora become predominant over time. The mechanism whereby viruses predispose to sinusitis may involve viral–bacterial synergy, induction of local inflammation that blocks the sinus ostia, increase of bacterial attachment to the epithelial cells, and disruption of the local immune defense. Conditions that favor the growth of anaerobic bacteria include reduction in oxygen tension and an increase in acidity within the sinus. These conditions are caused by the persistent edema and swelling, which reduce blood supply, and by the consumption of oxygen by the aerobic bacteria [14]. Another explanation for the slower emergence of

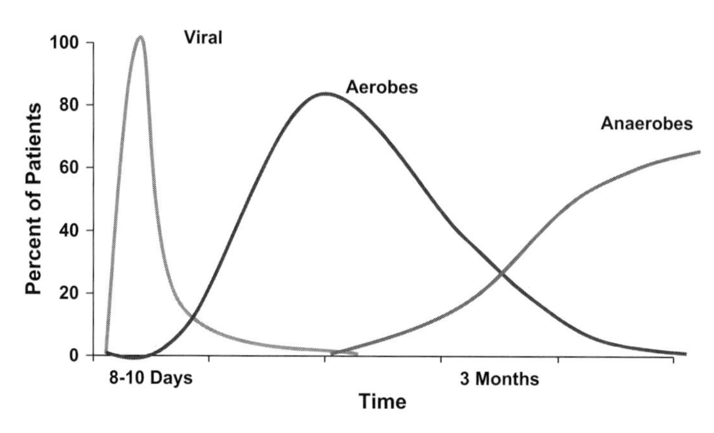

Fig. 2. The chronology of viral and bacterial causes of sinusitis.

anaerobes as pathogens is that the expression of some of their virulence factors (eg, as a capsule) is slow [15]. Some anaerobic and aerobic bacteria that are part of the normal oropharyngeal flora can possess in vitro interference capability with the growth of sinus pathogens. Higher numbers of interfering organisms were found in the nasopharynx of patients who were not prone to sinusitis than in those who were sinusitis prone [16].

Microbiology of acute and chronic sinusitis

Acute bacterial sinusitis

The most common bacteria recovered from pediatric and adult patients who have community-acquired, acute purulent sinusitis, using sinus aspiration by puncture or surgery, are shown in Table 1. These include *S pneumoniae, H influenzae, M catarrhalis,* group A beta-hemolytic streptococci, and *S aureus* [17–22]. Following routine vaccination of children in the United States with the seven-valent pneumococcal vaccine in 2000, the rate of *S pneumoniae* declined and that of *H influenzae* increased [23]. *S aureus* is a common pathogen in sphenoid sinusitis [24]; the other organisms are common in other sinuses.

The infection is polymicrobial in about one third of the cases. Enteric bacteria are recovered less commonly, and anaerobes are recovered from only a few cases of acute sinusitis. Appropriate methods for their recovery were rarely used in most studies of acute sinusitis, however. Anaerobic bacteria account for about 8% of isolates and are recovered more commonly from acute sinusitis associated with odontogenic origin, mostly as an extension of the infection from the roots of the premolar or molar teeth [8,25].

Pseudomonas aeruginosa and other gram-negative rods are common in sinusitis of nosocomial origin (especially in patients who have nasal tubes or catheters), the immunocompromised, and patients who HIV infection

Table 1
Microbiology of acute and chronic sinusitis

Bacteria	Maxillary[a]		Ethmoid[a]		Frontal[a]		Sphenoid[a]	
	Acute (N = not stated)	Chronic (N = 66)	Acute (N = 26)	Chronic (N = 17)	Acute (N = 15)	Chronic (N = 13)	Acute (N = 16)	Chronic (N = 7)
Aerobes								
S aureus	4	14	15	24	—	15	56	14
S pyogenes	2	8	8	6	3	—	6	—
S pneumoniae	31	6	35	6	33	—	6	—
H influenzae	21	5	27	6	40	15	12	14
M catarrhalis	8	6	8	—	20	—	—	—
Enterobacteriaceae	7	6	—	47	—	8	—	28
P aeruginosa	2	3	—	6	—	8	6	14
Anaerobes								
Peptostreptococcus	2	56	15	59	3	38	19	57
P acnes	—	29	12	18	3	8	12	29
Fusobacterium	2	17	4	47	3	31	6	54
Prevotella and *Porphyromonas*	2	47	8	82	3	62	6	86
B fragilis	—	6	—	—	—	15	—	—

[a] Because some patients had multiple isolates from the same specimen, the sum of percentages in each column exceeds 100%.

Data from Refs. [18–22,32].

or cystic fibrosis [26]. Anaerobic bacteria also can be recovered in these patients, however.

Chronic bacterial sinusitis

Although the etiology of the inflammation associated with chronic sinusitis is uncertain, bacteria are believed to play a major role in most cases [27,28]. Studies have described significant differences in the microbial pathogens present in chronic as compared with acute sinusitis. The usual pathogens in acute sinusitis (eg, *S pneumoniae*, *H influenzae*, *M catarrhalis*) are found with lower frequency [17–21,29–31]. *S aureus*, *S epidermidis*, and anaerobic gram-negative bacilli (AGNB) predominate in chronic sinusitis (see Table 1) [32]. The pathogenicity of some of the low-virulence organisms, such *S epidermidis*, a colonizer of the nasal cavity, is questionable [33,34]. Polymicrobial infection is common and may be synergistic in nature [15].

Gram-negative enteric rods also were reported in recent studies [35,36]. These include *P aeruginosa*, *Klebsiella pneumoniae*, *Proteus mirabilis*, *Enterobacter* spp, and *Escherichia coli*. Because these organisms are rarely found in cultures of the middle meatus obtained from normal individuals, their isolation from these symptomatic patients suggests a pathogenic role. Their presence also could result from selection pressure after administration of antimicrobial therapy. Nadel and colleagues [35] recovered gram-negative rods more commonly in patients who had previous surgery or those who had sinus irrigation. *P aeruginosa* also was more common in patients who received systemic steroids. Other studies have also noted this shift toward gram-negative organisms in patients who have been treated extensively and repeatedly [36–38]. The bacterial flora includes *Pseudomonas* spp, *Enterobacter* spp, methicillin-resistant *S aureus*, *H influenzae*, and *M catarrhalis*.

Role of anaerobes in chronic sinusitis

Numerous studies have examined the bacterial pathogens associated with chronic sinusitis. Most of these studies, however, did not use methods that are adequate for the recovery of anaerobic bacteria. That anaerobes play a role in chronic sinusitis is supported by the induction of chronic sinusitis in a rabbit by intrasinus inoculation of *Bacteroides fragilis* [39] and by the rapid production of serum IgG antibodies against this organism in the infected animals [40]. The pathogenic role of these organisms is supported also by the detection of IgG antibodies to two anaerobic organisms (*Fusobacterium nucleatum* and *Prevotella intermedia*) in sinus aspirates recovered from patients who had chronic sinusitis [41]. Antibody levels to these organisms declined in those who responded to therapy but did not decrease in those who did not respond (Fig. 3). The frequent involvement of anaerobes in chronic sinusitis may be related to the poor drainage and increased intranasal pressure that occur during inflammation. This increased pressure can reduce the oxygen tension in the

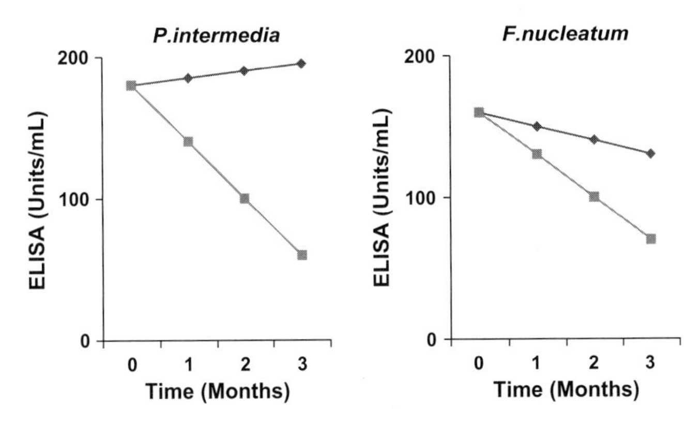

Fig. 3. Serum IgG antibodies to *Fusobacterium nucleatum* and *Prevotella intermedia* in 23 patients who had chronic sinusitis. (*Data from* Brook I, Yocum P. Immune responses to *Fusobacterium nucleatum* and *Prevotella intermedia* in patients with chronic maxillary sinusitis. Ann Otol Rhinol Laryngol 1999;108:294.)

inflamed sinus by decreasing the mucosal blood supply and depressing the mucociliary action [42]. The lowering of the oxygen content and pH of the sinus cavity supports the growth of anaerobic organisms by providing an optimal oxidation–reduction potential [14,42]. The mean oxygen tension in serous secretions obtained from acutely inflamed maxillary sinuses was 12.3% (compared with about 17% in the normal sinuses) [14]. The bacteria recovered from these aspirates were predominantly *S pneumoniae*. The oxygen tension in purulent secretion was zero, however, and an accumulation of carbon dioxide was found, particularly when anaerobic bacteria were recovered. It therefore is plausible that the reduced oxygen tension in the sinus during the serous phase better meets the requirements for the growth of the bacteria isolated in acute sinusitis, *S pneumoniae* and *H influenzae*, whereas the complete lack of oxygen in the purulent secretion supports the growth of the anaerobic organisms recovered in chronic sinusitis.

Anaerobes are recovered frequently from infections associated with complications of chronic sinusitis, including periorbital cellulitis, brain abscess, and subdural or epidural empyema [29,43,44]. This relationship further supports their role in complicated sinus infections.

Studies in children

Anaerobes were recovered in three studies, the only ones that used methods for their isolation [17,45,46]. Brook [17] studied 40 children who had chronic sinusitis, including involvement of maxillary sinuses in 15 cases, ethmoid sinuses in 13, and frontal sinuses in 7. Pansinusitis was present in five patients. A total of 121 isolates (97 anaerobic and 24 aerobic) were recovered. Anaerobes were recovered from all 37 culture-positive specimens, and in 14 cases (38%) they were mixed with aerobes. The predominant anaerobes were AGNB (36), gram-positive cocci (28), and *Fusobacterium* spp (13). The predominant aerobes were alpha-hemolytic streptococci (7), *S aureus* (7), and *Haemophilus* spp (4).

Brook and colleagues [45] correlated the microbiology of concurrent chronic otitis media with effusion and chronic maxillary sinusitis in 32 children. The origin was bacterial in two thirds of the patients. The most common isolates were *H influenzae* (9 isolates), *S pneumoniae* (7), *Prevotella* spp (8), and *Peptostreptococcus* spp (6). Microbiologic concordance between the ear and sinus was found in 22 culture-positive patients (69%).

Erkan and colleagues [46] studied 93 chronically inflamed maxillary sinuses in children. Anaerobes, which were isolated in 81of 87 culture-positive specimens (93%), were recovered alone in 61 cases (70%) and were mixed with aerobic or facultative bacteria in 20 cases (23%). The predominant anaerobic organisms were *Bacteroides* spp and anaerobic cocci; the predominant facultative species were *Streptococcus* spp and *S aureus*.

Studies in adults

Anaerobes were identified in chronic sinusitis whenever techniques for their cultivation were used [44]. A summary of 13 studies since 1974, including 1758 patients (133 of whom were children), is shown in Table 2 [17,30,31,38,44,46–54]. Anaerobes were recovered in 12% to 93%. The

Table 2
Isolation of anaerobes from patients who had chronic sinusitis

			Presence of anaerobes	
Reference	Country	No. patients	Patients (%)	Organisms (%)
Frederick and Braude, 1974 [47]	United States	83	75	52
Van Cauwenberge et al, 1976 [48]	Belgium	66	39	39
Karma et al, 1979 [49]	Finland	40 (adult)	—	19
Brook, 1981 [17]	United States	40 (pediatric)	100	80
Berg et al, 1988 [50]	Sweden	54 (adult)	≥33	42
Tabaqchali, 1988 [52]	United Kingdom	35	79	39
Brook, 1989 [18]	United States	72 (adult)	88	71
Fiscella and Chow, 1991 [51]	United States	15 (adult)	38	48
Erkan et al, 1994 [54]	Turkey	126 (adult)	88	71
		93 (pediatric)	93	74
Ito et al, 1995 [53]	Japan	10	60	82
Klossek et al, 1998 [55]	France	394	26	25
Finegold et al, 2002 [31]	United States	150 (adult)	56	48

predominant isolates were pigmented *Prevotella*, *Fusobacterium*, and *Peptostreptococcus* spp. The predominant aerobic bacteria were *S aureus, M catarrhalis*, and *Haemophilus* spp. The variability in recovery may result from differences in the methodologies used for transportation and cultivation, patient population, geography, and previous antimicrobial therapy. Finegold and colleagues [31] noted that among patients who had chronic maxillary sinusitis, recurrence of signs and symptoms was twice as frequent when their sinus cultures contained anaerobic bacterial counts above 10^3 colony-forming units per mL in the aspirate.

Brook [19–21] investigated the microbiology of chronic sinusitis including 13 patients who had frontal sinusitis, 7 who had with sphenoid sinusitis, and 17 who had ethmoid sinusitis. Anaerobic bacteria were recovered in more than two thirds of the patients. The predominant anaerobes included *Prevotella, Peptostreptococcus*, and *Fusobacterium* spp. The main aerobic organisms were gram-negative bacilli (*H influenzae, K pneumoniae, E coli*, and *P aeruginosa*).

Acute exacerbation of chronic sinusitis

Acute exacerbation of chronic sinusitis (AECS) represents a sudden worsening of the baseline manifestation of chronic sinusitis with either worsening or new symptoms. Typically, the acute (not chronic) symptoms resolve completely between occurrences. Brook and colleagues [56] evaluated the microbiology of maxillary AECS by performing repeated endoscopic aspirations in seven patients over a period of 125 to 242 days. Bacteria were recovered from all aspirates, and the number of isolates varied from two to four. The aerobes isolated were *H influenzae, S pneumoniae, M catarrhalis, S aureus*, and *K pneumoniae*. The anaerobes included pigmented *Prevotella* and *Porphyromonas, Peptostreptococcus*, and *Fusobacterium* spp, and *P acnes*. A change in the types of isolates was noted in all consecutive cultures obtained from the same patients as different organisms emerged and previously isolated bacteria were no longer found. An increase in antimicrobial resistance was noted in six instances. Brook [57] also compared the microbiology of maxillary AECS in 30 patients with the microbiology of chronic maxillary sinusitis in 32 patients. The study illustrates the predominance of anaerobic bacteria and the polymicrobial nature of both conditions (2.5–3 isolates/sinus). Aerobic bacteria that usually are found in acute infections (eg, *S pneumoniae, H influenzae*, and *M catarrhalis*) emerged in some of the episodes of AECS. Collectively, these findings highlight the importance of obtaining cultures from patients who have AECS for guidance in selection of appropriate antimicrobial therapy.

Nosocomial sinusitis

Nosocomial sinusitis often develops in patients who require extended periods of intensive care (postoperative patients, burn victims, patients with severe trauma) involving prolonged endotracheal or nasogastric intubation. *P aeruginosa* and other gram-negative rods are common in sinusitis of nosocomial origin, especially in patients who have nasal tubes or catheters, the immunocompromised, patients who have HIV infection, and patients who suffer from cystic fibrosis [26,58].

Nasotracheal intubation places the patient at a substantially higher risk for nosocomial sinusitis than orotracheal intubation. Approximately 25% of patients requiring nasotracheal intubation for more than 5 days develop nosocomial sinusitis [59]. In contrast to community-acquired sinusitis, the usual pathogens are gram-negative enteric bacteria (ie, *P aeruginosa*, *K pneumoniae*, *Enterobacter* spp, *P mirabilis*, *Serratia marcescens*) and gram-positive cocci (occasionally streptococci and staphylococci). Whether these organisms are actually pathogenic is unclear, because their recovery may represent only colonization of an environment with impaired mucociliary transport and presence of foreign body in the nasal cavity.

Evaluation of the microbiology of nosocomial sinusitis in nine neurologically impaired children revealed anaerobic bacteria, always mixed with aerobic and facultative bacteria, in six (67%) sinus aspirates and aerobic bacteria only in three (33%) [60]. There were 24 bacterial isolates; 12 were aerobic or facultative, and 12 were anaerobic. The predominant aerobic isolates were *K pneumoniae*, *E coli*, *S aureus*, *P mirabilis*, *P aeruginosa*, *H influenzae*, *M catarrhalis*, and *S pneumoniae*. The predominant anaerobes were *Prevotella* spp, *Peptostreptococcus* spp, *F nucleatum*, and *B fragilis*. Organisms similar to those recovered from the sinuses also were found in the tracheostomy site and gastrostomy wound aspirates in five of seven instances. This study demonstrates the uniqueness of the microbiologic features of sinusitis in neurologically impaired children, in whom facultative and anaerobic gram-negative organisms that can colonize other body sites are predominant.

Sinusitis in the immunocompromised host

Sinusitis occurs in a wide range of immunocompromised hosts including neutropenic patients, diabetic patients, patients in critical care units, and patients infected with HIV. Fungal and *P aeruginosa* are the most common forms of sinusitis in neutropenic patients. *Aspergillus* spp frequently are the causative organism, although Mucor, Rhizopus, Alternaria, and other molds have been implicated [61]. Fungi, *S aureus*, streptococci, and gram-negative enteric bacteria are the most common isolates in patients who have diabetes mellitus [62–64]. The causative organisms in patients who have HIV infection include *P aeruginosa*, *S aureus*, streptococci, anaerobes, and fungi (Aspergillus, Cryptococcus, and Rhizopus) [65]. Refractory parasitic sinusitis caused by Microsporidium, Cryptosporidium, and Acanthamoeba also has been described in patients who have advanced immunosuppression. Other causative agents include cytomegalovirus, atypical mycobacteria, and *Mycobacterium kansasii* [58].

Sinusitis of odontogenic origin

Odontogenic sinusitis is a well-recognized entity and accounts for approximately 10% to 12% of cases of maxillary sinusitis. Brook [8] studied the microbiology of 20 patients who had acute maxillary sinusitis and 28 patients who had chronic maxillary sinusitis associated with odontogenic infection. Polymicrobial infection was common, with 3.4 isolates per specimen, and in both acute and chronic infections, and 90% of the isolates were anaerobes. The predominant anaerobic bacteria were AGNB, *Peptostreptococcus* spp, and *Fusobacterium* spp. The predominant aerobes were α-hemolytic streptococci, microaerophilic streptococci, and *S aureus*.

The micro-organisms recovered from odontogenic infections generally reflect the indigenous oral flora. The association between periapical abscesses and sinusitis was established in a study of pus aspirates from five periapical abscesses of the upper jaw and their corresponding maxillary sinuses [25]. Polymicrobial flora was found in all instances; the number of isolates varied from two to five. Anaerobes were recovered from all specimens. The predominant isolates were *Prevotella*, *Porphyromonas*, and *Peptostreptococcus* spp and *F nucleatum*. The microbiologic findings from the periapical abscess were concordant with the maxillary sinus flora in all instances, suggesting contiguous spread of infection from the periapical abscess. The proximity of the maxillary molar teeth to the floor of the maxillary sinus allows such a spread.

Clinical presentation and diagnosis of bacterial sinusitis

Bacterial sinusitis is suspected, based on clinical symptoms and signs, when at least two major or one major and two minor criteria are present (Box 1) [66]. The most common presentation is a persistent (and unimproved) nasal discharge or cough (or both) lasting longer than 10 days [67]. A 10-day period separates simple viral upper respiratory tract infection (URTI) from bacterial sinusitis because most uncomplicated viral URTI last between 5 and 7 days—by day 10 most patients are improving.

The symptoms and signs of acute bacterial sinusitis can be divided further into nonsevere and severe forms (Box 2) [1]. The severe form carries a higher risk of complications and mandates earlier use of antimicrobial therapy. The combination of high fever and purulent nasal discharge lasting for at least 3 or 4 days points to a bacterial infection of the sinuses.

Patients who have acute bacterial sinusitis generally present with edema of the mucous membranes of the nose, mucopurulent nasal discharge, persistent postnasal drip, fever, and malaise. The quality of the nasal discharge varies: it can be thin or thick, clear mucoid, or purulent. Tenderness over the involved sinus is present, and so is pain, which can be induced over the affected sinus upon percussion. Cellulitis can be observed in the area overlying the affected sinus. Other occasional findings, especially in acute ethmoiditis,

Box 1. Major and minor clinical criteria suggestive of bacterial sinusitis

A strongly suggestive history requires the presence of two major criteria or one major and two or more minor criteria. A suggestive history requires the presence of one major criterion or two or more minor criteria.

Major criteria

Facial pain or pressure (requires a second major criterion to constitute a suggestive history)
Facial congestion or fullness
Nasal congestion or obstruction
Nasal discharge, purulence or discolored postnasal drainage
Hyposmia or anosmia
Fever (for acute sinusitis; requires a second major criterion to constitute a strong history)
Purulence on intranasal examination

Minor criteria

Headache
Fever (for subacute and chronic sinusitis)
Halitosis
Fatigue
Dental pain
Cough
Ear pain, pressure, or fullness

are periorbital cellulitis, edema, and proptosis. Failure to transilluminate the sinus and a nasal voice are also evident in many patients. Direct smear of the nasal secretions reveals mostly neutrophils and may aid in the detection of associated allergy if many eosinophils are present.

In patients who have subacute or chronic bacterial sinusitis, the symptoms are protracted and vary considerably. Fever may be absent or be of low grade. The patient may complain of malaise, easy fatigability, difficulty in mental concentration, anorexia, irregular nasal or postnasal discharge, frequent headaches, and pain or tenderness to palpation over the affected sinus. Cough and nasal congestion persist, and a sore throat (as a result of mouth-breathing) is common. The location of the facial pain can indicate the sinuses is involved. Often, maxillary bacterial sinusitis is associated with pain in the cheeks, frontal bacterial sinusitis with pain in with the forehead, ethmoid sinusitis with pain in the medial canthus, and sphenoid sinusitis with occipital pain. Other clues of chronic infection are sinus symptoms

Box 2. Severity of symptoms and signs in acute bacterial sinusitis

Nonsevere
Rhinorrhea (of any quality)
Nasal congestion
Cough
Headache, facial pain, and irritability (variable)
Low-grade or no fever

Severe
Purulent (thick, colored, opaque) rhinorrhea
Nasal congestion
Facial pain or headache
Periorbital edema (variable)
High fever (temperature $\geq$ 39°C)

that become worse or better with changes in motion or position. Disease in the upper molar teeth may be the source of maxillary sinusitis.

Further work-up and consideration for hospitalization include suspicion of nosocomial sinusitis (recent intubation, feeding or suction device), immunocompromised status, possible meningitis or other intracranial complications, or frontal or sphenoid sinusitis. Generally, plain-film radiographs are difficult to use in documenting the presence of infection and are less specific and sensitive than CT for analyzing the degree of sinus abnormalities. Because of this limitation, the use of plain-film radiography has declined, and it now has been replaced by CT. CT is especially advantageous for children, because their sinuses are smaller than those in adults and often are asymmetrical in shape and size, making them more difficult to evaluate [68]. Radiologically, clouding, opacity, and thickening of the mucosal interface ($\geq$ 4 mm) of the affected sinus usually are present. Fluid level often can be observed.

Management

Role of beta-lactamase–producing bacteria

Bacterial resistance to the antibiotics used for the treatment of sinusitis has increased consistently in recent years. Production of the enzyme beta-lactamase is one of the most important mechanisms of penicillin resistance. Beta-lactamase–producing bacteria (BLPB) may shield penicillin-susceptible organisms from the activity of penicillin, thereby contributing to their persistence [69]. The ability of BLPB to protect penicillin-sensitive micro-organisms has been demonstrated in vitro and in vivo [70]. The actual activity of the enzyme beta-lactamase and the phenomenon of shielding were demonstrated recently in fluids from acutely and chronically inflamed sinuses [71]. BLPB were isolated in sinus aspirates from 4 of 10 patients who had acute sinusitis and from 10 of 13 patients who had chronic sinusitis. The predominate BLPBs isolated in acute sinusitis were *H influenzae* and *M catarrhalis*, and those found in chronic sinusitis were *Prevotella* and *Fusobacterium* spp. Until recently, most *Prevotella* and *Fusobacterium* strains were considered susceptible to penicillin. Within the past 2 decades, however, penicillin-resistant strains have been reported with increasing frequency [72]. These species are the predominant gram-negative anaerobic bacilli [15] in the oral flora and are recovered most commonly in anaerobic infections in and around the oral cavity [17]. The recovery of BLPB is not surprising, because more than two thirds of the patients who had acute sinusitis and all of the patients who had chronic sinusitis received antimicrobial agents that might have selected for BLPB. These data suggest that therapy should be directed at the eradication of BLPB whenever present.

Antimicrobial therapy for acute bacterial sinusitis

Appropriate antibiotic therapy is of paramount importance for the prevention of septic complications [73]. Endoscopic examination and culture can assist in the selection of antimicrobial agents in the treatment of patients who do not respond [69]. Serial cultures of sinus secretions were obtained from patients who did not respond to antimicrobial therapy. Most of the bacteria isolated from the first culture were aerobic or facultative bacteria: *S Pneumoniae, H influenzae* non–type-b, and *M catarrhalis*. Repeated cultures generally yielded bacteria that were resistant to the antimicrobial agents prescribed for treatment. Failure to respond to therapy was associated with the emergence of resistant aerobic and anaerobic bacteria in subsequent aspirates (Fig. 4). The infection was eradicated in all instances after the administration of antimicrobial agents effective against these bacteria and, in several instances, after surgical drainage.

Amoxicillin is appropriate for the initial treatment of acute, uncomplicated, mild sinusitis (Box 3). Antimicrobial agents with more broad-spectrum activity may be indicated as initial therapy for patients who have more severe infection, comorbidity, risk factors for bacterial resistance, or who have not responded to amoxicillin therapy. These agents include amoxicillin and clavulanic acid, the newer quinolones (eg, levofloxacin, gatifloxacin, moxifloxacin), and some second- and third-generation cephalosporins (cefdinir, cefuroxime-axetil, and cefpodoxime proxetil). Telithromycin has been associated with severe hepatotoxicity and is contraindicated in patients who have myasthenia gravis. The Food and Drug Administration recently has removed its indication for telithromycin in the treatment of acute bacterial sinusitis and acute exacerbation of chronic bronchitis but

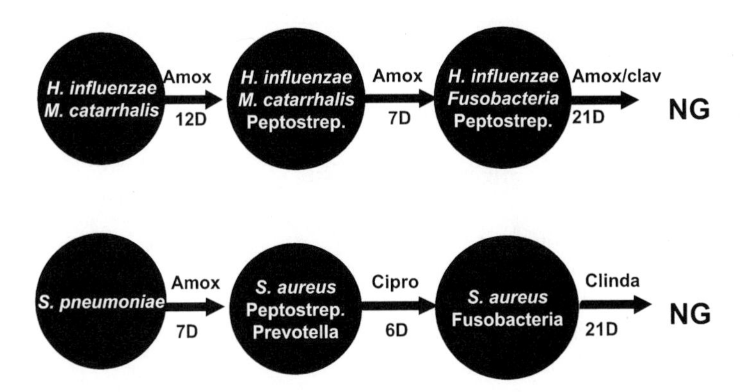

Fig. 4. Changes in the bacterial flora in two patients who had acute bacterial maxillary sinusitis that failed to respond to various antimicrobial regimens. Amox, amoxicillin; Amox/clav, amoxicillin/clavulanic-acid; Clinda, clindamycin; Cipro, ciprofloxacin; NG, no growth. (*Data from* Brook I, Frazier EH, Foote PA. Microbiology of the transition from acute to chronic maxillary sinusitis. J Med Microbiol 1996;45:373.)

has retained its approval for telithromycin in the treatment of moderate-to-severe community-acquired pneumonia. Patients who are allergic to penicillin may be treated with a macrolide, trimethoprim-sulfamethoxazole, tetracyclines, or clindamycin [74].

For a 10-day course of therapy, a bacteriologic cure rate higher than 80% to 90% may be expected. It has been estimated that spontaneous clearance may occur in approximately half of the patients [73,74]. The recommended length of therapy for acute bacterial sinusitis is at least 14 days, or 7 days beyond the resolution of symptoms, whichever is longer, but no controlled studies regarding the optimal duration of therapy are currently available.

Antimicrobial therapy for chronic bacterial sinusitis

Many of the pathogens found in chronically inflamed sinuses are resistant to penicillin through the production of beta-lactamase [18–21]. Retrospective studies suggest the superiority of therapy effective against both aerobic and anaerobic BLPB in chronic sinusitis [30,75]. These agents include the combination of a penicillin (eg, amoxicillin) and a beta-lactamase inhibitor (eg, clavulanic acid), clindamycin, the combination of metronidazole and a macrolide, or the newer quinolones (eg, levofloxacin, gatifloxacin, moxifloxacin). All of these agents (or similar ones) are available in oral and parenteral forms. Other effective antimicrobial agents available only in parenteral form include cefoxitin, cefotetan, and cefmetazole. If aerobic gram-negative organisms such as *P aeruginosa* are involved, an aminoglycoside, a fourth-generation cephalosporin (cefepime or ceftazidime), or a fluoroquinolone (only in postpubertal patients) is added. Parenteral therapy with a carbapenem (ie, imipenem, meropenem, or ertapenem) is more

Box 3. Empiric antimicrobial therapy in acute bacterial sinusitis

High-dose amoxicillin therapy is appropriate for

Mild illness
No history of recurrent acute sinusitis
Summer months
No recent antimicrobial therapy
No recent contact with patient(s) receiving antimicrobial therapy
Community experience shows high success rate of amoxicillin

More effective antimicrobial agents (amoxicillin and clavulanic acid, second- and third-generation cephalosporins, and the respiratory quinolones) are needed

1. When bacterial resistance is likely
   - Antibiotic use in the past month or close contact with a treated individual
   - Resistance common in community
   - Failure of previous antimicrobial therapy
   - Infection in spite of prophylactic treatment
   - Child in daycare facility
   - Winter season
   - Patient is a smoker or there is a smoker in family
2. In the presence of moderate-to-severe infection
   - Presentation with protracted (> 30 days) or moderate-to-severe symptoms
   - Complicated ethmoidal sinusitis
   - Frontal or sphenoidal sinusitis
   - Patient history of recurrent acute sinusitis
3. In the presence of comorbidity and at the extremes of life
   - Comorbidity (ie, chronic cardiac, hepatic, or renal disease, diabetes)
   - Immunocompromised patient
   - Age younger than 2 years or older than 55 years
4. Allergy to penicillin or amoxicillin

expensive but provides coverage for most potential pathogens including both anaerobes and aerobes. Therapy is given for at least 21 days and may be extended up to 10 weeks. Fungal sinusitis can be treated with surgical débridement of the affected sinuses and antifungal agents [76].

Surgical and adjuvant therapies

Symptomatic treatment is aimed at establishing good drainage by decongestants, nasal saline irrigation, humidification, and mucolytic agents. Systemic decongestants or antihistamines may be helpful, especially in allergic individuals. The short-term (3-day) use of topical α-adrenergic decongestants also can provide symptomatic relief, but their use should be restricted to older children and adults because of the potential for undesirable systemic effects in infants and young children. Topical glucocorticosteroids also may be useful in reducing nasal mucosal edema, mostly in patients who have seasonal allergic rhinitis complicating an acute URTI [77–80].

In contrast to acute sinusitis that generally is treated vigorously with antibiotics, surgical drainage is the mainstay of treatment for chronic sinusitis, especially in patients who have not responded to medical therapy. The surgeon's goals are to prevent persistence, recurrence, progression, and complications of chronic sinusitis. These goals are achieved by complete removal of diseased tissue, preservation of normal tissue, promotion of drainage (or obliteration if this is not possible), and consideration of the cosmetic outcome. In the past, it often was necessary to resort to radical procedures to cure chronic sinusitis. More recently, functional endoscopic sinus surgery has become the main surgical technique used; other procedures are reserved primarily for acute or chronic sinusitis complicated by orbital or intracranial involvement. Endoscopic surgery has success rates of 80% to 90% in both adults and children [81–83].

Complications

When not treated promptly and properly, sinus infection may spread by anastomosing veins or by direct extension to nearby structures (Fig. 5). Chandler and colleagues [84] categorized orbital complication into five separate stages according to severity. Contiguous spread could reach the orbital area, resulting in periorbital cellulitis, subperiosteal abscess, orbital cellulitis, and abscess. Orbital cellulitis may complicate acute ethmoiditis if a thrombophlebitis of the anterior and posterior ethmoidal veins leads to the spread of infection to the lateral or orbital side of the ethmoid labyrinth. Sinusitis also may extend to the central nervous system, causing cavernous sinus thrombosis, retrograde meningitis, and epidural, subdural, and brain abscesses [84,85]. Orbital symptoms frequently precede intracranial extension of the disease [43,86–92]. Other complications of acute and chronic sinusitis are sinobronchitis, maxillary osteomyelitis, and osteomyelitis of the frontal bone.

Brook and colleagues [86] reported eight children who had complications of sinusitis. Subdural empyema occurred in four patients; in one patient it was accompanied by cerebritis and brain abscess and in another by meningitis. Periorbital abscess was present in two children who had ethmoiditis. Alveolar abscess in the upper incisors was present in two children whose infection had

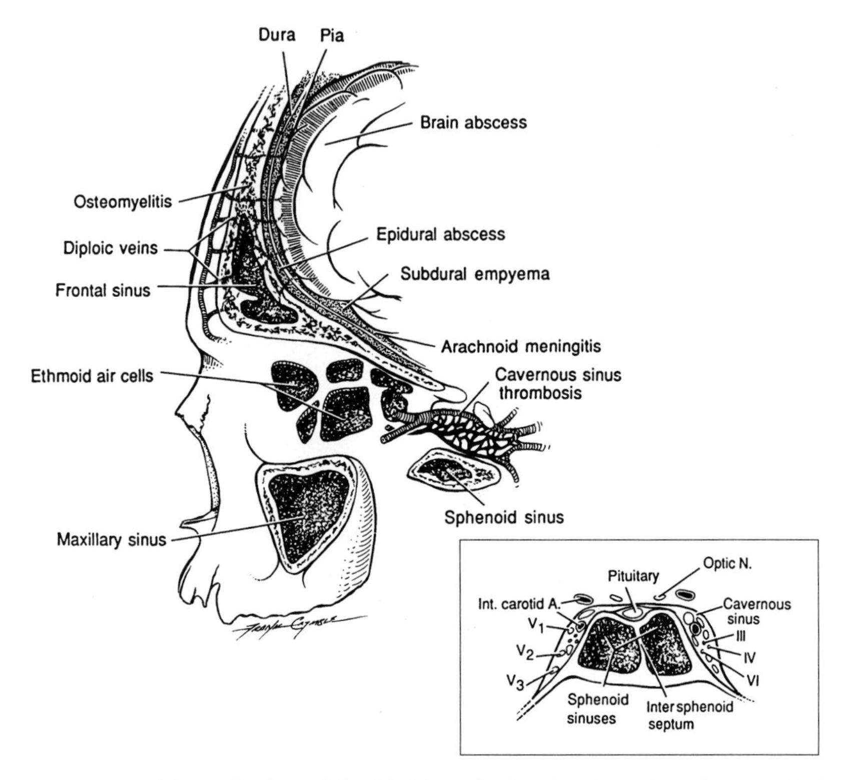

Fig. 5. Intracranial complications of sinusitis. The sagittal section shows the major routes for intracranial extension, either by contiguous spread or by the vascular supply. The coronal section demonstrates the structures adjoining the sphenoid sinus. (*From* Chow AW. Infections of the sinuses and parameningeal structures. In: Gorbach SL, Bartlett JG, Blacklow NR, editors. Infectious diseases. 3rd edition. Philadelphia: Lippincott Williams & Wilkins; 2004. p. 431; with permission.)

spread to the maxillary and ethmoid sinuses. Anaerobic bacteria were isolated from the infected sinuses in all the patients. Three of the four patients who had intracranial abscess did not respond initially to appropriate antimicrobial therapy directed against the organisms recovered from their abscesses. They improved only after both the subdural empyema and infected sinus were drained. Surgical drainage and appropriate antimicrobial therapy resulted in complete eradication of the infection in all patients.

The author has reported three children who had anaerobic osteomyelitis following chronic sinusitis [93]. One child developed frontal bone infection, another child had ethmoid sinusitis, and the third child had frontal and ethmoid osteomyelitis. All were associated with infection of the corresponding sinuses. Osteomyelitis of the frontal bone generally arises from spreading thrombophlebitis. A periostitis of the frontal sinus leads to an osteitis and a periostitis of the outer membrane, which gives rise to a tender, puffy swelling of the forehead.

Diagnosis is made by finding local tenderness and dull pain and is confirmed by CT and nuclear isotope scanning. The causative factors are anaerobic bacteria and *S aureus*. Management consists of surgical drainage and antimicrobial therapy. Surgical débridement is needed infrequently after a properly extended course of parenteral antimicrobial therapy [94]. Antibiotics should be given for at least 6 weeks. Monitoring for possible intracranial complication is warranted.

References

[1] Clement PAR, Bluestone CD, Gordts F, et al. Management of rhinosinusitis in children. Consensus Meeting, Brussels, Belgium, September 13, 1996. Arch Otolaryngol Head Neck Surg 1998;124:31–4.

[2] Dunham ME. New light on sinusitis. Contemp Pediatr 1994;1:102–17.

[3] Handelsman DJ, Conway AJ, Boylan LM, et al. Young's syndrome: obstructive azoospermia and chronic sinopulmonary infections. N Engl J Med 1984;310:3–9.

[4] Umetsu DT, Ambrosino DM, Quinti I, et al. Recurrent sinopulmonary infections and impaired antibody response to bacterial capsular polysaccharide antigen in children with selective IgG subclass deficiency. N Engl J Med 1985;313:1247–51.

[5] Berger M. Immunoglobulin G subclass determination in diagnosis and management of antibody deficiency syndromes. J Pediatr 1987;110:325–8.

[6] Lyon E, Miller C. Current challenges in cystic fibrosis screening. Arch Pathol Lab Med 2003; 127:1133–9.

[7] Bachert C, Patou J, Van Cauwenberge P. The role of sinus disease in asthma. Curr Opin Allergy Clin Immunol 2006;6:29–36.

[8] Brook I. Microbiology of acute and chronic maxillary sinusitis associated with an odontogenic origin. Laryngoscope 2005;115:823–5.

[9] Brook I. Aerobic and anaerobic bacteriology of purulent nasopharyngitis in children. J Clin Microbiol 1988;26:592–4.

[10] Savolainen S, Ylikoski J, Jousimies-Somer H. The bacterial flora of the nasal cavity in healthy young men. Rhinology 1986;24:249–55.

[11] Jousimies-Somer HR, Savolainen S, Ylikoski JS. Comparison of the nasal bacterial floras in two groups of healthy subjects and in patients with acute maxillary sinusitis. J Clin Microbiol 1989;27:2736–43.

[12] Brook I. Aerobic and anaerobic bacterial flora of normal maxillary sinuses. Laryngoscope 1981;91:372–6.

[13] Sande MA, Gwaltney JM. Acute community-acquired bacterial sinusitis—continuing challenges and current management. Clin Infect Dis 2004;39(Suppl 3):S151–8.

[14] Carenfelt C, Lundberg C. Purulent and non-purulent maxillary sinus secretions with respect to Po_2, Pco_2 and pH. Acta Otolaryngol 1977;84:138–44.

[15] Brook I. Role of encapsulated anaerobic bacteria in synergistic infections. Crit Rev Microbiol 1987;14:171–93.

[16] Brook I, Gober AE. Bacterial interference in the nasopharynx and nasal cavity of sinusitis prone and non-sinusitis prone children. Acta Otolaryngol 1999;119:832–6.

[17] Brook I. Bacteriologic features of chronic sinusitis in children. JAMA 1981;246:967–9.

[18] Brook I. Bacteriology of chronic maxillary sinusitis in adults. Ann Otol Rhinol Laryngol 1989;98:426–8.

[19] Brook I. Bacteriology of acute and chronic frontal sinusitis. Arch Otolaryngol Head Neck Surg 2002;128:583–5.

[20] Brook I. Bacteriology of acute and chronic sphenoid sinusitis. Ann Otol Rhinol Laryngol 2002;111:1002–4.

[21] Brook I. Bacteriology of acute and chronic ethmoid sinusitis. J Clin Microbiol 2005;43: 3479–80.
[22] Gwaltney JM Jr, Scheld WM, Sande MA, et al. The microbial etiology and antimicrobial therapy of adults with acute community-acquired sinusitis: a fifteen-year experience at the University of Virginia and review of other selected studies. J Allergy Clin Immunol 1992; 90:457–62.
[23] Brook I, Foote PA, Hausfeld JN. Frequency of recovery of pathogens causing acute maxillary sinusitis in adults before and after introduction of vaccination of children with the 7-valent pneumococcal vaccine. J Med Microbiol 2006;55:943–6.
[24] Lew D, Southwick FS, Montgomery WW, et al. Sphenoid sinusitis. A review of 30 cases. N Engl J Med 1983;309:1149–54.
[25] Brook I, Frazier EH, Gher ME Jr. Microbiology of periapical abscesses and associated maxillary sinusitis. J Periodontal 1996;67:608–10.
[26] Shapiro ED, Milmoe GJ, Wald ER, et al. Bacteriology of the maxillary sinuses in patients with cystic fibrosis. J Infect Dis 1982;146:589–93.
[27] Wald ER. Microbiology of acute and chronic sinusitis in children and adults. Am J Med Sci 1998;316:13–20.
[28] Biel MA, Brown CA, Levinson RM, et al. Evaluation of the microbiology of chronic maxillary sinusitis. Ann Otol Rhinol Laryngol 1998;107:942–5.
[29] Nord CE. The role of anaerobic bacteria in recurrent episodes of sinusitis and tonsillitis. Clin Infect Dis 1995;20:1512–24.
[30] Brook I, Thompson DH, Frazier EH. Microbiology and management of chronic maxillary sinusitis. Arch Otolaryngol Head Neck Surg 1994;120:1317–20.
[31] Finegold SM, Flynn MJ, Rose FV, et al. Bacteriologic findings associated with chronic bacterial maxillary sinusitis in adults. Clin Infect Dis 2002;35:428–33.
[32] Brook I. Acute and chronic frontal sinusitis. Curr Opin Pulm Med 2003;9:171–4.
[33] Gordts F, Halewyck S, Pierard D, et al. Microbiology of the middle meatus: a comparison between normal adults and children. J Laryngol Otol 2000;14:184–8.
[34] Jiang RS, Hsu CY, Jang JW. Bacteriology of the maxillary and ethmoid sinuses in chronic sinusitis. J Laryngol Otol 1998;112:845–8.
[35] Nadel DM, Lanza DC, Kennedy DW. Endoscopically guided cultures in chronic sinusitis. Am J Rhinol 1998;12:233–41.
[36] Bhattacharyya N, Kepnes LJ. The microbiology of recurrent rhinosinusitis after endoscopic sinus surgery. Arch Otolaryngol Head Neck Surg 1999;125:1117–20.
[37] Hsu J, Lanza DC, Kennedy DW. Antimicrobial resistance in bacterial chronic sinusitis. Am J Rhinol 1998;12:243–8.
[38] Brook I, Frazier EH. Correlation between microbiology and previous sinus surgery in patients with chronic maxillary sinusitis. Ann Otol Rhinol Laryngol 2001;110:148–51.
[39] Westrin KM, Stierna P, Carlsoo B, et al. Mucosal fine structure in experimental sinusitis. Ann Otol Rhinol Laryngol 1993;102(8 Pt 1):639–45.
[40] Jyonouchi H, Sun S, Kennedy CA, et al. Localized sinus inflammation in a rabbit sinusitis model induced by *Bacteroides fragilis* is accompanied by rigorous immune responses. Otolaryngol Head Neck Surg 1999;120:869–75.
[41] Brook I, Yocum P. Immune response to *Fusobacterium nucleatum* and *Prevotella intermedia* in patients with chronic maxillary sinusitis. Ann Otol Rhinol Laryngol 1999;108: 293–5.
[42] Aust R, Drettner B. Oxygen tension in the human maxillary sinus under normal and pathological conditions. Acta Otolaryngol 1974;78:264–9.
[43] Brook I. Brain abscess in children: microbiology and management. J Child Neurol 1995;10: 283–8.
[44] Finegold SM. Anaerobic bacteria in human disease. Orlando (FL): Academic Press Inc; 1977.

[45] Brook I, Yocum P, Shah K. Aerobic and anaerobic bacteriology of concurrent chronic otitis media with effusion and chronic sinusitis in children. Arch Otolaryngol Head Neck Surg 2000;126:174–6.
[46] Erkan M, Ozcan M, Arslan S, et al. Bacteriology of antrum in children with chronic maxillary sinusitis. Scand J Infect Dis 1996;28:283–5.
[47] Frederick J, Braude AI. Anaerobic infections of the paranasal sinuses. N Engl J Med 1974; 290:135–7.
[48] Van Cauwenberge P, Verschraegen G, Van Renterghem L. Bacteriological findings in sinusitis (1963-1975). Scand J Infect Dis Suppl 1976;(9):72–7.
[49] Karma P, Jokipii L, Sipila P, et al. Bacteria in chronic maxillary sinusitis. Arch Otolaryngol 1979;105:386–90.
[50] Berg O, Carenfelt C, Kronvall G. Bacteriology of maxillary sinusitis in relation to character of inflammation and prior treatment. Scand J Infect Dis 1988;20:511–6.
[51] Fiscella RG, Chow JM. Cefixime for the treatment of maxillary sinusitis. Am J Rhinol 1991; 5:193–7.
[52] Tabaqchali S. Anaerobic infections in the head and neck region. Scand J Infect Dis Suppl 1988;57:24–34.
[53] Ito K, Ito Y, Mizuta K, et al. Bacteriology of chronic otitis media, chronic sinusitis, and paranasal mucopyocele in Japan. Clin Infect Dis 1995;20(Suppl 2):S214–9.
[54] Erkan M, Aslan T, Ozcan M, et al. Bacteriology of antrum in adults with chronic maxillary sinusitis. Laryngoscope 1994;104(3 Pt 1):321–4.
[55] Klossek JM, Dubreuil L, Richet H, et al. Bacteriology of chronic purulent secretions in chronic rhinosinusitis. J Laryngol Otol 1998;112:1162–6.
[56] Brook I, Foote PA, Frazier EH. Microbiology of acute exacerbation of chronic sinusitis. Laryngoscope 2004;114:129–31.
[57] Brook I. Bacteriology of chronic sinusitis and acute exacerbation of chronic sinusitis. Arch Otolaryngol Head Neck Surg 2006;132:1099–101.
[58] Del Borgo C, Del Forno A, Ottaviani F, et al. Sinusitis in HIV-infected patients. J Chemother 1997;9:83–8.
[59] Arens JF, LeJeune FE Jr, Webre DR. Maxillary sinusitis, a complication of nasotracheal intubation. Anesthesiology 1974;40:415–6.
[60] Brook I, Shah K. Sinusitis in neurologically impaired children. Otolaryngol Head Neck Surg 1998;119:357–60.
[61] Gillespie MB, O'Malley BW Jr, Francis HW. An approach to fulminant invasive fungal rhinosinusitis in the immunocompromised host. Arch Otolaryngol Head Neck Surg 1998;124: 520–6.
[62] Jackson RM, Rice DH. Acute bacterial sinusitis and diabetes mellitus. Otolaryngol Head Neck Surg 1987;97:469–73.
[63] Talmor M, Li P, Barie PS. Acute paranasal sinusitis in critically ill patients: guidelines for prevention, diagnosis and treatment. Clin Infect Dis 1997;25:1441–6.
[64] Brook I. Microbiology of nosocomial sinusitis in mechanically ventilated children. Arch Otolaryngol Head Neck Surg 1998;124:35–8.
[65] Godofsky EW, Zinreich J, Armstrong M, et al. Sinusitis in HIV-infected patients. A clinical and radiographic review. Am J Med 1992;93:163–70.
[66] Lanza DC, Kennedy DW. Adult rhinosinusitis defined. Otolaryngol Head Neck Surg 1997; 117:51–7.
[67] Wald ER, Guerra N, Byers C. Upper respiratory tract infections in young children: duration of and frequency of complications. Pediatrics 1991;87:129–33.
[68] Aalokken TM, Hagtvedt T, Dalen I, et al. Conventional sinus radiography compared with CT in the diagnosis of acute sinusitis. Dentomaxillofac Radiol 2003;32:60–2.
[69] Brook I, Frazier EH, Foote PA. Microbiology of the transition from acute to chronic maxillary sinusitis. J Med Microbiol 1996;45:372–5.

[70] Brook I. The role of beta-lactamase-producing bacterial in the persistence of streptococcal tonsillar infection. Rev Infect Dis 1984;6:601–7.
[71] Brook I, Yocum P, Frazier EH. Bacteriology and beta-lactamase activity in acute and chronic maxillary sinusitis. Arch Otolaryngol Head Neck Surg 1996;122:418–22.
[72] Brook I. Beta-lactamase producing bacteria in head and neck infection. Laryngoscope 1988; 98:428–31.
[73] Wald ER, Chiponis D, Leclesma-Medina J. Comparative effectiveness of amoxicillin and amoxicillin-clavulanate potassium in acute paranasal sinus infection in children: a double-blind, placebo-controlled trial. Pediatrics 1998;77:795–800.
[74] Brook I, Gooch WM III, Jenkins SG, et al. Medical management of acute bacterial sinusitis. Recommendations of a clinical advisory committee on pediatric and adult sinusitis. Ann Otol Rhinol Laryngol 2000;109:1–20.
[75] Brook I, Yocum P. Management of chronic sinusitis in children. J Laryngol Otol 1995;109: 1159–62.
[76] Decker CF. Sinusitis in the immunocompromised host. Curr Infect Dis Rep 1999;1:27–32.
[77] Nuutinen J, Ruoppi P, Suonpaa J. One dose beclomethasone dipropionate aerosol in the treatment of seasonal allergic rhinitis. A preliminary report. Rhinology 1987;25:121–7.
[78] Chalton R, Mackay I, Wilson R, et al. Double blind placebo controlled trial of betamethasone nasal drops for nasal polyposis. Br Med J 1985;291:788.
[79] Brown SL, Graham SG. Nasal irrigations: good or bad? Curr Opin Otolaryngol Head Neck Surg 2004;12:9–13.
[80] Parnes SM, Chuma AV. Acute effects on anti-leukotrienes on sinonasal polyposis and sinusitis. Ear Nose Throat J 2000;79:18–20.
[81] Gross CW, Gurucharri MJ, Lazar RH, et al. Functional endoscopic sinus surgery (FESS) in the pediatric age group. Laryngoscope 1989;99:272–5.
[82] Kennedy DW. Prognostic factors, outcomes and staging in ethmoid sinus surgery. Laryngoscope 1992;102:1–18.
[83] Stankiewicz JA. Complications of endoscopic intranasal ethmoidectomy. Laryngoscope 1987;97:1270–3.
[84] Chandler JR, Langenbrunner DJ, Stevens EF. The pathogenesis of orbital complications in acute sinusitis. Laryngoscope 1970;80:1414–28.
[85] Brook I. Microbiology of intracranial abscesses and their associated sinusitis. Arch Otolaryngol Head Neck Surg 2005;131:1017–9.
[86] Brook I, Friedman E, Rodriguez WJ, et al. Complications of sinusitis in children. Pediatrics 1980;66:568–72.
[87] Baker AS. Role of anaerobic bacteria in sinusitis and its complications. Ann Otol Rhinol Laryngol Suppl 1991;154:17–22.
[88] Brook I, Frazier EH. Microbiology of subperiosteal orbital abscess and associated maxillary sinusitis. Laryngoscope 1996;106:1010–3.
[89] Clayman GL, Adams GL, Paugh DR, et al. Intracranial complications of paranasal sinusitis: a combined institutional review. Laryngoscope 1991;101:234–9.
[90] Arjmand EM, Lusk RP, Muntz HR. Pediatric sinusitis and subperiosteal orbital abscess formation: diagnosis and treatment. Otolaryngol Head Neck Surg 1993;109:886–94.
[91] Gerald J, Harris MD. Subperiosteal abscess of the orbit age as a factor in the bacteriology and response to treatment. Ophthalmology 1994;101:585–95.
[92] Dill SR, Cobbs CG, McDonald CK. Subdural empyema: analysis of 32 cases and review. Clin Infect Dis 1995;20:372–86.
[93] Brook I. Anaerobic osteomyelitis in children. Pediatr Infect Dis 1986;5:550–6.
[94] Stankiewicz JA, Newell DJ, Park AH. Complications of inflammatory diseases of the sinuses. Otolaryngol Clin North Am 1993;26:639–55.

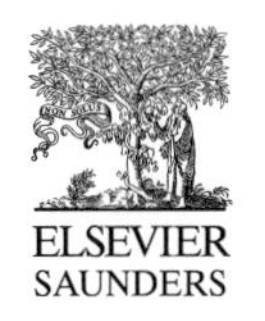

ELSEVIER
SAUNDERS

Infect Dis Clin N Am 21 (2007) 449–469

INFECTIOUS
DISEASE CLINICS
OF NORTH AMERICA

Pharyngitis and Epiglottitis

Maria L. Alcaide, MD[a,b], Alan L. Bisno, MD[a,c,*]

[a]*Division of Infectious Diseases, Department of Medicine, University of Miami Miller School of Medicine, 1400 NW 10th Avenue, 090-A Dominion Tower #812, Miami, FL 33136, USA*
[b]*Medical Service, Infectious Diseases Section (111-1), Miami Veterans Affairs Healthcare System, 1201 NW 16th St., Miami, FL 33125, USA*
[c]*Medical Service (111), Miami Veterans Affairs Healthcare System, 1201 NW 16th St., Miami, FL 33125, USA*

Pharyngitis

Sore throat accounts for 1% to 2% of all patient visits to office-based primary care practitioners, hospital outpatient departments, and emergency departments in the United States [1]. Data from the National Medical Care Survey indicate approximately 7.3 million annual visits for children [2] and 6.7 such visits for adults [3]. Thus, familiarity with the principles of diagnosis and management of this disorder is essential for primary care physicians seeing patients of all ages.

Etiology

The hallmarks of acute pharyngitis are sore throat of varying degrees of clinical severity, pharyngeal erythema, and fever. Most cases of pharyngitis are of viral origin, and with few exceptions these illnesses are both benign and self-limited. A large proportion of cases of pharyngitis is associated with rhinovirus [4] and coronavirus colds or with influenza. The most important cause of bacterial pharyngitis is the beta-hemolytic group A streptococcus (*Streptococcus pyogenes*, GAS). There are other uncommon or rare types of pharyngitis, and for some of these treatment is also required or available.

The recognized microbial causes of pharyngitis are listed in Table 1, which shows the syndromes of respiratory illness caused by the various agents [5–10]. It still is not possible to determine the cause in a sizable

* Corresponding author. Medical Service (111), Miami Veterans Affairs Healthcare System, 1201 NW 16th St., Miami, FL 33125.

E-mail address: abisno@med.miami.edu (A.L. Bisno).

doi:10.1016/j.idc.2007.03.001

Table 1
Microbial causes of acute pharyngitis

Pathogen	Associated disorder(s)
Bacterial	
Streptococcus, group A	Pharyngitis, tonsillitis, scarlet fever
Streptococcus, groups C, G	Pharyngitis, tonsillitis
Mixed anaerobes	Vincent's angina
Neisseria gonorrhoeae	Pharyngitis, tonsillitis
Corynebacterium diphtheriae	Diphtheria
Arcanobacterium haemolyticum	Pharyngitis, scarlatiniform rash
Yersinia enterocolitica	Pharyngitis, enterocolitis
Yersinia pestis	Plague
Francisella tularensis	Tularemia, oropharyngeal form
Treponema pallidum	Secondary syphilis
Viral	
Rhinovirus	Common cold
Coronavirus	Common cold
Adenovirus	Pharyngoconjunctival fever
Herpes simplex type 1 & 2	Pharyngitis, gingivostomatitis
Parainfluenza	Cold, croup
Coxsackie A	Herpangina, hand-foot-mouth disease
Epstein-Barr virus	Infectious mononucleosis
Cytomegalovirus	CMV mononucleosis
Human immunodeficiency virus	Primary HIV infection
Influenza A, B	Influenza
Mycoplasmal	
Mycoplasma pneumoniae	Pneumonia, bronchitis, pharyngitis
Chlamydophilal	
Chlamydophila psittaci	Acute respiratory disease, pneumonia
Chlamydophila pneumoniae	Pneumonia, pharyngitis

Modified from Bisno AL. Pharyngitis. In: Mandell GL, Dolan R, Bennett JE, editors. Principles and practice of infectious diseases. 6th edition. New York: Churchill Livingstone; 2006. p. 752; with permission.

proportion of cases. A major task of the primary care physician is to identify those patients with acute pharyngitis who require specific antimicrobial therapy and to avoid unnecessary and potentially deleterious treatment in the great majority who suffer from a benign, self-limited, usually viral infection. In most cases this distinction can be made easily by attention to the epidemiologic setting, history, and physical findings augmented by performance of a few simple and readily available laboratory studies.

Epidemiology

The results of epidemiologic investigations are influenced by the season of the year, the age of the population, the severity of illness, and the diagnostic methods used to detect cases. Most cases of pharyngitis occur during the colder months of the year, during the respiratory disease season. Viral agents such as rhinoviruses tend to have annual periods of peak prevalence in the fall and spring; coronaviruses have been found most often in the winter. Influenza appears in epidemics, which in the United States usually occur between December and April. In military recruits, adenoviruses cause the syndrome of acute respiratory disease during the colder months. In civilians, acute respiratory disease occurs in the winter, and epidemics of pharyngoconjunctival fever occur in the summer. Streptococcal pharyngitis occurs during the respiratory disease season, with peak rates of infection in winter and early spring. Spread among family members in the home is a prominent feature of the epidemiologic behavior of most of these agents, with children being the major reservoir of infection [11].

Bacterial infections

Group A streptococci

As shown in Table 1, a number of bacteria may cause acute pharyngitis, but most of these are rare or unusual causes of the syndrome. Moreover, the benefit of antimicrobial therapy for some of these agents (ie, *Arcanobacterium haemolyticum*, non–group A beta hemolytic streptococci) is unclear. Thus, GAS is the only commonly occurring cause of sore throat for which antimicrobial therapy is definitely indicated.

GAS is estimated to be the cause of 15% to 30% of cases of acute tonsillopharyngitis occurring during the cooler months of the year in school-aged children [12] and of approximately 10% of cases in adults [13,14], but there is considerable variability from study to study [15]. Nationally, however, approximately 53% of children [2] and 73% of adults [3] who have sore throat receive antimicrobial agents, and a substantial proportion receives antimicrobial agents not recommended as treatments of choice for GAS pharyngitis. The following discussion provides recommendations by which such unnecessary and/or inappropriate therapy may be minimized.

Clinical manifestations

The characteristic clinical findings are summarized in Table 2. The presence of marked odynophagia, exudative tonsillopharyngitis (Fig. 1), anterior cervical adenitis, fever, and leukocytosis is highly suggestive of GAS pharyngitis. None of the signs and symptoms listed in the table is specific for "strep throat," however. Moreover, patients vary widely in the severity of their symptoms. Many cases are milder and nonexudative. Only approximately half of children presenting with sore throats and positive throat cultures have tonsillar or pharyngeal exudates [12]. Patients who have had a tonsillectomy may have milder symptoms. Children less than 3 years of age may have coryza and crusting of the nares; exudative pharyngitis caused by GAS is rare in this age group. On the other hand, the presence of cough, coryza (in children older than 3 years), hoarseness, diarrhea, conjunctivitis, and/or anterior stomatitis is highly indicative of viral rather than streptococcal infection.

Table 2
Clinical presentation of streptococcal tonsillopharyngitis

Common findings in GAS infection[a]	Findings not suggesting GAS infection
Symptoms	
Sudden onset sore throat	Coryza
Pain on swallowing	Hoarseness
Fever	Cough
Headache	Diarrhea
Abdominal pain	
Nausea and vomiting	
Signs	
Tonsillopharyngeal erythema	Conjunctivitis
Tonsillopharyngeal exudates	Anterior stomatitis
Soft palate petechiae ("doughnut" lesions)	Discrete ulcerative lesions
Beefy red, swollen uvula	
Anterior cervical adenitis	
Scarlatiniform rash	

Abbreviation: GAS, group A streptococci.

[a] These findings are noted primarily in children older than 3 years of age and adults. Symptoms and signs in younger children can be different and less specific.

From Dajani A, Taubert K, Ferrieri P, et al. Treatment of acute streptococcal pharyngitis and prevention of rheumatic fever: a statement for health professionals. Committee on Rheumatic Fever, Endocarditis, and Kawasaki Disease of the Council on Cardiovascular Disease in the Young, the American Heart Association. Pediatrics 1995;96:759; with permission.

Scarlet fever results from infection with a streptococcal strain that elaborates streptococcal pyrogenic exotoxins (erythrogenic toxins) to which the patient is not immune. Although this disease usually is associated with pharyngeal infections, it may follow streptococcal infections at other sites such as wound infections or puerperal sepsis. Nowadays, the clinical syndrome is similar in most respects to that associated with nontoxigenic strains, save for

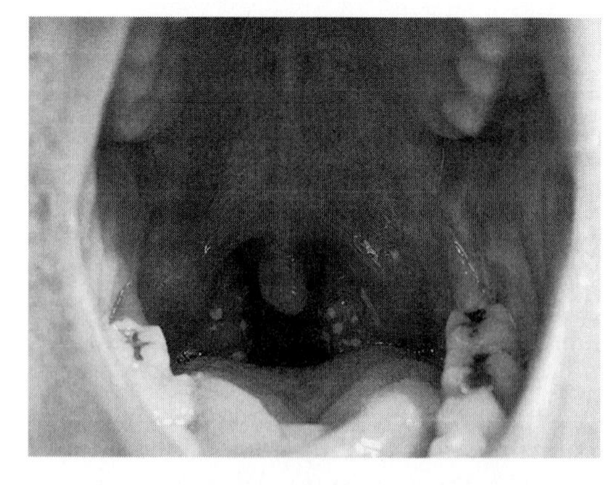

Fig. 1. Streptococcal pharyngitis. Note white exudates on erythematous swollen tonsils. (*From* Nimishikavi S, Stead L. Images in clinical medicine. Streptococcal pharyngitis. N Engl J Med 2005;352(11):e10; with permission Copyright © 2005, Massachusetts Medical Society.)

the scarlatinal rash. The latter must be differentiated from those of viral exanthems, drug eruptions, staphylococcal and streptococcal toxic shock syndrome, and Kawasaki disease.

Diagnosis

When confronted with a patient who has acute pharyngitis, the clinician must decide whether the likelihood of GAS infection is high enough to warrant a confirmatory diagnostic test. Patients lacking the suggestive clinical and epidemiologic findings or manifesting signs and symptoms indicative of viral pharyngitis (see Table 2) need not be tested or treated with antimicrobial agents. Attempts have been made to incorporate clinical and epidemiologic features of acute pharyngitis into scoring systems that attempt to predict the probability that a particular illness is caused by GAS [14,16–19]. These clinical scoring systems are helpful in identifying patients at such low risk of streptococcal infection that further testing is usually unnecessary. Selective use of diagnostic studies for GAS will increase the proportion of positive test results and also the percentage of patients with positive tests who are truly infected rather than merely streptococcal carriers. The signs and symptoms of streptococcal and nonstreptococcal pharyngitis overlap too broadly, however, to allow the requisite diagnostic precision on clinical grounds alone. Although some have suggested otherwise [1,20], empiric antimicrobial treatment based on clinical and epidemiologic grounds alone has been found suboptimal in cost effectiveness [21] and by prospective analyses [18]. Therefore, if the clinician is unable to rule out strep throat on clinical and epidemiologic grounds, further testing is required (see later discussion) [22].

A properly performed and interpreted throat culture is the gold standard for the diagnosis of GAS pharyngitis. It has a sensitivity of 90% or higher, as judged by studies employing duplicate throat cultures. Obtaining definitive results of the throat culture takes 18 to 48 hours. In the minority of patients who are severely ill or toxic at presentation and in whom clinical and epidemiologic evidence leads to a high index of suspicion, oral antimicrobial therapy may be initiated while awaiting the results of the throat culture. If oral therapy is prescribed, the throat culture serves as a guide to the necessity of completion of a full antimicrobial course or, alternatively, of recalling the patient for an injection of penicillin G benzathine. Early initiation of antimicrobial therapy results in faster resolution of the signs and symptoms, but two facts should be kept in mind. First, GAS pharyngitis usually is a self-limited disease; fever and constitutional symptoms are markedly diminished within 3 or 4 days after onset even without antimicrobial therapy. Thus, antimicrobial therapy initiated within the first 48 hours of onset will hasten symptomatic improvement only modestly. Second, it has been shown that therapy can be postponed safely up to 9 days after the onset of symptoms and still prevent the occurrence of the major nonsuppurative sequela, acute rheumatic fever [23].

The issues alluded to in the previous discussion may be obviated in part by the use of rapid antigen detection tests (RADT), which can confirm the presence of GAS carbohydrate antigen on a throat swab in a matter of minutes. Currently available commercial test kits yield results that are highly specific for the presence of GAS. Thus, a positive RADT can be considered equivalent to a positive throat culture, and therapy may be initiated without further microbiologic confirmation. Unfortunately, the sensitivity of most of these tests ranges between 70% and 90% when compared with the blood agar plate culture [24]. For this reason it is necessary to back up negative RADTs with a conventional throat culture. One possible exception to the need for such backup relates to adults, in whom the prevalence of GAS pharyngitis is relatively low and the risk of a first attack of acute rheumatic fever in North America is minimal [25,26].

A positive RADT or throat culture does not differentiate between the presence of acute streptococcal infection and chronic GAS carriage [27]. In the appropriate clinical setting, however, a positive test should be considered as confirmatory of strep throat. Follow-up throat cultures are not indicated routinely for asymptomatic patients who have received a complete course of therapy for GAS pharyngitis, because most such patients are streptococcal carriers. Exceptions include patients who have a history of rheumatic fever, patients who develop acute pharyngitis during outbreaks of either acute rheumatic fever or poststreptococcal acute glomerulonephritis, and outbreaks of GAS pharyngitis in closed or semiclosed communities. Follow-up throat cultures also may be indicated when "ping-pong" spread of GAS has been occurring within a family.

Antimicrobial therapy

Treatment of GAS pharyngitis is recommended to prevent acute rheumatic fever, prevent suppurative complications [28], shorten the clinical course (although only modestly) [28], and reduce transmission of the infection in family and school units. There is no definitive evidence that such therapy can prevent acute glomerulonephritis. A number of antibiotics have been shown to be effective in therapy of GAS pharyngitis. These include penicillin and its congeners (such as ampicillin and amoxicillin), numerous cephalosporins, macrolides, and clindamycin. Penicillin, however, remains the treatment of choice because of its proven efficacy, safety, narrow spectrum, and low cost. Amoxicillin often is used in place of oral penicillin V in young children; the efficacy appears equal, and this choice is related primarily to superior palatability of the suspension. Erythromycin is a suitable alternative for patients allergic to penicillin, although increases in GAS resistance to this agent have been reported in certain localized areas of the United States. First-generation cephalosporins also are acceptable for penicillin-allergic patients who do not manifest immediate-type hypersensitivity to beta-lactam antibiotics.

There is debate regarding the relative efficacy of cephalosporins vis-a-vis penicillin [29] in eradicating GAS from the pharynx and about the utility of shorter courses of certain antimicrobial agents in treating strep throat. For a further discussion of this topic, the reader is referred to the Infectious Diseases Society of America (IDSA) practice guideline [25]. Penicillin, however, remains the preferred therapy according to guidelines published by the American Heart Association [30], American Academy of Pediatrics [31], and IDSA (Table 3) [25]. The IDSA guideline also offers guidance in management of patients who have recurrent episodes of culture- or RADT-positive acute GAS pharyngitis.

Preliminary investigations have demonstrated that once-daily amoxicillin therapy is effective in the treatment of group A beta hemolytic streptococcus pharyngitis [32–34]. In the most careful of these studies, Feder and colleagues [32] randomly assigned 152 children to receive amoxicillin, 750 mg once daily, or penicillin V, 250 mg three times daily. Compliance was monitored by urine antimicrobial activity, and serotyping was performed to distinguish treatment failures from new acquisitions. The two regimens

Table 3
Recommendations for antimicrobial therapy of group A streptococcal pharyngitis

Antimicrobial agents	Dosage	Duration[a]
Oral regimens		
Penicillin V[b]	Children: 250 mg b.i.d. or t.i.d.	10 days
	Adolescents and adults: 250 mg t.i.d. or q.i.d. or 500 mg b.i.d.	10 days
For patients allergic to penicillin[f]		
Erythromycin	Varies with formulation[e]	10 days
First-generation cephalosporins	Varies with agent	10 days
Intramuscular regimens		
Benzathine penicillin G	1.2×10^6 U	1 dose
	6.0×10^5 U[c]	1 dose
Mixtures of benzathine and procaine penicillin G	Varies with formulation[d]	1 dose

[a] Although shorter courses of azithromycin and some cephalosporins have been reported to be effective for treating group A streptococcal upper respiratory tract infections, evidence is not sufficient to recommend these shorter courses for routine therapy at this time.

[b] Amoxicillin often is used in place of oral penicillin V for young children; efficacy seems to be equal. The choice is related primarily to acceptance of the taste of the suspension.

[c] For patients who weigh < 27 kg.

[d] Dose should be determined on basis of the benzathine component. For example, mixtures of 9×10^5 U of benzathine penicillin G and 3×10^5 U of procaine penicillin G contain less benzathine penicillin G than is recommended for treatment of adolescents or adults.

[e] Available as stearate, ethyl succinate, estolate, or base. Cholestatic hepatitis, rarely, may occur in patients, primarily adults, receiving erythromycin estolate; the incidence is greater among pregnant women, who should not receive this formulation.

[f] These agents should not be used to treat patients with immediate-type hypersensitivity to beta-lactam antibiotics.

From Bisno AL, Gerber MA, Gwaltney JM Jr, et al. Practice guidelines for the diagnosis and management of group A streptococcal pharyngitis. Infectious Diseases Society of America. Clin Infect Dis 2002;35(2):120; with permission.

were equally effective in eradicating GAS from the pharynx. If additional investigations confirm these results, once-daily amoxicillin therapy, because of its low cost and relatively narrow spectrum, could become an alternative regimen for the treatment of group A beta-hemolytic streptococcal pharyngitis.

Suppurative complications of GAS pharyngitis include peritonsillar infection, retropharyngeal abscess, cervical lymphadenitis, mastoiditis, Lemierre syndrome, sinusitis, and otitis media. Such complications have become relatively rare since the advent of effective chemotherapy.

Peritonsillar infection may take the form of cellulitis or abscess (quinsy) and is the most common form of deep oropharyngeal infection. Although peritonsillar abscesses may occur as complications of GAS pharyngitis, the abscesses themselves frequently contain a variety of other oral flora including anaerobes, with or without GAS [35–37]. They occur more frequently in adolescents and adults than in young children. Pharyngeal pain is usually severe, and dysphagia is common. On examination, there is inflammation and swelling of the peritonsillar area with medial displacement of the tonsil, and patients speak with a "hot potato" voice. Trismus may be present. Peritonsillar cellulitis may be treated with antibiotics alone, but abscesses require drainage by direct aspiration or by incision and drainage. Given the polymicrobial nature of these infections, parenteral antibiotics such as clindamycin, penicillin with metronidazole, or ampicillin-sulbactam are frequently employed. Their superiority over penicillin has not been demonstrated definitively, however.

Lemierre syndrome (postanginal septicemia) is caused by an acute oropharyngeal infection with secondary septic thrombophlebitis of the internal jugular vein and, often, bacteremic spread to lungs or elsewhere [38]. The most common causative organism is *Fusobacterium necrophorum*. The clinical findings include acute presentation with fever, swelling and tenderness at the angle of the jaw, and neck rigidity. Dysphagia and dysphonia can occur. The peritonsillar area is inflamed only early in the disease. Emergency medical treatment with intravenous antibiotics such as clindamycin, penicillin with metronidazole or ampicillin-sulbactam is usually sufficient, but at times ligation of the internal jugular vein is required.

Acute rheumatic fever and poststreptococcal acute glomerulonephritis are the delayed nonsuppurative sequelae of GAS pharyngitis. Although the former occurs only after GAS upper respiratory infection, the latter may occur after infection of the throat or skin (streptococcal pyoderma). Discussion of these entities is beyond the scope of this article.

Streptococci other than group A

Non–group A beta-hemolytic streptococci are classified biochemically by species. For clinical purposes, however, they usually are identified by their expression of the Lancefield cell-wall antigens. Certain of these strains clearly are capable of causing acute pharyngitis when ingested in high inocula. Streptococci of serogroup G have been linked to common-source outbreaks of pharyngitis, usually related to a food product. One unusual species of group C organisms, *Streptococcus equi* subspecies *zooepidemicus*, has given rise to common-source epidemics of pharyngitis, usually caused by consumption of unpasteurized dairy products. Several of these outbreaks have been associated with poststreptococcal acute glomerulonephritis [39].

Groups C and G streptococci are common commensals of the human pharynx. They form large colonies similar to those of GAS and belong to the species *Streptococcus dysgalactiae* subspecies *equisimilis*. Physicians who do not back up negative RADTs with throat cultures will not identify these organisms.

The extent to which they cause sporadically occurring episodes of true acute pharyngitis is unclear, but several careful studies suggest that group C streptococci may cause episodes of pharyngitis that mimic GAS infection [40,41]. Moreover, a community-wide outbreak of group G streptococcal pharyngitis occurred in Connecticut during the winter of 1986–1987 [42]. Because of the difficulty in differentiating benign colonization from true infection with groups C or G streptococci, the benefit, if any, of antimicrobial therapy in sporadically occurring cases is unknown. Should therapy be elected, agents listed in Table 3 would be appropriate, but probably for a shorter duration, because non–group A streptococci never have been shown to cause acute rheumatic fever.

Arcanobacterium haemolyticum. *Arcanobacterium* (formerly *Corynebacterium*) *haemolyticum* is a gram-positive bacillus that is a relatively uncommon cause of acute pharyngitis and tonsillitis. Symptomatic infection with this organism closely mimics acute streptococcal pharyngitis. Rarely, *A haemolyticum* produces a membranous pharyngitis that can be confused with diphtheria. Two features of pharyngeal infection with this organism are notable. It has a predilection for adolescents and young adults, and it frequently provokes a generalized rash that may resemble that of scarlet fever [43–45]. The organism is detected more readily on human- than sheep-blood agar plates and thus may not be identified in the routine throat culture. Thus, the clinician should suspect *A haemolyticum* infection in a teenager or young adult who has an acute pharyngitis and scarlatiniform rash but a negative culture or RADT for GAS. Should antimicrobial therapy of a patient who has *A haemolyticum* pharyngitis be elected, a macrolide or, alternatively, a beta-lactam antimicrobial agent may be prescribed.

Neisseria gonorrhoeae. *Neisseria gonorrhoeae* is an uncommon, sexually transmitted cause of acute pharyngitis seen in persons who practice receptive oral sex. The risk of acquisition by this means is highest in men who have sex with men (MSM). Rates of pharyngeal gonorrhea in MSM have been reported as being as high as 15%. A recent study in San Francisco found *N gonorrhoeae* in the pharynx of 5.5% of MSM and concluded that the pharynx was the most common site of infection in this population [46]. Because of this high prevalence, the United States Centers for Disease Control and Prevention (CDC) guidelines for sexually transmitted diseases recommend a yearly pharyngeal test for *N gonorrhoeae* in MSM who receive oral intercourse [47]. Although the presence of gonorrhea in the pharynx is common, the occurrence of symptomatic pharyngitis is rare. In the above-mentioned San Francisco study, there was no association between the presence of *N gonorrhoeae* and pharyngeal symptoms.

When symptomatic oral infection does occur, pharyngitis and tonsillitis are the most common manifestations. Sore throat with an erythematous pharynx, bilateral tonsillar enlargement, at times with grayish-yellowish exudate, and occasionally with cervical lymphadenopathy have been reported [48]. Gingivitis and glossitis also have been described. The diagnosis should be confirmed by culture on Thayer-Martin medium. Currently, ceftriaxone (125 mg in a singular intramuscular dose) is the only CDC recommended therapy for uncomplicated pharyngeal gonorrhea. Concomitant therapy for chlamydia is recommended if this infection has not been ruled out.

Corynebacterium diphtheriae. Pharyngeal diphtheria is caused by *Corynebacterium diphtheriae*. Humans are the only reservoir of the organism. Asymptomatic carriers account for 3% to 5% of the population in endemic areas, and transmission occurs through respiratory secretions. Although diphtheria has become extremely rare in the United States and other developed countries with effective childhood immunization programs, there are reasons for the primary care physician and infectious disease specialist to be familiar with this disease. First, there have been a few indigenous cases in the United States in the last 10 years in unimmunized or underimmunized individuals in the lower socioeconomic groups [49]. Second, a large proportion of adults in North America and Western Europe lack protective serum levels of antitoxic immunity and are at risk for acquiring the infection when traveling to endemic areas. In 2003, a fatal case occurred in a Pennsylvania resident who traveled to Haiti to assist in building a church [50]. Epidemics of diphtheria involving thousands of cases occurred in the 1990s among residents of the newly independent countries of the former Soviet Union. Third, early diagnosis and treatment are important predictors of ultimate prognosis.

Respiratory diphtheria is typically caused by toxin-producing ("toxigenic") strains of *C diphtheriae* and rarely by toxigenic strains of *Corynebacterium ulcerans*. The main pathogenic factor is an exotoxin capable of producing a severe local reaction of the respiratory mucosa with the formation of a dense necrotic coagulum and pseudomembranes. These pseudomembranes can lead to airway obstruction resulting in suffocation and death. The toxin is also responsible for severe cardiac and neurologic complications [51].

The incubation period of 2 to 4 days is followed by malaise, sore throat, and low-grade fever. The most notable physical finding is the grayish-brown diphtheritic pseudomembrane that may involve one or both tonsils or may extend widely to involve the nares, uvula, soft palate, pharynx, larynx, and tracheobronchial tree. It is firmly adherent to the mucosa, and its removal provokes bleeding. In severe cases, there is swelling of the soft tissues of the neck ("bull neck"), cervical adenopathy, profound malaise, prostration, and stridor. Cardiac complications manifested as myocarditis with cardiac dysfunction occur in 10% to 25% of cases, usually when the pharyngeal manifestations are improving. Neurologic complications can occur also and are related directly to the severity of the primary infection, the immunization history, and the time between the onset of symptoms and institution of treatment.

The diagnosis of diphtheria requires a high index of suspicion and specific laboratory techniques. Diagnosis should be suspected on epidemiologic grounds and in the presence of pharyngitis with pseudomembranes, especially if extending to the uvula and soft palate and bleeding when dislodged. Plating on Loeffler's or Tindale's selective media can identify black colonies with metachromatic granules, but definitive diagnosis requires demonstration of toxin production by immunoprecipitation, polymerase chain reaction (PCR), or immunochromatography. Because successful treatment is inversely related to the duration of the disease, therapy should be started once the diagnosis seems likely on clinical grounds and while awaiting laboratory confirmation.

Treatment of diphtheria includes diphtheria antitoxin and antibiotics. Equine diphtheria antitoxin is only available through the National Immunization Program of the CDC. The therapeutic dose and mode of administration are recommended by the American Academy of Pediatrics according to the duration and extension of the disease [52]. Antibiotics are effective in decreasing local infection, decreasing toxin production, and decreasing spread. Intramuscular penicillin G, switched to oral penicillin V once the patient is able to swallow, and erythromycin are the antibiotics of choice. Respiratory diphtheria (in contrast to cutaneous diphtheria) does not induce protective immunity, so diphtheria toxoid should be administered to patients during convalescence. Prevention of transmission is crucial and is accomplished by strict isolation. Close contacts should be cultured and started on prophylactic antibiotics while awaiting culture results; if not fully immunized, they should receive diptheria toxoid. Both penicillin and erythromycin are efficacious in eradicating the carrier state, but erythromycin has been shown to be superior in some reports.

C ulcerans is an animal pathogen that causes bovine mastitis but can be transmitted to humans through the consumption of raw milk. It can produce diphtheritic toxin and a clinical disease undistinguishable from *C diphtheriae*.

Atypical bacteria

Mycoplasma pneumoniae and *Chlamydophila pneumoniae* are known causes of lower respiratory tract infections; they also can be found in the throats of patients who have symptomatic pharyngitis and of asymptomatic carriers. Although these agents probably cause some cases of acute pharyngitis, either as primary pathogens or copathogens, the frequency with which this occurs is still unclear. The pharyngeal manifestations that have been described include erythema, tonsillar enlargement, and, less often, exudate with cervical lymphadenopathy. In a recent Italian study, 133 children who had acute tonsillopharyngitis were tested for *M pneumoniae* and *C pneumoniae* with acute- and convalescent-phase titers and PCR on nasopharyngeal aspirates. Thirty-six of the children (27%) had serologically confirmed acute *M pneumoniae* infection, and 10 (7.5%) had serologically confirmed *C pneumoniae* infection. Five of the latter also had a positive nasopharyngeal PCR for this organism [53]. The children were assigned randomly to receive azithromycin plus symptomatic treatment or symptomatic treatment alone and were followed for 6 months. In the short term, there was no difference in the outcomes of children with or without atypical infection. A significantly decreased rate of recurrent upper and lower respiratory infections occurred in patients with atypical infections who were randomized to azithromycin, however. These results require confirmation.

Viral infections

Infectious mononucleosis

Clinical manifestations. Infectious mononucleosis (IM) or "glandular fever" is caused by the Epstein-Barr virus (EBV). The virus is present in the oropharyngeal secretions of patients who have IM and is spread by person-to-person contact. Infection with EBV is frequent in childhood but usually is asymptomatic. Clinical manifestations are more common when the infection is acquired in adolescence or young adulthood. Thus, most cases of IM occur between ages 15 and 24 years. Symptoms develop after an incubation period of 4 to 7 weeks. Following a 2- to 5-day prodromal period of chills, sweats, feverishness, and malaise, the disease presents with the classic triad of severe sore throat accompanied by fever as high as 38°C to 40°C and lymphadenopathy. Pharyngitis with associated tonsillitis occurs in 70% to 90% of the patients. Tonsillar exudates are present in approximately one third of cases, and palatal petechiae may also be present Lymphadenopathy is bilateral, particularly posterior cervical, but can involve axillary and inguinal areas. About 10% of patients have a rash of variable morphology, but administration of ampicillin or amoxicillin provokes a pruritic maculopapular eruption in 90% of patients. Hepatomegaly is present in 10% to 15% of patients who have IM, and splenomegaly occurs in almost half of the patients. This classic clinical presentation of IM occurs in most of the children and young adults. Older adults may not exhibit pharyngitis or lymphadenopathy, and disease can be manifested only with fever and more prominent hepatic abnormalities (typhoidal presentation) [54]. EBV infection can be complicated by a variety of neurologic and oncologic conditions that are beyond the scope of this article.

The hematologic findings include leukocytosis with 60% to 70% lymphocytosis and thrombocytopenia that usually is mild but occasionally may be severe. The lymphocytosis usually is found at presentation and peaks 2 to 3 weeks after onset of the disease. The presence of more than 10% atypical lymphocytes in peripheral blood is one of the characteristic features of IM and supports the diagnosis.

The differential diagnosis at initial presentation includes GAS pharyngitis, other respiratory viral infections (see Table 1), cytomegalovirus infection, and, if suggested by epidemiologic history, the acute retroviral syndrome (see later discussion). Rarely, entities such as toxoplasmosis, hepatitis A, human herpesvirus 6, and rubella must be considered. In most cases, the diagnosis is readily confirmed if suspected. Initial diagnostic studies should include throat culture or RADT for GAS and a serologic test for the presence of heterophile antibodies. The latter are antibodies directed against antigens in erythrocytes from different animal species. They are present in approximately 90% of affected adolescents and adults within the first 1 to 3 weeks of illness and may persist for up to 1 year. Spot and slide tests that use horse or purified bovine erythrocytes and allow rapid screening are commercially available. When combined with a compatible clinical presentation, a positive rapid test for heterophile antibodies can be considered diagnostic of IM. False-negative tests can occur in up to 10% of patients, however, especially in children and older adults and in the early stages of the disease.

Approximately 10% of patients who have a classic mononucleosis syndrome have negative tests for heterophile antibodies. In such patients, EBV-specific antibodies should be assayed. The most useful of these for general clinical purposes is the IgM antibody to viral capsid antigen. This test is present at clinical presentation and persists for 4 to 8 weeks. Antibody to Epstein-Barr nuclear antigen first appears 3 to 4 weeks after onset and persists for life [55].

Many patients who have heterophile-negative IM are found by the aforementioned tests to be infected with EBV. In the majority of the remainder, serologic studies confirm infection with cytomegalovirus, which can produce a syndrome closely mimicking that induced by EBV.

IM is predominantly a self-limited disease, and studies have failed to detect any benefit of using antiviral agents. Most symptoms resolve within 3 weeks of onset. Physical activity is tailored to patient tolerance. Because of the risk of splenic rupture, contact sports and heavy lifting should be avoided until the spleen returns to normal size, usually in approximately 3 to 4 weeks. The use of corticosteroids has been studied in clinical trials, but no clear benefit has been demonstrated [56,57]. Steroids, however, may be useful in the management of severe complications such as airway obstruction, hemolytic anemia, severe thrombocytopenia, and aplastic anemia.

HIV

Within days to weeks after initial infection with HIV type 1, 50% to 90% of patients develop a constellation of symptoms known as the "acute retroviral syndrome." Fever, sore throat, lymphadenopathy, maculopapular rash, myalgia, arthralgias, and mucocutaneous ulcerations are the landmarks of the syndrome [58–61]. A nonexudative pharyngitis is present in 50% to 70% of patients. Other oropharyngeal findings include ulcers and thrush. Oral ulcers, which occur in 10% to 20% of the patients, appear in the first days of the illness and last for approximately 1 week. Their distribution is usually in the inner lips and in the floor of the mouth, but tonsils, soft palate, and uvula also can be involved.

Fever occurs in almost 100% of patients who have acute retroviral syndrome, and it is usually high. Lymphadenopathy occurs in 40% to 70% of the patients, is nontender, usually develops after 1 week of illness, and involves cervical, axillary, and inguinal regions. Skin rash, which occurs in 40% to 50% of patients, usually is maculopapular, disseminated, and almost invariably involves the neck and upper trunk. The rash usually spares the distal extremities, although palms and soles can be affected.

The clinical findings of fever, pharyngitis, and lymphadenopathy may simulate IM. Atypical lymphocytosis, although infrequent, also could lead to a misdiagnosis of mononucleosis. Acute retroviral syndrome can be differentiated from mononucleosis, however, by its more acute onset, the absence of exudate or prominent tonsillar hypertrophy, the frequent occurrence of rash (rare in mononucleosis except after treatment with ampicillin or amoxicillin), and the presence of oral ulcerations (Table 4) [62].

It is important for the clinician to recognize that the ELISA commonly used to diagnose HIV-1 infection are negative in the first 3 to 4 weeks after infection and therefore are not useful in this setting. Tests for p24 antigen or, preferably, quantitative assays for plasma HIV RNA by branched chain

Table 4
Differentiating clinical features of infectious mononucleosis and acute retroviral infection

	Infectious mononucleosis	Acute HIV infection
Onset	Insidious	Acute
Exudate	Often present	Absent
Maculopapular rash	Rare, unless provoked by antibiotics	40%–50%
Oral ulcerations	Absent	10%–20%
Diarrhea	Rare	Common

Data from Refs. [52,55,59].

DNA or PCR should be performed. The viral load can be anticipated to be very high during this acute phase of infection. An HIV antibody test always should be performed later in time to confirm the diagnosis.

Treatment of acute retroviral syndrome with highly active antiretroviral medication has been controversial, current recommendations consider the use of antiretroviral medications in the setting of acute HIV infection to be optional [63]. Potential benefits of antiretroviral therapy in acute HIV would be to decrease the severity of acute disease and to decrease viral replication. Studies have demonstrated improvement of laboratory markers of disease progression when highly active antiretroviral therapy is used in acute HIV infection [64,65]. These results would suggest a decrease in progression and transmission of the disease. Treating acute HIV infection, however, also can have potential risks, including known side effects to medications, possible development of resistance, and adverse effects on quality of life. If the patient and clinician elect to start antiretroviral medications, the goal should be suppression of viral replication.

Other viral infections

Whereas most respiratory viruses can cause symptoms indistinguishable from the common cold or acute pharyngitis, some viruses may produce more distinctive clinical syndromes.

Adenovirus. Adenovirus is a common cause of viral pharyngitis. It is manifested clinically as an upper respiratory infection with fever, cough, rhinorrhea, and sore throat, usually more pronounced than in the common cold. The pharynx is erythematous and frequently may have exudates that mimic streptococcal pharyngitis [66]. A distinctive syndrome associated with adenovirus infection in children is pharyngoconjunctival fever. The disease occurs in outbreaks and is characterized by conjunctivitis, pharyngitis, rhinitis, cervical adenitis, and high fever. Although adenoviral infections commonly occur in winter months, pharyngoconjuntival fever has been implicated in outbreaks in summer camps [67] and associated with contaminated swimming pools and ponds. Several types of adenovirus also have been implicated in outbreaks of influenza-like illnesses with sore throat, rhinorrhea, and tracheobronchitis, known as acute respiratory disease of army recruits [68,69]. These infections are self limited, and symptomatic treatment alone is recommended.

Coxsackie virus. Most enteroviral infections occur in the summer and fall and present as febrile illnesses with sore throat, cough, or coryza. Distinctive manifestations of enteroviral infection are herpangina and hand-foot-and-mouth disease. Herpangina most often is caused by coxsackie A and is most frequent in infants or young children. It usually presents acutely with fever, sore throat, odynophagia, diffuse pharyngeal erythema, and a vesicular enanthem. Headache and vomiting can be preceding symptoms. The oral lesions consist of 1- to 2-mm gray-white papulovesicles that progress to ulcers on an erythematous base and may be present on the soft palate, uvula, and anterior tonsillar pillars [70]. They are moderately painful and usually number less than a dozen. Hand-foot-and-mouth disease also is caused by coxsackie A. It is characterized by a febrile vesicular stomatitis with associated exanthema. The oral findings include small, painful vesicles in the buccal mucosa and tongue that can coalesce and form ulcerative bullae. The lesions are similar to those seen in herpangina, but there is an associated peripheral rash involving hands and feet that can extend proximally. These coxsackie diseases are self limited, and treatment is symptomatic.

Herpes simplex virus. Several studies have documented primary human herpes simplex (HSV) type 1 infection as a cause of pharyngitis in college students [71,72]. HSV2 occasionally can cause a similar illness as a consequence of oral–genital contact [73]. This form of pharyngitis represents primary infection in immunocompetent patients but can occur as a reactivation of latent virus in immunocompromised hosts. Although the characteristic presentation consists of small vesicles and ulcerations in the posterior pharynx and tonsils, HSV also may produce pharyngeal erythema and exudates at times indistinguishable from strep throat. Lesions may extend to the palate, gingiva, tongue, lip, and face. General symptoms include fever, malaise, inability to eat, and cervical lymphadenopathy. Treatment of HSV oral infection with antiherpetic medication is efficacious in reducing the duration of signs and symptoms as well as viral shedding. Acyclovir, valcyclovir, and famciclovir are all useful in treating HSV infection.

Symptomatic treatment of pharyngitis

Acetaminophen or nonsteroidal anti-inflammatory drugs are effective analgesics and antipyretics. Treatment should be started as soon as symptoms develop and is useful in both viral and bacterial diseases. Oral hydration and gargles with salt water may help alleviate the pharyngeal complaints. Oral cough suppressants, decongestants, and antihistamines are helpful, depending on the symptoms present. Lozenges containing local anesthetics are widely available over the counter and seem to provide temporary relief of sore throat [74,75]. Several authors have reported that adjuvant therapy with dexamethasone decreases the duration of throat pain in patients who have severe odynophagia [76–78]. The regimens used and the magnitude of the effect varied among the studies. No adverse effects have been reported, but duration of follow-up often has been limited. One randomized, double-blind, placebo-controlled trial of adjuvant dexamethasone therapy in children found efficacy only in patients who had RADT-positive pharyngitis, and the benefit was judged to be only "of marginal clinical importance" [79]. The authors do not recommend use of corticosteroids in the therapy of GAS pharyngitis.

Epiglottitis

Acute epiglottitis or supraglottitis is an inflammatory process of the epiglottis and adjacent structures that can lead to life-threatening acute respiratory obstruction. In the past, epiglottitis occurred most frequently in children between 2 and 4 years of age and was associated mainly with *Haemophilus influenzae* type B (Hib) infection. Since the initiation of the childhood vaccination programs, epiglottitis caused by this organism is much less common. Nevertheless, there are still cases of Hib epiglottitis in both immunized and nonimmunized children, and the possibility of an infection with this pathogen cannot be excluded completely in vaccinated patients [80,81]. Bacteria associated with epiglottitis nowadays include *Streptococcus pneumoniae, Staphylococcus aureus*, and beta hemolytic streptococci. Multiple agents including other bacteria, viruses, and fungi have been implicated in rare cases. The typical presentation in children includes fever, irritability, sore throat, and rapidly progressive stridor with respiratory distress. The affected child adopts a forward-leaning position, drooling oral secretions while trying to breathe. Adults usually present with sore throat and a milder disease, although airway compromise can occur also. Physical examination of patients suspected of having epiglottitis requires careful inspection of the oropharyngeal and suprapharyngeal area. The diagnosis requires direct visualization of an erythematous and swollen epiglottis under laryngoscopy. Because of the risk of airway obstruction, this procedure should be performed in children only when skilled personnel and equipment to secure the airway are available [82]. Once the airway has been secured, culture of the surface of the epiglottis along with blood cultures should be obtained to guide antibiotic therapy. Management focuses on two important aspects: close monitoring of the airway with intubation if necessary and treatment with intravenous antibiotics. Because of the aforementioned possibility of failure of vaccination, antibiotics should be directed against Hib in every patient regardless of immunization status. Cefotaxime, ceftriaxone, or ampicillin/sulbactam are appropriate choices. Steroids are used commonly in the management of acute epiglottitis although no randomized trial has been done to support this practice. When a case of Hib epiglottitis is diagnosed, the American Academy of Pediatrics recommends that postexposure prophylaxis with rifampin be given to household contacts when there is at least one child in the household younger than 4 years of age, a child in the household younger than 12 months of age who has not received the primary series of Hib vaccine, or an immunosuppressed child, regardless of that child's Hib immunization status [83].

Summary

Acute pharyngitis is an extremely common disorder that usually runs a benign course. In almost all cases, the primary care physician must discriminate between a viral sore throat, which requires only symptomatic management, and GAS pharyngitis, which requires specific antimicrobial therapy. This distinction is important so that GAS pharyngitis can be treated appropriately to minimize the risk of suppurative and nonsuppurative complications. Equally important is minimizing unnecessary and potentially deleterious overtreatment of viral infections with antimicrobial agents. This article has outlined the epidemiologic, clinical, and laboratory findings that assist in decision making. The clinician also must be alert to the occurrence of rare but serious upper respiratory infections that may be life threatening and require special forms of therapy (eg, diphtheria, parapharyngeal suppurative processes, acute epiglottitis).

References

[1] Snow V, Mottur-Pilson C, Cooper RJ, et al. Principles of appropriate antibiotic use of acute pharyngitis in adults. Ann Intern Med 2001;134:506–8.
[2] Linder JA, Bates DW, Lee GM, et al. Antibiotic treatment of children with sore throat. JAMA 2005;294(18):2315–22.
[3] Linder JA, Stafford RS. Antibiotic treatment of adults with sore throat by community primary care physicians: a national survey, 1989–1999. JAMA 2001;286(10):1181–6.
[4] Gwaltney JM. Clinical significance and pathogenesis of viral respiratory infections. Am J Med 2002;112(Suppl 6A):13S–18S.
[5] Banham TM. A collaborative study of the aetiology of acute respiratory infection in Britain 1961-4. A report of the Medical Research Council working party on acute respiratory virus infections. BMJ 1965;2(5457):319–26.
[6] Gwaltney JM Jr. Virology of middle ear. Ann Otol Rhinol Laryngol 1971;80(3):365–70.
[7] Hamre D, Connelly AP Jr, Procknow JJ. Virologic studies of acute respiratory disease in young adults. IV. Virus isolations during four years of surveillance. Am J Epidemiol 1966; 83(2):238–49.
[8] Monto AS, Ullman BM. Acute respiratory illness in an American community. The Tecumseh study. JAMA 1974;227(2):164–9.
[9] Evans AS, Dick EC. Acute pharyngitis and tonsillitis in University of Wisconsin students. JAMA 1964;190:699–708.
[10] Glezen WP, Clyde WAJ, Senior RJ, et al. Group A streptococci, mycoplasmas, and viruses associated with acute pharyngitis. JAMA 1967;202:455–60.
[11] Gwaltney JMJ, Bisno AL. Pharyngitis. In: Mandell GL, Bennett JE, Dolin R, editors. Principles and practice of infectious diseases. Philadelphia: Churchill Livingstone; 2000. p. 656–62.
[12] Kaplan EL, Top FH Jr, Dudding BA, et al. Diagnosis of streptococcal pharyngitis: differentiation of active infection from the carrier state in the symptomatic child. J Infect Dis 1971; 123:490–501.
[13] McIsaac WJ, White D, Tannenbaum D, et al. A clinical score to reduce unnecessary antibiotic use in patients with sore throat. Can Med Assoc J 1998;158(1):75–83.
[14] Komaroff AL, Pass TM, Aronson MD, et al. The prediction of streptococcal pharyngitis in adults. J Gen Intern Med 1986;1:1–7.
[15] Peter GS, Bisno AL. Group A streptococcal pharyngitis in adults. In: Pechere JC, Kaplan EL, editors. Streptococcal pharyngitis. Basel (Switzerland): Karger; 2004.
[16] Centor RM, Witherspoon JM, Dalton HP, et al. The diagnosis of strep throat in adults in the emergency room. Med Decis Making 1981;1(3):239–46.
[17] Wald ER, Green MD, Schwartz B, et al. A streptococcal score card revisited. Pediatr Emerg Care 1998;14(2):109–11.

[18] McIsaac WJ, Kellner JD, Aufricht P, et al. Empirical validation of guidelines for the management of pharyngitis in children and adults. JAMA 2004;291(13):1587–95.
[19] Stillerman M, Bernstein SH. Streptococcal pharyngitis: evaluation of clinical syndromes in diagnosis. Am J Dis Child 1961;101:476–89.
[20] Cooper RJ, Hoffman JR, Bartlett JG, et al. Principles of appropriate antibiotic use for acute pharyngitis in adults: background. Ann Emerg Med 2001;37(6):711–9.
[21] Neuner JM, Hamel MB, Phillips RS, et al. A cost-effectiveness analysis of diagnosis and management of adults with pharyngitis. Ann Intern Med 2003;139:113–22.
[22] Bisno AL. Diagnosing strep throat in the adult patient: do clinical criteria really suffice? Ann Intern Med 2003;139(2):150–1.
[23] Catanzaro FJ, Stetson CA, Morris AJ, et al. The role of streptococcus in the pathogenesis of rheumatic fever. Am J Med 1954;17:749–56.
[24] Gerber MA, Shulman ST. Rapid diagnosis of pharyngitis caused by group A streptococci. Clin Microbiol Rev 2004;17(3):571–80.
[25] Bisno AL, Gerber MA, Gwaltney JM Jr, et al. Practice guidelines for the diagnosis and management of group A streptococcal pharyngitis. Infectious Diseases Society of America. Clin Infect Dis 2002;35(2):113–25.
[26] Humair JP, Revaz SA, Bovier P, et al. Management of acute pharyngitis in adults: reliability of rapid streptococcal tests and clinical findings. Arch Intern Med 2006;166(6):640–4.
[27] Gerber MA. Treatment failures and carriers: perception or problems? Pediatr Infect Dis J 1994;13:576–9.
[28] Del Mar CB, Glasziou PP, Spinks AB. Antibiotics for sore throat. Cochrane Database Syst Rev 2006;(4):CD000023.
[29] Bisno AL. Are cephalosporins superior to penicillin for treatment of acute streptococcal pharyngitis? Clin Infect Dis 2004;38(11):1535–7.
[30] Dajani A, Taubert K, Ferrieri P, et al. Treatment of acute streptococcal pharyngitis and prevention of rheumatic fever: a statement for health professionals. Committee on Rheumatic Fever, Endocarditis, and Kawasaki Disease of the Council on Cardiovascular Disease in the Young, the American Heart Association. Pediatrics 1995;96(4 Pt 1):758–64.
[31] Committee on Infectious Diseases. Group A streptococcal infections. In: Pickering LK, editor. 2003 red book. Elk Grove Village (IL): American Academy of Pediatrics; 2003. p. 573–84.
[32] Feder HMJ, Gerber MA, Randolph MF, et al. Once-daily therapy for streptococcal pharyngitis with amoxicillin. Pediatrics 1999;103(1):47–51.
[33] Gopichand I, Williams GD, Medendorp SV, et al. Randomized, single-blinded comparative study of the efficacy of amoxicillin (40 mg/kg/day) versus standard-dose penicillin V in the treatment of group A streptococcal pharyngitis in children. Clin Pediatr (Phila) 1998; 37(6):341–6.
[34] Shvartzman P, Tabenkin H, Rosentzwaig A, et al. Treatment of streptococcal pharyngitis with amoxycillin once a day. BMJ 1993;306:1170–2.
[35] Brook I. Microbiology and management of peritonsillar, retropharyngeal, and parapharyngeal abscesses. J Oral Maxillofac Surg 2004;62(12):1545–50.
[36] Shoemaker M, Lampe RM, Weir MR. Peritonsillitis: abscess of cellulitis? Pediatr Infect Dis J 1986;5:435–9.
[37] Snow DG, Campbell JB, Morgan DW. The microbiology of peritonsillar sepsis. J Laryngol Otol 1991;105(7):553–5.
[38] Chirinos JA, Lichtstein DM, Garcia J, et al. The evolution of Lemierre syndrome: report of 2 cases and review of the literature. Medicine (Baltimore) 2002;81(6):458–65.
[39] Baracco GJ, Bisno AL, et al. Group C and group G streptococcal infections: epidemiologic and clinical aspects. In: Fischetti VA, Novick RP, Ferreti JJ, editors. Gram positive pathogens. Washington, DC: ASM Press; 2006. p. 222–9.
[40] Turner JC, Hayden FG, Lobo MC, et al. Epidemiologic evidence for Lancefield group C beta-hemolytic streptococci as a cause of exudative pharyngitis in college students. J Clin Microbiol 1997;35(1):1–4.

[41] Meier FA, Centor RM, Graham L Jr, et al. Clinical and microbiological evidence for endemic pharyngitis among adults due to group C streptococci. Arch Intern Med 1990;150: 825–9.
[42] Gerber MA, Randolph MF, Martin NJ, et al. Community-wide outbreak of group G streptococcal pharyngitis. Pediatrics 1991;87(5):598–603.
[43] Karpathios T, Drakonaki S, Zervoudaki A, et al. *Arcanobacterium haemolyticum* in children with presumed streptococcal pharyngotonsillitis or scarlet fever. J Pediatr 1992; 121:735–7.
[44] Mackenzie A, Fuite LA, Chan FT, et al. Incidence and pathogenicity of *Arcanobacterium haemolyticum* during a 2-year study in Ottawa. Clin Infect Dis 1995;21:177–81.
[45] Miller RA, Brancato F, Holmes KK. *Corynebacterium hemolyticum* as a cause of pharyngitis and scarlatiniform rash in young adults. Ann Intern Med 1986;105:867–72.
[46] Morris SR, Klausner JD, Buchbinder SP, et al. Prevalence and incidence of pharyngeal gonorrhea in a longitudinal sample of men who have sex with men: the EXPLORE study. Clin Infect Dis 2006;43(10):1284–9.
[47] Workowski KA, Berman SM. Sexually transmitted diseases treatment guidelines, 2006. MMWR Recomm Rep 2006;55(RR-11):1–94.
[48] Balmelli C, Gunthard HF. Gonococcal tonsillar infection–a case report and literature review. Infection 2003;31(5):362–5.
[49] Centers for Disease Control and Prevention (CDC). Status report on the Childhood Immunization Initiative: reported cases of selected vaccine-preventable diseases–United States, 1996. MMWR Morb Mortal Wkly Rep 1997;46(29):665–71.
[50] Centers for Disease Control and Prevention (CDC). Fatal respiratory diphtheria in a U.S. traveler to Haiti–Pennsylvania, 2003. MMWR Morb Mortal Wkly Rep 2004;52(53):1285–6.
[51] MacGregor RR. Corynebacteria diphtheriae. In: Mandell GL, Bennett JE, Dolan R, editors. Principles and practice of infectious diseases. 6th edition. Philadelphia: Elsevier Churchill Livingstone; 2005. p. 2457–65.
[52] Committee on Infectious Diseases. Diphtheria. In: Pickering LK, editor. Red book: 2006 report of the Committee on Infectious Diseases. Elk Grove (IL): American Academy of Pediatrics; 2006. p. 263–6.
[53] Esposito S, Bosis S, Begliatti E, et al. Acute tonsillopharyngitis associated with atypical bacterial infection in children: natural history and impact of macrolide therapy. Clin Infect Dis 2006;43(2):206–9.
[54] Auwaerter PG. Infectious mononucleosis in middle age. JAMA 1999;281(5):454–9.
[55] Johannsen EC, Schooley RT, Kaye KM. Epstein-Barr Virus (infectious mononucleosis). In: Mandell GL, Bennett JE, Dolin R, editors. Principles and practice of infectious diseases. 6th edition. Philadelphia: Elsevier Churchill Livingstone; 2005. p. 1801–20.
[56] Straus SE, Cohen JI, Tosato G, et al. NIH conference. Epstein-Barr virus infections: biology, pathogenesis, and management. Ann Intern Med 1993;118(1):45–58.
[57] Candy B, Hotopf M. Steroids for symptom control in infectious mononucleosis. Cochrane Database Syst Rev 2006;3:CD004402.
[58] Kahn JO, Walker BD. Acute human immunodeficiency virus type 1 infection. N Engl J Med 1998;339(1):33–9.
[59] Cooper DA, Gold J, Maclean P, et al. Acute AIDS retrovirus infection. Definition of a clinical illness associated with seroconversion. Lancet 1985;1(8428):537–40.
[60] Hare C, Kahn J. Primary HIV infection. Curr Infect Dis Rep 2004;6:65–71.
[61] Sun HY, Chen MJ, Hung CC, et al. Clinical presentations and virologic characteristics of primary human immunodeficiency virus type-1 infection in a university hospital in Taiwan. J Microbiol Immunol Infect 2004;37(5):271–5.
[62] Gaines H, von Sydow M, Pehrson P, et al. Clinical picture of HIV infection presenting as a glandular-fever-like illness. BMJ 1988;297:1363–8.
[63] Smith DE, Walker BD, Cooper DA, et al. Is antiretroviral treatment of primary HIV infection clinically justified on the basis of current evidence? AIDS 2004;18(5):709–18.

[64] Hoen B, Dumon B, Harzic M, et al. Highly active antiretroviral treatment initiated early in the course of symptomatic primary HIV-1 infection: results of the ANRS 053 trial. J Infect Dis 1999;180(4):1342–6.
[65] Malhotra U, Berrey MM, Huang Y, et al. Effect of combination antiretroviral therapy on T-cell immunity in acute human immunodeficiency virus type 1 infection. J Infect Dis 2000;181(1):121–31.
[66] Dominguez O, Rojo P, de Las HS, et al. Clinical presentation and characteristics of pharyngeal adenovirus infections. Pediatr Infect Dis J 2005;24(8):733–4.
[67] Centers for Disease Control and Prevention (CDC). Outbreak of pharyngoconjunctival fever at a summer camp–North Carolina, 1991. MMWR Morb Mortal Wkly Rep 1992; 41(19):342–4.
[68] Hendrix RM, Lindner JL, Benton FR, et al. Large, persistent epidemic of adenovirus type 4-associated acute respiratory disease in U.S. army trainees. Emerg Infect Dis 1999; 5(6):798–801.
[69] Kolavic-Gray SA, Binn LN, Sanchez JL, et al. Large epidemic of adenovirus type 4 infection among military trainees: epidemiological, clinical, and laboratory studies. Clin Infect Dis 2002;35(7):808–18.
[70] Scott LA, Stone MS. Viral exanthems. Dermatol Online J 2003;9(3):4.
[71] McMillan JA, Weiner LB, Higgins AM, et al. Pharyngitis associated with herpes simplex virus in college students. Pediatr Infect Dis J 1993;12:280–4.
[72] Glezen WP, Fernald GW, Lohr JA. Acute respiratory disease of university students with special reference to the etiologic role of *Herpesvirus hominis*. Am J Epidemiol 1975;101: 111–21.
[73] Young EJ, Vainrub B, Musher DM, et al. Acute pharyngotonsillitis caused by herpesvirus type 2. JAMA 1978;239:1885–6.
[74] Fischer J, Pschorn U, Vix JM, et al. Efficacy and tolerability of ambroxol hydrochloride lozenges in sore throat. Randomised, double-blind, placebo-controlled trials regarding the local anaesthetic properties. Arzneimittelforschung 2002;52(4):256–63.
[75] Schachtel BP, Homan HD, Gibb IA, et al. Demonstration of dose response of flurbiprofen lozenges with the sore throat pain model. Clin Pharmacol Ther 2002;71(5):375–80.
[76] Wei JL, Kasperbauer JL, Weaver AL, et al. Efficacy of single-dose dexamethasone as adjuvant therapy for acute pharyngitis. Laryngoscope 2002;112(1):87–93.
[77] Olympia RP, Khine H, Avner JR. Effectiveness of oral dexamethasone in the treatment of moderate to severe pharyngitis in children. Arch Pediatr Adolesc Med 2005;159(3): 278–82.
[78] Niland ML, Bonsu BK, Nuss KE, et al. A pilot study of 1 versus 3 days of dexamethasone as add-on therapy in children with streptococcal pharyngitis. Pediatr Infect Dis J 2006;25(6): 477–81.
[79] Bulloch B, Kabani A, Tenenbein M. Oral dexamethasone for the treatment of pain in children with acute pharyngitis: a randomized, double-blind, placebo-controlled trial. Ann Emerg Med 2003;41(5):601–8.
[80] Gonzalez VH, Wald ER, Rose E, et al. Epiglottitis and Haemophilus influenzae immunization: the Pittsburgh experience–a five-year review. Pediatrics 1995;96(3 Pt 1): 424–7.
[81] McEwan J, Giridharan W, Clarke RW, et al. Paediatric acute epiglottitis: not a disappearing entity. Int J Pediatr Otorhinolaryngol 2003;67(4):317–21.
[82] Rafei K, Lichenstein R. Airway infectious disease emergencies. Pediatr Clin North Am 2006; 53(2):215–42.
[83] Committee on Infectious Diseases. Haemophilus influenzae. In: Pickering LK, editor. Red book: 2006 report of the committee on infectious diseases. Elk Grove Village (IL): American Academy of Pediatrics; 2006. p. 310–3.

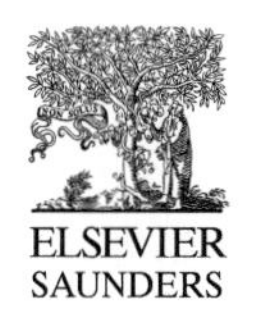

ELSEVIER
SAUNDERS

Infect Dis Clin N Am 21 (2007) 471–502

INFECTIOUS
DISEASE CLINICS
OF NORTH AMERICA

Dental Caries and Periodontitis: Contrasting Two Infections That Have Medical Implications

Walter Loesche, DMD, PhD[a,b,*]

[a]*Department of Biological and Materials Science, School of Dentistry, University of Michigan, Room 3209, Ann Arbor, MI 48109, USA*
[b]*Department of Microbiology and Immunology, School of Medicine, University of Michigan, Ann Arbor, MI, USA*

What a difference a century makes! At the beginning of the twentieth century almost every adult and child experienced painful tooth infections (dental caries) that resulted in about 60% of the population eventually losing all 32 teeth. Dental schools were newly opened at most medical centers to deal with this seeming overwhelming public health problem. Now, at the beginning of the twenty-first century, dental caries is no longer a public health problem; nine dental schools have closed their doors, and most others have downsized. Today all individuals can expect to retain most, if not all, of their teeth for a lifetime. What happened?

A caries epidemic, caused by *Streptococcus mutans*, had been contained by a variety of factors that appeared in the late twentieth century, not the least of which was fluoride in drinking water and in dentifrices. This epidemic had been triggered in the late nineteenth century by the widespread availability of low-cost sugar (sucrose) in the diet. Candies permitted the long-term bioavailability of sucrose in the oral cavity, which allowed one group of bacteria, namely the mutans streptococci, to expand their niche on the tooth surfaces. This expansion was associated with acid production and prolonged pH drops on the tooth surfaces, which caused the teeth to dissolve and resulted in widespread destruction of the tooth surfaces known as "dental caries."

There are more than 500 bacterial species resident in the human oral cavity [1,2], but only a few aciduric species contribute to the caries process [3], and

* Department of Biological and Materials Science, School of Dentistry, University of Michigan, Room 3209, Ann Arbor, MI 48109.
E-mail address: wloesche@umich.edu

0891-5520/07/$ - see front matter
doi:10.1016/j.idc.2007.03.006

a limited number of proteolytic species contribute to the other infection of the teeth, periodontal disease [4]. The scientists in the nineteenth century could not have comprehended this diversity of flora or the specific role of a limited number of bacterial species in decay and periodontal disease. Accordingly they concluded that dental infections were caused by the overgrowth of bacteria on the tooth surfaces [5] and essentially were bacteriologically nonspecific. The aim of treatment was to have a "clean tooth." This belief has had an enduring effect on dental treatment, because to this day plaque control is the dominant goal of clinical dentistry and serves as the basis for a successful business model, namely periodic cleaning of the teeth over a lifetime.

Such is the influence of myths, because there is little evidence that plaque control truly prevents either dental caries or periodontal disease [6,7]. On the contrary, more than 1000 publications in the last 45 years indicate that both dental caries and periodontal disease are diagnosable and treatable chronic infections.

Medical implications of dental infections

The teeth are not isolated from the rest of the body. In 1989 Finnish investigators reported that poor dental health could be associated with both acute myocardial infarctions [8] and cerebrovascular accidents [9]. These investigators developed a measurement of dental disease, called the "total dental index," that documented the number of missing, decayed, and/or periodontally involved teeth. Subsequently, in a 7-year prospective study, the total dental index ($P = .007$) and the number of previous myocardial infarctions ($P = .003$) were associated with a risk of developing a new and often fatal myocardial infarction [10]. Traditional risk factors such as diabetes, hypertension, smoking, total cholesterol levels, high-density lipoprotein cholesterol levels, triglyceride levels, socioeconomic status, gender, and age were not significant predictors of a coronary event. This is the only longitudinal study that has shown that dental infections actually predicted an adverse medical outcome and as such would indicate that dental infections are a true risk factor for acute myocardial infarction.

Other studies have confirmed this link between dental disease and coronary heart disease. A prospective cohort design study involving data for 9760 men in the United States who were examined three times between 1971 and 1987 found a slight but significant relationship between either periodontitis or edentulism (missing all teeth) and coronary heart disease after adjusting for 13 known risk factors [11]. A representative sample of 1384 Finnish men, 45 to 64 years old, showed that the number of missing teeth, along with hypertension, geographic area, and educational level, were independent explanatory factors for the presence of ischemic heart disease [12]. In United States military veterans, a significant association between periodontal disease and coronary heart disease and stroke could be demonstrated after adjusting for various cardiovascular risk factors [13]. The dental parameter(s) measured in these studies were not a rigorous indicator of disease (ie, in some cases, the subjects simply were asked if they had periodontal disease [14] or how many teeth they had lost before age 35 years [12]). The analyses were always post facto. One group of investigators looking at the same National Health and Nutrition Examination Survey (NHANES) data set found a connection [11], but another group reported no connection [15] between dental disease and coronary artery disease.

Other medical conditions have been associated with dental diseases (Table 1). Preterm birth of low birth weight infants has been highly associated with maternal periodontal disease and especially with plaque levels of the gram-negative species, *Treponema denticola, Porphyromonas gingivalis, Tannerella forsythia*, and *Actinobacillus actinomycetemcomitans* [16]. An intervention study involving topical chlorhexidine applications to the mother's teeth in the second trimester significantly reduced the number of preterm births [17], whereas a larger study using traditional débridement procedures was without any effect [18].

Perhaps the most tantalizing association was the reported loss of teeth before age 35 years and the subsequent development of Alzheimer's disease [19]. This study compared a variety of medical, demographic, social, and other variables as predictors of subsequent dementia, including Alzheimer's disease, among a large cohort of Scandinavian twins. Among identical twins, the twin with dementia was four times more likely to have worse oral health, as measured by the number of teeth lost before age 35 years.

Possible mechanisms linking dental infections and medical conditions

Periodontal disease

Although no direct link between dental disease and cardiovascular pathology has been demonstrated, there is evidence that dental infections contribute to the overall inflammatory milieu of the host by causing asymptomatic bacteremias [20], endotoxemia [21], a generalized increase in white blood cell counts [22], a generalized increase in inflammatory

Table 1
Medical conditions in which dental infections may be contributory

Medical condition	Dental risk indicator
Preterm births	Periodontal infections (gram-negative anaerobes)
Cerebral vascular accident	Periodontal infections (gram-negative anaerobes)
Coronary artery disease	Periodontal infections (gram-negative anaerobes); Tooth loss
Diabetes	Periodontal infections (gram-negative anaerobes)
Alzheimer's disease	Tooth loss before age 35 years

mediators, such as C-reactive protein (CRP) [23], and possibly specific effects on coagulation [24].

Periodontal infections raise the serum levels of CRP [23,25]. Among subjects participating in the NHANES study, those who had periodontal disease had significantly higher levels of CRP than subjects without periodontal disease [23]. Thirty-eight percent of the subjects who had periodontal disease had CRP levels of 10 mg/L or higher, the level which indicates significant inflammatory disease. CRP can be provoked by lipopolysaccharides (LPS), and almost all of the periodontopathogens are gram-negative anaerobes [4]. The presence of bacteria that possess a trypsinlike enzyme, benzoyl-DL-arginine naphthylamide (BANA), was associated with significantly higher CRP plasma levels after controlling for other risk factors for elevated CRP levels [26]. Higher levels of endotoxin (LPS) can be detected in the blood stream of subjects who had periodontal disease than in subjects who do not have periodontal disease 5 to 10 minutes after chewing gums [21]. The DNA of periodontopathogens as well as medically important pathogens can be detected in atheromas removed at endarterectomy [27,28].

The gram-negative bacteria penetrate the gingival epithelium in small numbers, and their LPS, either attached to cell remnants, or free in the tissues or blood stream, activates a variety of cells, especially monocytes, releasing cytokines (Fig. 1). These cytokines act on the liver, producing an acute-phase response that is dominated by CRP. Thus periodontal infections contribute to the individual's CRP pool. This finding suggests that

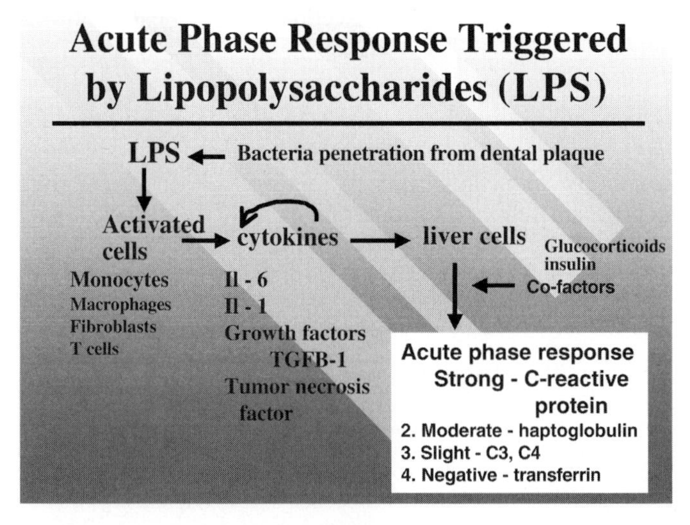

Fig. 1. Role of lipopolysaccharide (LPS) from gram-negative bacteria in gingival tissues triggering the acute-phase response with release of various proinflammatory cytokines. C3, complement 3; C4, complement 4: Il, interleukin; TGFB, transforming growth factor.

treatment of periodontal disease could result in reductions in serum CRP levels, and, indeed, intervention studies have shown that significant reduction in CRP levels occurs as a result of periodontal treatment [29–31].

Missing teeth

The relationship between missing teeth and medical conditions is equivocal. If the teeth were lost because of pulpal or periodontal inflammation, then the loss of the teeth would remove this provocation to the host, and one might expect to see the dental contributions to the inflammatory milieu diminish. This situation seems to be true in older individuals, in whom there is no connection between missing teeth and medical conditions [32]; but in individuals under the age of 50 years, missing teeth can be associated with several medical conditions (see Table 1) [33]. This evidence suggests that the inflammatory challenge from these teeth was so great that most of the cardiovascular damage occurred before their extraction.

Missing teeth can contribute to medical diseases through malnutrition. Edentulous individuals, even those who have dentures and other prosthetic devices, do not masticate as well as individuals who have a natural dentition. Elderly persons (60 years of age or older) who had reduced numbers of functional teeth tended to report difficulty chewing, avoidance of stringy foods (including meat), of crunchy foods (including vegetables), and of dry solid foods (including breads), and difficulty in swallowing. These difficulties could cause food choices high in empty calories, leading to obesity, diabetes, and high cholesterol levels. Removable prostheses did not seem to prevent these consequences and did not seem to be equivalent to natural teeth in masticatory potential [34]. Any impairment in mastication could contribute to systemic disease simply by contributing to some form of malnutrition.

The myth of plaque control

Legacy of the nonspecific plaque hypothesis

Dental decay is caused by the dissolution of tooth mineral (hydroxyapatite, $Ca_{10}[PO_4]_6[OH]_2$) by acids derived from bacterial fermentation of sucrose and other dietary carbohydrates. The connection between dietary carbohydrates and bacteria was the basis of a nineteenth-century theory regarding the causation of caries known as the "chemoparasitic theory" [5]. Miller, its chief proponent, was unable to find any consistent microbial association with the carious lesion and concluded that decay was bacteriologically nonspecific (ie, the nonspecific plaque hypothesis) [35]. He noted that decay occurred almost uniformly in the retentive areas of the tooth, such as the occlusal fissures on the tops of the teeth, and in the approximal surfaces where the teeth made contact with each other. He advocated keeping these areas clean of plaque accumulations, which translated clinically to tooth brushing with abrasive powders and dentifrices and to annual or biannual dental cleanings by the dentist called "dental prophys." No preventive benefit of this nonspecific plaque approach was ever shown until the 1960s, when fluoride was added to toothpastes.

Before 1960 the nonspecific plaque approach actually contributed to the prevalence of dental caries in that sucrose was added to toothpaste to improve its taste. The toothpaste therefore provided a nutrient that selected for the mutans streptococci and allowed this cariogen to become dominate on the tooth surfaces. The prevalence of dental decay and missing teeth was so high in the twentieth century that it was the major cause of young men being rejected for military service in World War I, World War II, and the Korean War [5]. This staggering amount of dental morbidity led to a national effort in the 1960s to increase dental manpower with new schools and the enlargement of existing facilities. Projections indicated that almost all individuals, if they lived long enough, would be edentulous (toothless), and that the cost of dental health would rival those of medically important diseases such as diabetes. (Fortunately, the dire projections about edentulousness did not materialize, but the cost of dental care was more than $50 billion dollars per year in 2005.)

Another legacy of the nonspecific plaque hypothesis delayed the understanding of dental infections, especially periodontal infections. Periodontal disease was considered a "dirty mouth syndrome," which meant that there was no need to distinguish between plaques that caused decay and those that caused periodontal disease. It now is known that two distinct plaque communities reside on the tooth surfaces, one above the gingival margin (gum line) that is called the "supragingival plaque," and one that resides below the gingival margin and is called the "subgingival plaque" (Table 2). The supragingival plaque flora has access to dietary and salivary nutrients and tends to be composed of gram-positive, facultative organisms dominated by Streptococci and Actinomyces, organisms that have specific mechanisms

Table 2
Contrasting characteristics of dental caries and periodontal disease

Characteristic	Dental caries	Periodontal disease
Location on tooth	Supragingival	Subgingival
Dominant bacterial species	Streptococci, *Actinomyces*, *Veillonella* spp	Spirochetes, *Prevotella*, *Porphyromonas* spp
Dominant types	Adherent species	Motile species
Gram stain	Gram positive	Gram negative
Oxygen sensitivity	Facultative	Anaerobes
Nutrient sources	Diet	Gingival crevicular fluid
	Saliva	Host/Inflammatory molecules
	Retained foods	Retained foods
Metabolic activity	Saccharolytic	Proteolytic
Growth rate (doubling time)	4–5 hours	Days to weeks

for adhering to the tooth surfaces. When exposed to frequent pulses of sucrose, as occurs during snacking, this plaque selects for the mutans streptococci and causes dental decay.

The subgingival plaque, although derived from bacterial species that initially colonized the supragingival plaque, tends to become anaerobic because of the low pressure of oxygen tensions in the area below the gingival margin. In periodontal disease, the space beneath the gingiva enlarges to form a pocket around the tooth that can harbor almost a billion bacteria, such as spirochetes. The dominant bacteria are proteolytic, and many derive their nutrients from the host by cell sloughing, from a secretion called the gingival crevicular fluid, and, in periodontal disease, from tissue breakdown and inflammatory molecules that leak from the tissue into the pocket.

The specific-plaque hypothesis

Dental decay in the twenty-first century is a controllable infection and should be preventable in many individuals. Almost 50% of young children are caries free, and the level of edentia among individuals over 65 years of age has dropped from 50% to about 20%. It has been found that periodontal disease reflects the host's response to a limited number of anaerobic species and that it can be diagnosed and treated. These changes reflect a new understanding of the microbiology of dental plaque, the specific-plaque hypothesis, which was proposed in 1976 to account for the unique role of *S mutans* in dental caries [35]. In recent years it has been expanded to include periodontal infections [4] and also tongue conditions associated with oral malodor [36]. The specific-plaque hypothesis states that there is a nondiseased plaque which is associated with good dental health and that environment influences cause a rearrangement of this normal flora that can lead to either a cariogenic or a periodontopathic plaque.

Dental decay

Dental decay has been known since the beginning of recorded history but was not an important health problem until sucrose became a major component of the human diet in the late nineteenth century. When sucrose is consumed frequently, a group of organisms known as the mutans streptococci, the most prominent of which are *S mutans* and *Streptococcus sobrinus*, emerge as prominent organisms in the supragingival plaque. Because most studies did not distinguish between *S mutans* and *S sobrinus* (they both ferment mannitol and sorbitol), these organisms are referred to as the "mutans streptococci" in the text, except when *S mutans* is specifically identified.

S mutans was isolated from human carious lesions in 1924 but was neglected until the 1960s when it was reidentified as the causative agent of a transmissible caries infection in rodent models [3,5]. In the rodent models, all of Koch's postulates for infectivity were fulfilled. It proved difficult, however, to show that the mutans streptococci were human dental pathogens, because they seem to be a member of the normal flora on the teeth, and it was difficult to show that an increase in the mutans streptococci actually preceded and/or coincided with the clinical lesion.

Dental decay is measured clinically as a cavitation on the tooth surface. Cavitation, however, is a late event in the pathogenesis of decay, being preceded by a clinically detectable subsurface lesion known as a "white spot." From a diagnostic and treatment perspective, the lesion should be detected at the white spot stage. This identification usually cannot be made without rigorous descriptive criteria (not all white spots are caused by the decay process); also, the white spot stage in the caries-prone fissures and approximal surfaces of the tooth cannot be visualized directly during a dental examination.

For many years dental epidemiologists ignored the white spot lesion in their documentation of dental decay, relying instead on the number of teeth (T) or tooth surfaces (S) that had obvious decay (D), contained a dental restoration or filling (F), or were missing (M). These "DMF" teeth (DMFT) and "DMF" surface (DMFS) scores did not distinguish the relative proportions of the score resulting from decay, versus fillings and extractions. This insensitivity of the DMFT and DMFS scores in quantifying the actual decay, independent of morbidity, led to unimpressive associations in early clinical studies between the mutans streptococci and DMFT or DMFS scores. When the comparison was limited to individuals who had decayed teeth, or when the plaque samples were taken from a decayed tooth site, a significant association between the mutans streptococci and decay was always evident, however [37].

This association is seen clearly in individuals who developed xerostomia secondary to radiation treatment of head and neck cancer. The mutans streptococci and lactobacilli normally are present in low numbers in the plaque of these individuals. When the salivary flow decreases, the pH in the plaque drops, leading to a selection for aciduric (acid-tolerant) bacteria, such as the mutans streptococci and lactobacilli. New decayed lesions become obvious within 3 months after radiotherapy, and the patient may average one or more new decayed surfaces per postradiation month. During the development of decay, the proportions of first the mutans streptococci and then lactobacilli increase significantly [5]. This sequence of events indicates that the mutans streptococci are involved with the initiation of decay, whereas the lactobacilli are associated with the progression of the lesion.

The mutans streptococci colonize the teeth shortly after eruption [38,39], but the size of their niche is limited by infrequent exposure to sucrose. In most adults the mutans streptococci remain in the background and do not cause decay, but if the host changes his/her dietary habits and begins to snack regularly on sugar-containing foods, these frequent sucrose pulses cause the mutans streptococci to grow and expand its niche on the tooth surface. The pH of the plaque becomes acidic for longer periods during the day, and aciduric species like the mutans streptococci and possibly lactobacilli increase proportionally in the plaque at the expense of the nonaciduric bacterial species such as *Streptococcus sanguis*.

The salivary buffers are unable to maintain the plaque pH near 7.0, and when the pH drops to around 5.0, the tooth itself begins to buffer, releasing calcium and phosphate ions. If this mineral is not replaced, a net loss of tooth substance occurs, giving rise to the white spot lesion. Bacteriologic studies of the white spot lesion show the dominance of the mutans streptococci in the plaque flora, as well as lactobacilli and unidentified aciduric species [40–43]. When the lesion progresses to the stage of cavitation, the organisms penetrate into the enamel crystals and underlying dentine. The lactobacilli may now be the dominant species, because these organisms are capable of growth at pH levels below 5.0. When the lesion reaches the advanced clinical stage, mutans streptococci may no longer be able to survive, and only secondary cariogens, such as the lactobacilli and opportunistic organisms, can be found.

This model predicts that a bacterial succession occurs during the progression of a carious lesion and that the flora of the advanced lesion may bear little resemblance to the flora of the incipient lesion. Thus it was necessary to sample the plaque during the initial lesion or white spot stage to find the causative agents of decay. When this sampling was done, the mutans streptococci dominated in the plaque flora. For the lesion to progress to the stage of cavitation, however, lactobacilli may be necessary [44].

Pathogenesis

The nineteenth-century microbiologists noted that decay occurred at retentive sites on the teeth. It now is known that the retentive sites were caries-prone because they provided the microenvironment that selects for the mutans streptococci and lactobacilli. The attributes of mutans streptococci and the lactobacilli that enable them to be successful on retentive sites are among the virulence factors that make these organisms specific dental pathogens. First, however, the unique role of sucrose in the carious process is discussed.

Sucrose in the diet

Evidence from epidemiologic observations and animal experiments indicates that, shortly after sucrose is introduced into the diet, a notably higher incidence of decay occurs. Dietary components are normally high molecular weight polymers (such as starch and proteins) that are in the mouth for short periods. They have a minimal effect on plaque growth except when food is retained between and on the teeth. Sucrose, because it is a low molecular weight disaccharide that can be sequestered rapidly and used by the plaque flora, changes this pattern. Plaque organisms capable of fermenting sucrose have a decided advantage over the nonsucrose fermenters in that they can proliferate during periods of sucrose ingestion, which is often between meals, and thereby become the dominant plaque organisms.

The magnitude of the bioavailability of sucrose to the plaque flora determines its cariogenicity. Sucrose taken in the form of a candy produces a rapid drop in the plaque pH to 5.0 or lower, whereas sucrose ingested during meals is admixed with others foods during mastication, eliciting sufficient saliva to buffer the plaque pH so that decay does not occur [5]. In fact, as much as three quarters of a pound of sucrose consumed daily at meals for 2 years was not associated with an increase in dental decay in young institutionalized adults [45]. When the same or lesser amounts of sucrose were ingested between meals, however, subjects developed new decay at the rate of about four to seven tooth surfaces per year (Table 3). This study would be unethical by today's standards, because individuals were fed excessive amounts of sugar (1200 calories/d) that sent some of them into a rampant caries situation and also led to excessive weight gain.

The ad lib ingestion of sucrose between meals leads to the presence of sucrose in the saliva for most of the waking day. Because this sucrose is available for microbial fermentation in the plaque, plaque pH is low for long periods each day. The salivary buffers are overwhelmed, and, as lactic acid diffuses into the tooth, enamel dissolves, releasing calcium and phosphate ions from sites beneath the surface enamel. Normally, the bathing saliva replenishes these minerals, but because the duration of the flux from the enamel is so great, repair does not occur, and cavitation results. Thus, sucrose consumption per se does not cause decay, but the frequent ingestion of sucrose, by prolonging the time period during which the plaque

Table 3
Effect of bioavailability of dietary sucrose to plaque flora on caries activity

Diet group	Year of study	Daily sucrose consumption (g/person)		Carious surfaces per year
		At meals	Between meals	
Sucrose (n = 57)	1	90	—	0.44
	2	330	—	0.49
	3	330	—	0.96
	4	190	—	0.84
Toffee, male (n = 48)	1	90	—	0.38
	2	180	120	4.29
	3	180	120	4.58[a]
	4	110	—	0.33
Toffee, female (n = 39)	1[b]	90	—	0.23
	2	180	120	6.90
	3	180	120	7.41
	4	110	—	0.36

Adapted from: Gustafsson BE, Quensel CE, Lanke LS, et al. The Vipeholm dental caries study; the effect of different levels of carbohydrate intake on caries activity in 436 individuals observed for five years. Acta Odontol Scand 1954;11(3-4):244; with permission.

[a] Root surface cries accounted for about 25% of total.

[b] Tooth brushed daily in about 50% of women.

flora can break down sucrose to acids, is cariogenic. This between-meal eating of sucrose overcame the natural defense mechanisms of the host in regard to salivary remineralization of the tooth surfaces.

Sucrose metabolism in the mutans streptococci

The reaction between mutans streptococci and sucrose is unique. Plaque bacteria that ferment sucrose produce acids, which lower the pH value to below 5.0. When germ-free animals were fed a high-sucrose diet, however, only *S mutans* and *S sobrinus* caused decay [46]. This finding suggested that acid production is not the exclusive determinant of decay and that mutans streptococci possess other attributes that are responsible for its virulence. The mutans streptococci subsequently were shown to metabolize sucrose in a remarkably diverse fashion that is not matched by any other known plaque organism (Box 1). The major pathway involves energy metabolism, in which invertase splits sucrose into its component glucose and fructose molecules, which then are converted to lactic acid by the glycolytic pathway. If there is excess sucrose and a lowering pH, the mutans streptococci can shunt the extra glucose and fructose to intercellular polysaccharides or mannitol.

Intracellular polysaccharide formation

The mutans streptococci, as well as most saccharolytic plaque species, experience a feast-or-famine situation as to availability of fermentable dietary nutrients. These organisms have adapted by forming storage polysaccharides. When a soluble dietary carbohydrate, such as sucrose, is in excess, the mutans streptococci have the capacity to convert internalized

Box 1. Sucrose metabolism by the mutans streptococci

Extracellular

Glucosyltransferase
- → Alpha 1–6 dextrans + fructose
- → Alpha 1–3-mutans + fructose

Fructosyltransferase
- Levans + glucose
- Inulin + glucose

Intracellular

Sucrose phosphotransferase
- Invertase → glucose + fructose
- Glucose-6-P → alpha 1–4 intracellular glucans
- Glucose-6-P → lactic acid
- Glucose-6-P ↔ mannitol

glucose or fructose to an intracellular alpha 1-4 polysaccharide polymer. When the external sucrose pulse is depleted, the bacteria then can draw on this stored polysaccharide for energy metabolism. In this way, the pH in the plaque can be reduced for 30 to 60 minutes after the sucrose is cleared from the mouth, thereby providing a sustained challenge to the integrity of the enamel surface. If the sucrose pulse is taken at bedtime, such as was done in the first 60 years of the twentieth century when sucrose was added to dentifrices, the pH drop in the plaque could last for hours, because there was little salivary flow to neutralize the plaque acids.

Extracellular polysaccharide formation

Many plaque bacteria form intracellular polysaccharides, so this characteristic cannot reflect the unique relationship between mutans streptococci, sucrose, and dental decay. The mutans streptococci have enzymes, called "glucosyltransferases," that split sucrose outside the cell and transfer the glucose moiety to a glucose polymer, forming an extracellular polysaccharide known as a "glucan." *S mutans* forms several complex glucans that differ in their core linkage, amount of branching, and molecular weight. The first glucan identified had a core linkage consisting of an alpha1-6 bond that classified it as a dextran [47]. Later, a unique glucan having an alpha 1-3 core linkage was identified and given the name "mutan" [48,49]. *S mutans* also has enzymes that split sucrose and transfer the fructose moiety to a fructose polymer known as a "fructan." Other plaque bacteria can use sucrose to synthesize one or more of these polymers, but none can form a mutan. Only *S mutans* can form all of them, a fact that led to an inquiry into the relationship between polymer production and caries formation.

In vitro experiments showed that the glucans enable the mutans streptococci, especially *S sobrinus*, to adhere to surfaces. This finding suggested that in vivo these adhesive polymers would enable the mutans streptococci to adhere to the tooth surface and to accumulate on these surfaces, thereby causing decay in the underlying surface. Animal experiments, in which rodents were infected with mutants of the mutans streptococci that lacked the ability to form either dextran or mutan, indicated that the absence of mutan was associated with a greater reduction in smooth surface decay than was the absence of dextran [49–51]. In each instance, the amount of pit-and-fissure decay was not affected significantly by these mutations. Decay on smooth surfaces seems to depend on the retentive polymers, whereas in sites where retention is provided by the anatomy of the teeth (pits, fissures, and contact points between teeth), these polymers are not as important.

Aciduricity

This finding suggests that any acidogenic organism that can survive in these retentive sites may cause pit-and-fissure decay. Most plaque species cannot survive in these stagnant environments. In germ-free rats, only the mutans streptococci, *Lactobacillus casei*, and *Streptococcus faecalis* can cause fissure decay. These three organisms are aciduric compared with other plaque bacteria; that is, they produce acids, and they are relatively resistant to the resulting low pH caused by acid accumulation. Lactobacilli are the most aciduric of the plaque bacteria, and this trait allows these organisms to predominate by the time the carious lesion has extended into the dentin.

Aciduricity best explains the involvement of both the mutans streptococci and lactobacilli in human decay. A retentive site is colonized initially by organisms present in saliva. If the mutans streptococci are among the initial colonizers, even as a low percentage ($< 1\%$) of the initial inoculum, they would be selected for if a low pH value in the site is not well buffered by saliva. Frequent ingestion of sucrose-containing products predisposes toward lower pH values and thus selects for the mutans streptococci. When the pH remains in the vicinity of 5.0 to 5.5, tooth mineral is solubilized, thereby buffering the plaque and maintaining an environment suitable for growth of the mutans streptococci. Eventually, enough mineral is lost so that a cavitation occurs in the enamel, and if this cavitation enlarges so that it extends into the dentin, a semiclosed system is formed in which the pH value drops below 5.0. These acidic conditions favor the growth of lactobacilli, and these organisms succeed as the predominant flora in the carious lesion. The importance of aciduricity was shown when a mutant of *S mutans* with decreased aciduricity was unable to cause caries in germfree rats [52].

Sorbitol/mannitol fermentation

The mutans streptococci can be distinguished from other oral streptococci by their ability to ferment sorbitol and mannitol. This fermentation is an unusual nutrient requirement, because these hexanols are unlikely to occur in the oral environment during the evolutionary history of the oral flora. In fact sorbitol, because of its humectant qualities and slight sweetness, has been added to the diet only recently as a sugar substitute in candies, chewing gums, and dentifrices. Therefore it is peculiar that the mutans streptococci would possess the enzymes to ferment these sugar alcohols. In addition to the mutans streptococci, however, these sugar alcohols are fermented by *L caseii* and certain yeasts such as *Candida albicans*, which been associated with decay and are aciduric.

The enzymes involved in sorbitol and mannitol fermentation are inducible and reversible. That is, they can form sorbitol and mannitol from glucose and fructose as well as the reverse reaction converting these sugar alcohols into glucose-6-P and fructose-6-P. It is likely that the normal function of these enzymes is to form sorbitol and mannitol in the plaque when there is excess sucrose in the environment. When *S mutans* and *L casei* are exposed to very high levels of either glucose or sucrose in vitro, mannitol can be detected [53]. The advantage to the organisms is the regeneration of

NAD without the formation of lactic acid. Thus, these organisms, when experiencing the luxury of excess glucose, fructose, or sucrose, can divert some of the fructose-6-phosphate from the glycolytic pathway and use it as a hydrogen acceptor for NADH to prevent lactic acid formation and a further pH drop. This ability suggests that the operation of the mannitol/sorbitol pathway in reverse is connected somehow with the aciduricity of these organisms and contributes to their cariogenicity.

Microbiologic diagnosis

A microbiologic diagnosis for a mutans streptococci/lactobacilli infection is rarely obtained, primarily because the acute pain that brings the patient to the dentist is almost always relieved by a dental restoration or extraction. Thus, the knowledge of an underlying mutans streptococci infection would not change the treatment. Microbiologic diagnosis, however, would be advantageous in the management of the patient to prevent or minimize future decay. Also, because decay usually occurs within a year after a tooth erupts or a new restoration is placed, it would be prudent to monitor the mutans streptococci levels during these intervals.

Scandinavian investigators have empirically determined that a *S mutans* level of 10^6 colony-forming units/mL in stimulated saliva can be associated with future caries activity [54–56]. They have designed simple chairside tests that can, in a semiquantitated manner, provide information on the salivary levels of *S mutans*. All of these tests rely on the facts that *S mutans* is resistant to 5 ug/mL of bacitracin and that it will grow in the presence of 20% sucrose. In liquid media containing these additives, mutans streptococci form adherent colonies on the side of glass, plastic strips, or any other solid surfaces that are present. In a practical application of these tests, the clinician initiates anti–mutans streptococci treatment (as discussed later) in individuals who have 10^6 colony-forming units of mutans streptococci per mL saliva. Individuals who should be screened include children seen at the first dental examination and children undergoing orthodontic treatment (because they would be apt to develop decay around the margins of the bands). Likewise an individual who is having dental bridges or implants placed would be at risk of developing new decay around the margins of these restorations. A mutans-positive patient would need to be treated to lower his/her salivary mutans streptococci levels before the placement of the dental devices or restorations.

Prevention and treatment

Conventional dental therapy has not incorporated any microbiologically based strategy into its armamentarium. Instead, treatments based on response to symptoms and plaque control have prevailed. The bankruptcy of this approach was demonstrated by the overwhelming dental morbidity observed in the first half of the twentieth century. Then, beginning around

1960, something happened that brought the caries epidemic under control. The most obvious change was the availability of fluoride in drinking water and in dentifrices.

The fluoride effect

The mechanisms by which fluoride prevents decay are multiple, and the relative contributions of each mechanism are not fully understood [5]. The 30% to 50% reduction in decay that follows water fluoridation generally is attributed to the fluoride replacing hydroxyl groups in the tooth crystal, thereby forming fluorapatite. Fluorapatite is less soluble in acid than hydroxyapatite, so a tooth containing fluorapatite dissolves slowly in the low pH value found in plaque and, accordingly, remineralizes faster in the intervals between sugar ingestion. These explanations do not account completely for the proved efficacy of topically applied fluorides.

The fluoride ion (F^-) inhibits the bacterial enzyme enolase, thereby interfering with production of phosphoenolpyruvate. Phosphoenolpyruvate is a key intermediate of the glycolytic pathway and is the source of energy and phosphate needed for sugar uptake. In vitro 10 to 100 ppm of F^- inhibits acid production by most plaque bacteria, but these high levels are never achieved in vivo. At acidic pH values (5.5 or below), however, low levels of F^- (1–5 ppm) inhibit the oral streptococci. These levels are found in plaque, especially in individuals who drink fluoridated water or who use fluoridated dentifrices. If this fluoride is derived from the tooth, an antibacterial mode of action that involves a depot effect can be postulated for systemic (water) and topical fluoride administration.

The depot effect comes about in this manner. Water fluoridation promotes the formation of fluorapatite, whereas topical fluorides cause a net retention by the enamel of fluoride as fluorapatite or as more labile calcium salts. Microbial acid production in the plaque may solubilize this enamel-bound fluoride, which at the prevailing low pH in the plaque microenvironment could become inhibitory for the acid-producing microbes. Such a sequence would discriminate against the mutans streptococci and lactobacilli because they, as a result of their aciduric nature, are most likely the numerically dominant acid producers at the plaque–enamel interface. The fluoridated tooth thus contains a depot of a potent antimicrobial agent that is released at an acid pH value and is most active at this pH value. This hypothesis attributes some of the success of water fluoridation and topical fluorides to an antimicrobial effect.

Neutral 1.0% sodium fluoride given daily to adults, who normally would experience rampant caries secondary to a xerostomia following irradiation for jaw cancer, has resulted in few or no caries [57]. Controls, who were given a placebo as well as the best available hygiene instruction, averaged more than two new decayed surfaces per postradiation month. When the control patients were placed on the daily fluoride regimen, their decay rate dropped to almost zero. In another study, 5- to 6-year-old children who had 10 or more carious tooth surfaces were given the necessary dental restorations and either 1.2% F^- as a neutral sodium fluoride gel or a placebo gel [5]. The gels were taken unsupervised at home, twice daily for 1 week. After 2 years, the fluoride group had about 40% less decay than the placebo group. Eleven of these 20 children who formerly had rampant caries had no new decay in their permanent teeth. In these studies of patients who had xerostomia and children who had rampant caries, the initially high proportions of mutans streptococci were decreased by the fluoride treatments, which resulted in reduced decay.

Sucrose substitutes that aid in caries control

Eating foods that contain sucrose between meals can be highly cariogenic, as was demonstrated in the Vipeholm study. Dietary counseling that instructs patients to avoid between-meal snacks may help decrease the incidence of dental decay, but only if the patients are compliant. Another dietary approach to caries control is to recommend that patients eat snack foods that contain compounds that provide the hedonistic appeal of sucrose but are not fermented by the plaque flora to the low pH levels associated with enamel demineralization.

The least acidogenic sucrose substitutes are the polyols, such as sorbitol, mannitol, and xylitol. Few plaque bacteria can ferment these substances, and those that can (the mutans streptococci and *L casei* ferment sorbitol and mannitol) do not lower the pH to values that can dissolve the tooth [58]. Xylitol, the only polyol with a sweet taste comparable to that of sucrose and the only one that cannot be fermented by the mutans streptococci, has been shown to be anticariogenic when substituted for sucrose in either foods or chewing gum [59]. In a study of chewing gum, young adults who consumed about 6 to 7 g of xylitol gum per day had, after 1 year, an 80% reduction in caries increment compared with a control group who consumed 6 to 7 g of sucrose gum per day [59]. This intensive use of a xylitol chewing gum was shown to decrease salivary and plaque levels of the mutans streptococci [60]. When the between-meal sucrose supply is reduced, the levels of the mutans streptococci declines, because the low plaque pH values that selected for them are not as dominant a factor in the plaque microecology. Thus, xylitol products can satisfy the craving for sweets, discriminate against the mutans streptococci, and significantly reduce the incidence of dental decay [59,61].

The substitution of xylitol-containing snacks for sucrose-containing snacks collapses the niche for mutans streptococci on the teeth, causing a decline in decay. Other oral and throat streptococci also depend on sucrose to maintain a sizable presence in the oral and throat flora. When sucrose usage is restricted because of the use of xylitol products, these other streptococci, including *S pneumoniae*, also decline in number. This decline has been associated with a clinically significantly reduction in ear infections caused by *S pneumoniae* among young Finnish children [62].

Interference with transmission from mother to infant

Vertical transmission of the mutans streptococci from caregiver, usually the mother, to the infant is detectable shortly after tooth eruption [38,63]. In animal models, if this colonization is delayed, the magnitude of the carious destruction is reduced greatly. This finding suggests that a viable preventive strategy would be to treat mothers who are infected with the mutans streptococci to prevent its spread to their children. The first such effort was a Swedish study in which mothers were treated with dental restorations, topical fluorides, oral hygiene instructions, dietary counseling, and topical chlorhexidine [64]. This regimen was repeated at intervals of 2 to 4 months as necessary until their children were 3 years old. The test mothers as a group showed approximately 10-fold fewer mutans streptococci during the test period. At the age of 3 years, 70% of the children in the control group carried mutans streptococci, compared with 41% in the test group ($P < .01$). Fifty-two percent of the children who carried mutans streptococci had caries at this age, compared with 3% of the children without this organism. These children were followed until they were 7 years old [65]. Significantly more children of control mothers than of test mothers carried mutans streptococci (95% versus 46%, $P < .01$). Twenty-three percent of the test children were caries free, compared with 9% of the control children ($P < .01$). The mean caries experience of the test children also was significantly lower than that of the control children (dms 5.2 and 8.6, respectively; $P < .05$). The results show that reduction of the mutans streptococci in the mother during the emergence of the primary teeth in her child has a long-term influence on colonization by these bacteria and the caries experience in the child.

The regimen used in this study was expensive and not very practical. Others have used the chewing of xylitol gum to determine whether the transmission from mother to infant can be interrupted. One hundred sixty-nine mother–child pairs participated in a 2-year study exploring whether the mothers' xylitol consumption could be used to prevent mother–child transmission of mutans streptococci [66]. All mothers showed high salivary levels of mutans streptococci during pregnancy. The mothers in the xylitol group ($n = 106$) were asked to chew xylitol-sweetened gum (65% weight of xylitol/weight of gum) at least two or three times a day, starting 3 months after delivery. In the two control groups, the mothers received chlorhexidine ($n = 30$) or fluoride ($n = 33$) varnish treatments at 6, 12, and 18 months after delivery. The salivary mutans streptococci levels of the mothers remained high and were not significantly different among the three study groups. Clear differences were seen in the children, however: 9.7% of the children in the xylitol group, 28.6% in the chlorhexidine varnish group, and 48.5% in the fluoride varnish group showed a detectable level of mutans streptococci at age 2 years. The reduction in the xylitol group was still evident in the children after 3 and 6 years [67]. In another study, less caries was observed in children of mothers who chewed gums with xylitol as the single sweetener during the time of eruption of the children's first primary teeth than in those who used gums containing fluoride, sorbitol, and lower amounts of xylitol [68]. This finding suggests that by providing xylitol snacks, such as chewing gums, to mothers infected with the mutans streptococci, cariogenic infection in their children can be reduced. This intervention strategy is best exploited by physicians.

Periodontal disease

Periodontal disease involves a group of bacteria that are metabolic opposites of those involved in the caries process. Dental caries reflects an acellular response of the teeth to the bacterial challenge. Periodontal disease reflects a cellular inflammatory response of the gingiva and surrounding connective tissue to the bacterial accumulations on the teeth. These inflammatory responses are divided into two clinical groupings: gingivitis and periodontitis. Gingivitis is extremely common and is manifested clinically as bleeding of the gingival or gum tissues without evidence of bone loss or deep periodontal pockets. Periodontitis occurs when the plaque-induced inflammatory response in the tissue results in actual loss of collagen attachment of the tooth to the bone and in loss of bone, resulting in deep periodontal pockets that, in some cases, can extend the entire length of the tooth root (15–20 mm). Periodontitis is not as prevalent as once thought: a recent survey of American adults revealed that only 5% of the population surveyed had one tooth site with pocket depths measuring 6 mm or more [69]. This finding is in agreement with recent population surveys in other countries which show that from 5% to 15% of the population has periodontitis [70].

Etiology and pathogenesis

Although clinical treatment is based on the principle that periodontal disease is the host's response to bacterial overgrowth in the pocket, considerable evidence indicates that these clinical entities are specific bacterial infections [4]. These infections are unusual in that obvious bacterial invasion of the tissues is rarely encountered. Rather, bacteria in the subgingival plaque elaborate various compounds, such as hydrogen sulfide, ammonia, amines, endotoxins, enzymes (such as collagenases), and antigens, some portion of which penetrate the gingiva and elicit an inflammatory response. This inflammatory response, although overwhelmingly protective, seems to be responsible for a net loss of periodontal supporting tissue and leads to pocket formation, loosening of the teeth, and eventual tooth loss. Neutrophils are important in this inflammatory response, and if they are absent, as in various neutropenias, or compromised as a result of chemotherapy, an aggressive form of periodontitis is encountered. T4 helper cells play a role in this defense, as shown by the periodontitis encountered in patients who have AIDS [71]. This inflammatory response also can result in inflammatory mediators entering the systemic circulation and augmenting the levels of CRP, prostaglandin, and other molecules, thereby contributing to systemic diseases.

Gingivitis

The simplest form of gingivitis is associated with the accumulation of supragingival plaque along the gingival margins of the teeth. This form of gingivitis has been studied extensively in human volunteers, and the sequence of events is well described. In these studies, individuals are brought to a state of health and then refrain from all forms of oral hygiene for a 3- to 4-week period [72]. The initial colonizers of the teeth are streptococci, which proliferate and in turn become colonized by other bacteria present in saliva, such as various *Actinomyces* species and Veillonella. The greatest growth of the plaque occurs at the gingival margin, where plaque accumulations usually are visible after several days. This plaque may, in some instances, provoke a bleeding gingivitis in which spirochetes and *Actinomyces viscosus* are prominent members of the plaque flora [73,74]. If this plaque remains undisturbed, the flora gradually shifts toward an anaerobic, gram-negative flora that includes black-pigmented species and several types of spirochetes. The increase in these anaerobic organisms can be explained by the low oxidation–reduction potential of the aged plaque [75] and by nutrients derived from the inflammatory exudate at the site.

The gingivitis may resolve by itself or fester subclinically for an indeterminate period; however, the potential for the formation of a periodontal pocket (periodontitis) exists at any time. When pockets are detected clinically, they often are associated with calcified plaque deposits, called "calculus," present on the tooth surfaces. For many years, calculus was thought to be the causative agent of periodontitis, because inflammation usually subsided when it was removed and the tooth surfaces were cleaned mechanically. Calculus, however, is always covered by plaque, and removal of calculus would be synonymous with removal of plaque.

Periodontitis

Periodontitis comprises an early-onset form mainly seen in young individuals and a chronic form seen in adults over age 35 years. The early-onset form is now called "aggressive periodontitis," and the adult form is called "adult periodontitis" [76]. Both entities are associated with an overgrowth of anaerobic bacteria resulting in obvious plaque accumulations, with one exception, a rare form of aggressive periodontitis seen in teenagers that formerly was called "localized juvenile periodontitis" (LJP).

Aggressive periodontitis: localized juvenile periodontitis

LJP is different from other periodontal infections because it is not associated with plaque accumulations or calculus (in fact, the absence of such associations led early investigators to consider it a degenerative condition called "periodontosis"), is localized to certain anterior or front teeth and first molars, and is seen following puberty. It occurs in about 0.1% to 0.5% of teenagers but often is clustered within families. This familial background suggested a genetic predisposition that subsequently has been identified as a neutrophil defect associated with reduced chemotaxis. A familial tendency also can be explained by the vertical transmission of periodontopathic bacteria from parents to child [77–79]. Bacterial examinations of subgingival plaque from affected teeth and adjacent healthy teeth revealed that the diseased teeth were colonized by an essentially gram-negative flora [80] dominated by organisms subsequently identified as various *Capnocytophaga* and *Wolinella* species and *A actinomycetemcomitans* [81,82].

A selective medium for *A actinomycetemcomitans* containing bacitracin and vancomycin was developed [83], and its use quickly led to the conclusion that *A actinomycetemcomitans* was the causative agent of LJP [82,84]. *A actinomycetemcomitans* is more prevalent in tooth sites associated with LJP and is less prevalent in healthy sites in the same mouth and in periodontally healthy individuals. It often is found among other family members in a household with an LJP individual, and indeed among siblings at risk of LJP there are data suggesting that colonization by *A actinomycetemcomitans* precedes the development of a pocket and subsequent bone loss.

This evidence, however, was biased toward *A actinomycetemcomitans*, because in most studies no other periodontopathic species were sought [4]. A longitudinal study in the United States examined 14,013 adolescents in grades 8 through 12, over a 6-year period, for the development of attachment loss [85]. From this group a subset of 248 adolescents chosen because they had attachment loss of 3 mm or more on two or more teeth were compared with a randomly selected group that had no attachment loss. The control group was matched with the putative LJP group in gender, race, age, geographic location, and urban status. The plaque was colleted from two sites in each subject and was examined for the presence of several periodontopathogens by using DNA probes. The individuals showing attachment loss had significantly higher levels of *P gingivalis, T denticola*, and *Prevotella intermedia.* There was no relationship between *A actinomycetemcomitans* and disease progression. Other studies also found anaerobes rather than *A actinomycetemcomitans* were associated with LJP, and indeed antibiotics directed against anaerobes, such as metronidazole, are effective in the treatment of LJP [86].

When the periodontitis extends beyond the molars/incisors in individuals under 35 years of age, the clinical condition is called "aggressive periodontitis." In the longitudinal study cited previously, *P gingivalis* and *T denticola* were significantly elevated in teenagers who had aggressive periodontitis as compared with the healthy controls and the LJP subjects [85]. All forms of aggressive periodontitis, including those in genetically susceptible individuals (eg, persons who have Down or Papillon-Lefevre syndrome) can be considered anaerobic infections [4].

Adult periodontitis

The periodontitis found in adults older than 35 years may be the most common infection among Americans [87]. Bacteriologic investigations of adult periodontitis were hampered by the labor-intensive cost of anaerobic culturing procedures and by the inability of these procedures to grow the majority of organisms. For instance spirochetes, which may be the numerically dominant group in most subgingival plaques, are so fragile that they are destroyed by most dispersal procedures used to disrupt the plaque samples. Even today, most of the more than 500 species that can be identified by DNA analysis [1] cannot be cultured. This inability suggests that any statement describing the causative agents of periodontitis may be premature. The pattern discerned, however, indicates that an anaerobic flora is involved (see Table 2), and although the actual causative agents may not be known, the monitoring of the known flora seems adequate to diagnose and treat patients successfully.

It has been difficult to assign causative significance to any single plaque species by using cultural methods. Cultural studies miss uncultivable species, such as the spirochetes, that may account for more than 40% of the flora [4,88]. Cultural studies also reveal a bewildering array of species, many of them either newly described or as yet unspeciated. What is most frustrating is that none of these putative periodontopathic species predominate in all disease-associated plaques. Despite these problems in assigning virulence to any one species, it is clear that the bacterial communities at disease sites are different from the communities at healthy and successfully treated periodontal sites. The diseased sites are dominated by anaerobes and in particular by spirochetes and black-pigmented species, such as *P gingivalis* and *P intermedia*. This pattern was identified in several studies that looked at large numbers of plaque samples.

The author and colleagues reported on both the prominent cultivable flora and microscopic counts of more than 400 plaque samples taken from 120 patients, including untreated patients who had aggressive periodontitis and adult periodontitis as well as successfully treated patients [89]. Only the spirochetes were significantly elevated in plaques taken from untreated patients compared with the values observed in the treated patients. *P gingivalis* was significantly increased in the patients who had aggressive periodontitis. Subsequently, using DNA probes, polyclonal antibodies, and microscopic and cultural methods, the author and colleagues examined more than 200 plaques removed from teeth that were scheduled to have periodontal surgery or to be extracted [90]. *P gingivalis, T denticola, T forsythia,* and spirochetes were present in 80% to 100% of the plaques.

In a cross-sectional study involving more than 1300 residents of Erie County, New York, *T forsythia* and *P gingivalis*, but not *A actinomycetemcomitans*, were associated significantly with attachment loss [91] and alveolar bone loss [92]. In a prospective study involving 415 of these subjects who were monitored for 2 to 5 years, the prevalence of *T forsythia, P gingivalis,* and *P intermedia* at the baseline examination was able to predict subsequent bone and/or tooth loss [93]. Of these species, subjects colonized by *T forsythia* were at seven times greater risk for increased pocket depths [94]. When whole-genomic probes of 40 plaque species were applied to more than 13,000 plaques removed from 185 individuals, only three species—*T forsythia*, *T denticola*, and *P gingivalis*—could be associated with either increased pocket depth or bleeding on probing [95]. Others using the whole-genomic approach have found these species to be associated with periodontal infections in Chinese [96] and Brazilian [97,98] subjects.

These data and others [4] indicate that periodontal infections are associated with anaerobic species, of which *T forsythia, P gingivalis*, and *T denticola* are invariably found, occasionally with other species such as *P intermedia, A actinomycetemcomitans*, and *Eubacterium* species. These findings indicate that aggressive periodontitis and adult periodontitis are essentially the same polymicrobial infection caused by the overgrowth of a finite number of bacterial species in the subgingival plaque. *A actinomycetemcomitans* is rarely found. Thus, although aggressive periodontitis looks different from adult periodontitis (Fig. 2), there are no obvious bacteriologic differences. The subjects who had aggressive periodontitis had an anaerobic infection, based on three or more of four plaque samples being BANA positive. (The BANA test, as discussed later, measures an enzyme that is possessed by *T denticola, P gingivalis*, and *T forsythia*.) The spirochetes in

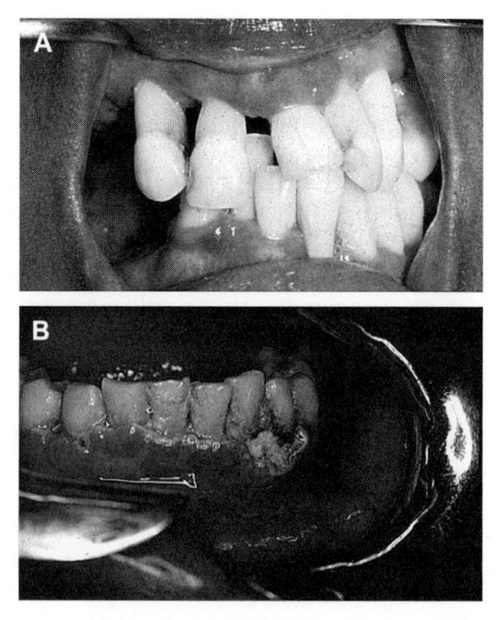

Fig. 2. (*A*) Aggressive periodontitis in a 22-year-old woman. (*B*) Adult periodontitis in a 54-year-old man.

the subjects' plaques averaged 43% of the microscopic count. In subjects who had adult periodontitis, the spirochetes averaged 38% of the microscopic count, and all subjects had an anaerobic infection.

P gingivalis, T denticola, and *T forsythia* are among the few subgingival plaque bacteria that can hydrolyze the synthetic trypsin substrate BANA [99]. These organisms possess a wide array of enzymes, such as a collagenase, peptidases, hyaluronidase, and a keratinolytic enzyme, and produce noxious end products, such as butyrate, NH_3, H_2S, and endotoxin, that could cause an inflammatory response if they entered the periodontal tissue. This inflammatory response in turn could lead to tissue breakdown products, such as arginine-containing peptides, entering the pocket environment where they could serve as nutrients for bacteria such as the BANA-positive species. Therefore the collective overgrowth of these anaerobic BANA-positive species may represent a polymicrobial infection that depends for nutrients on tissue-breakdown molecules leaking into the pocket. Coincidentally, these inflammatory mediators and markers could diffuse into the systemic circulation, accounting for the association between periodontal infections and medical conditions.

Microbiologic diagnosis

Microbiologic diagnosis is not commonly used in the management of periodontal disease. Dark-field and phase-contrast microscopy have been used to identify spirochetes and other motile organisms in plaque samples. Because spirochetes are detectable in most plaques, it is necessary to establish some critical value for the diagnosis of a spirochetal infection. The author's experience suggests that any plaque sample composed of 20% or more of spirochetes permits the diagnosis of an anaerobic infection [100].

A microscopic examination cannot distinguish the species of bacteria present unless one uses an immunologic staining reagent specific for the organism in question. Such immunodiagnostic reagents have been used in the research laboratory to detect and quantitate the levels of *P gingivalis, P intermedia, T denticola,* and *A actinomycetemcomitans* in the plaque, but no standard products are available commercially. Cultural methods can provide information about the levels of *A actinomycetemcomitans*, black-pigmented species, *Campylobacter* species, and other periodontopathogens. Also, because viable organisms are available, antibiotic sensitivities of the isolated organisms can be determined, and this information may be useful in certain instances. Cultural methods, however, would not be adequate for the enumeration of most anaerobic species unless special efforts are made to maintain anaerobiosis.

Other diagnostic reagents are being developed to detect in plaque specific microbes or metabolites or enzymes unique to inflammation or infection. For example, specific microbes can be demonstrated in plaque by the use of DNA probes [95,101], but no commercial DNA probes are available that would provide standardization of these probes. Future diagnostic procedures may rely on the detection of hydroxyproline, a collagen degradation product; prostaglandin, an inflammatory mediator; and enzymes derived from either the host or the microbes.

A trypsinlike enzyme is present in *T denticola*, *P gingivalis*, and *T forsythia* and is absent from at least 60 other subgingival plaque organisms [99]. The ability of subgingival plaque to hydrolyze BANA was associated with elevated levels and proportions of spirochetes and with probing depths greater than 6 mm. Subsequently, BANA hydrolysis was shown to be related to the *T denticola* and *P gingivalis* content of the plaque and to the clinical diagnosis of health or disease [102]. When these identification procedures were performed on the same plaque samples, the DNA probes and immunologic reagents were significantly more likely to detect *P gingivalis, T forsythia, A actinomycetemcomitans,* and *T denticola* than was the traditional cultural approach [90]. When the probes and immunologic reagents were compared with the BANA test, the probes and antibodies were slightly more accurate (88% versus 83%) [103]. All three approaches were essentially comparable, indicating that reliable noncultural methods are available to aid in the microbiologic diagnosis of periodontal infections. Because the BANA test detects an enzyme found in three anaerobic species, it may be used to detect an anaerobic periodontal infection.

Prevention and treatment

Gingivitis

Gingivitis can be prevented by good oral hygiene, by professional débridement of the teeth, and, if needed, by short-term use of products containing chlorhexidine, stannous fluoride, or other antimicrobial agents. Mouth rinses, gels, and toothpastes, when used in conjunction with tooth brushing and flossing, are probably adequate to deliver any antimicrobial agents to subgingival sites that are 1 to 4 mm in depth. At probing depths greater than 3 mm, there may not be sufficient penetration of the agent to the bottom of the pocket, and infection may persist. Subgingival scaling (débridement) by a professional is indicated, and additional benefits usually can be obtained by the use of irrigating devices containing an antimicrobial agent.

There rarely is any need to use systemic antimicrobial agents to treat gingivitis associated with pocket depths of 1 to 4 mm, with the exception of an increasingly rare and painful condition known as "acute necrotizing ulcerative gingivitis" (ANUG) and formerly known as "trench mouth." Cases of ANUG that are refractory to mechanical débridement and topical antimicrobial agents respond quickly and dramatically to systemic metronidazole [104]. The recognition of metronidazole's efficacy in ANUG led to the discovery that metronidazole has bactericidal activity against anaerobes [105]. ANUG is characterized by tissue invasion by spirochetes and possibly other anaerobes and by elevated plaque levels of spirochetes and *P intermedia* [106]. ANUG thus resembles periodontitis in being an anaerobic infection. It also resembles a form of acute gingivitis that is observed in patients who have HIV and that also be treated successfully with metronidazole [71].

Periodontitis

Clinical dentistry has been about 80% to 85% successful in treating periodontitis by débridement and surgical procedures [107,108]. Surgery, however, is labor intensive, costly, painful, and/or perceived as an elective by many individuals. Therefore many periodontitis infections go untreated and possibly contribute to the medical conditions described previously. Most bacteriologic studies implicate anaerobes as the etiologic agents of aggressive and adult periodontitis, and this finding suggests the use of a drug such as metronidazole, which is specific for anaerobes. Unlike other antimicrobial agents, metronidazole would leave behind in the plaque facultative *Streptococcus* and *Actinomyces* species that have been associated with periodontal health [89,95].

Six double-blind studies have demonstrated that metronidazole, given for periods as short as 1 week, can improve periodontal health significantly [109]. In all cases, metronidazole was given in conjunction with professional débriding of the teeth (ie, scaling) and root planing, and patients receiving this intervention were compared with patients who received scaling and root planing plus a placebo. Thus the improvements seen with metronidazole were better than those obtained with the "standard of care." Maximal benefits were obtained when the metronidazole was given after the débridement [110]. The best clinical response often was noted in patients who had more advanced disease, with pocket depths of 6 mm or more; there was only a moderate benefit when the pocket depths were from 4 to 6 mm. In these advanced cases some teeth that initially were scheduled for extraction were found on re-examination no longer to need extraction.

These studies raised the question as to how to measure the efficacy of any type of periodontal treatment. The traditional method is to measure the amount of pocket reduction that occurs following treatment. Normally débridement can reduce pockets about 1 to 2 mm, and periodontal surgery should eliminate pockets. Surgery, however, should be the last resort. In their metronidazole studies, the author and colleagues determined whether metronidazole could reduce the need for periodontal surgery. In three double-blind studies, the unsupervised use of metronidazole for 1 week, when combined with the standard débridement procedures, was able to reduce significantly the number of teeth needing surgery when compared with the débridement procedures plus placebo treatment. In the largest of the studies, about 90% of the teeth initially recommended for either surgery or extraction did not need either surgery of extraction [111]. The initial treatment benefits were sustained, because most patients showed no increase in surgical needs after 6.4 years [112]. Surgical needs over this time period were reduced when metronidazole was taken, unsupervised, for 1 week after the first- and second-year examinations. About 15% of the patients relapsed (ie, more than five teeth needed surgery or extraction). The predictive factors for these patients was smoking at baseline, and, surprisingly, being most compliant in having their teeth cleaned at the scheduled 3-month intervals. Patients who returned sporadically to have their teeth cleaned had significantly less surgical needs.

The observation that some teeth in the patients who received the most sessions of scaling and root planing were most likely to need surgery raises questions concerning the role of débridement in periodontal treatment. It has been dogma in dentistry that a "clean tooth is a healthy tooth," and that plaque control is essential for dental health. A recent study, however, indicated that patients who were most reliable in returning to have their teeth cleaned by the dentist over a 15-year period lost more teeth to periodontal disease than patients who were less compliant in returning for dental cleanings [113]. These studies suggest that a clean tooth is not a healthy tooth in some patients, probably those in whom the underlying infection was not controlled adequately.

It is possible that the nonresponsive teeth in these patients were undertreated, resulting in a persistent anaerobic infection. Teeth that do not respond to scaling and root planing remain colonized by the BANA-positive species *P gingivalis, T forsythia*, and *T denticola* [114,115]. BANA-positive teeth are significantly likely to lose attachment in the 1- to 2-year period following after scaling, root planing, and 1 week of metronidazole use [116]. Teeth that remain infected continue to deteriorate and may serve to infect other teeth, especially if they are instrumented frequently by the clinician during a dental cleaning.

The fact that deterioration was most evident in the multirooted teeth [112] suggests that inadequate access to the root surface is an important aspect of the adverse effect of débridement. Because furcations (the place were multiple roots on a single tooth intersect) cannot be débrided adequately, it is likely that some periodontopathic bacteria remain on the root surfaces and that any bacteria that have invaded the root surface can grow out from this reservoir and repopulate the root. The use of dental instruments such as scalers in these furcations can cause bleeding that could provide nutrients for host-dependent microbes such as *P gingivalis* (hemin and menadione), *T denticola* (spermine, ceruloplasmin) and *T forsythia* (acetylmuramic acid). The dental instrument would be contaminated with these organisms and could spread them to other teeth, because the normal debridement protocol begins with the molars (the teeth most likely to be infected) and moves in an anterior direction to the teeth less likely to be infected.

These findings indicate that periodontal infections should be treated with a combination of débridement and antimicrobial agents, as is done elsewhere in medicine when infections are diagnosed on accessible surfaces. The myth that a clean tooth is a healthy tooth is wrong about 20% of the time and is an error that does not need to be tolerated, especially if dental infections are risk factors for serious medical conditions.

Summary

Dental decay and periodontal disease are diagnosable and treatable bacterial infections. They are distinctly different infections, with dental decay occurring on the supragingival surfaces of the teeth, and periodontal infections occurring in the gingival tissue approximating the subgingival plaque. The bacteria involved and the pathophysiology of these infections are distinctly different.

Dental decay is a sucrose-mediated bacterial overgrowth of aciduric bacterial species, which includes the mutans streptococci and the *Lactobacilli* species. The mutans streptococci quickly sequester dietary sucrose, especially when it is present between meals, forming intracellular and extracellular polysaccharides and sufficient acid to lower the pH at the tooth–plaque interface to pH 5. At that pH, the tooth acts as a buffer and dissolves. If the lost calcium and phosphate ions are not replaced by their supersaturated levels in the saliva, decay results. At this stage, the *Lactobacilli* and other aciduric species become prominent in the plaque. This infection can be treated by the use of sucrose substitutes (eg, xylitol) in snacks such as candies and chewing gums. Also, any fluoride in the plaque, whether delivered by drinking water or dentifrices, can exert an antimicrobial effect at a low pH on the aciduric organisms.

Periodontal infections, in contrast, involve the overgrowth of anaerobic species in the subgingival plaque, initially because of poor oral hygiene but eventually because these organisms can grow on nutrients released by the host from inflamed tissues. Although the infection is polymicrobial, three bacterial species, *T forsythia, P gingivalis*, and *T denticola,* are conspicuous in plaque samples taken from sites of tissue inflammation and destruction. These anaerobic organisms can be identified indirectly in plaque samples by the detection of the BANA enzyme. These infections can be treated by débriding the tooth surfaces, followed immediately by 1 to 2 weeks of systemic metronidazole.

The realization that dental decay and periodontal disease are treatable bacterial infections comes at a time when tooth loss and periodontal disease have been implicated as contributing to serious medical conditions, such as cardiovascular disease, preterm births, and Alzheimer's disease, among others. If further study shows that these dental infections are contributory to the medical problems, then they are modifiable risk factors, and the management of dental decay and periodontal disease using infectious disease principles could reduce the prevalence of these medical conditions.

References

[1] Paster BJ, Boches SK, Galvin JL, et al. Bacterial diversity in human subgingival plaque. J Bacteriol 2001;183(12):3770–83.
[2] Kazor CE, Mitchell PM, Lee AM, et al. Diversity of bacterial populations on the tongue dorsa of patients with halitosis and healthy patients. J Clin Microbiol 2003;41(2): 558–63.
[3] Loesche WJ. Role of Streptococcus mutans in human dental decay. Microbiol Rev 1986; 50(4):353–80.
[4] Loesche WJ, Grossman NS. Periodontal disease as a specific, albeit chronic, infection: diagnosis and treatment. Clin Microbiol Rev 2001;14(4):727–52.
[5] Loesche W. Dental caries: a treatable infection. 1st edition. Grand Haven (MI): Automated Diagnostic Documentation Inc; 1993.
[6] Hujoel PP, Cunha-Cruz J, Banting DW, et al. Dental flossing and interproximal caries: a systematic review. J Dent Res 2006;85:298–305.
[7] Hujoel PP, Cunha-Cruz J, Loesche WJ, et al. Personal oral hygiene and chronic periodontitis: a systematic review. Periodontol 2000, 2005;37:1–6.
[8] Mattila KJ, Nieminen MS, Valtonen VV, et al. Association between dental health and acute myocardial infarction. BMJ 1989;298(6676):779–81.
[9] Syrjanen J, Peltola J, Valtonen V, et al. Dental infections in association with cerebral infarction in young and middle-aged men. J Intern Med 1989;225(3):179–84.
[10] Mattila KJ, Valtonen VV, Nieminen M, et al. Dental infection and the risk of new coronary events: prospective study of patients with documented coronary artery disease. Clin Infect Dis 1995;20(3):588–92.
[11] DeStefano F, Anda RF, Kahn HS, et al. Dental disease and risk of coronary heart disease and mortality. BMJ 1993;306(6879):688–91.
[12] Paunio K, Impivaara O, Tiekso J, et al. Missing teeth and ischaemic heart disease in men aged 45-64 years. Eur Heart J 1993;14(Suppl K):54–6.
[13] Beck J, Garcia R, Heiss G, et al. Periodontal disease and cardiovascular disease. J Periodontol 1996;67(10 Suppl):1123–37.
[14] Joshipura KJ, Rimm EB, Douglass CW, et al. Poor oral health and coronary heart disease. J Dent Res 1996;75(9):1631–6.
[15] Hujoel PP, Drangsholt M, Spiekerman C, et al. Periodontal disease and coronary heart disease risk. JAMA 2000;284(11):1406–10.
[16] Offenbacher S, Jared HL, O'Reilly PG, et al. Potential pathogenic mechanisms of periodontitis associated pregnancy complications. Ann Periodontol 1998;3(1):233–50.
[17] Lopez NJ, Da Silva I, Ipinza J, et al. Periodontal therapy reduces the rate of preterm low birth weight in women with pregnancy-associated gingivitis. J Periodontol 2005;76(11–s): 2144–53.
[18] Michalowicz BS, Hodges JS, DiAngelis AJ, et al. Treatment of periodontal disease and the risk of preterm birth. N Engl J Med 2006;355(18):1885–94.
[19] Gatz M, Mortimer JA, Fratiglioni L, et al. Potentially modifiable risk factors for dementia in identical twins. Alzheimers Dement 2006;2:110–7.
[20] Durack DT. Prevention of infective endocarditis. N Engl J Med 1995;332(1):38–44.
[21] Geerts SO, Nys M, De MP, et al. Systemic release of endotoxins induced by gentle mastication: association with periodontitis severity. J Periodontol 2002;73(1):73–8.
[22] Kweider M, Lowe GD, Murray GD, et al. Dental disease, fibrinogen and white cell count; links with myocardial infarction? Scott Med J 1993;38(3):73–4.
[23] Slade GD, Ghezzi EM, Heiss G, et al. Relationship between periodontal disease and C-reactive protein among adults in the Atherosclerosis Risk in Communities study. Arch Intern Med 2003;163(10):1172–9.
[24] Herzberg MC, Meyer MW. Effects of oral flora on platelets: possible consequences in cardiovascular disease. J Periodontol 1996;67(10 Suppl):1138–42.

[25] Noack B, Genco RJ, Trevisan M, et al. Periodontal infections contribute to elevated systemic C-reactive protein level. J Periodontol 2001;72(9):1221–7.
[26] Bretz WA, Weyant RJ, Corby PM, et al. Systemic inflammatory markers, periodontal diseases, and periodontal infections in an elderly population. J Am Geriatr Soc 2005; 53(9):1532–7.
[27] Haraszthy VI, Zambon JJ, Trevisan M, et al. Identification of periodontal pathogens in atheromatous plaques. J Periodontol 2000;71(10):1554–60.
[28] Mastragelopulos N, Haraszthy VI, Zambon JJ, et al. [Detection of periodontal pathogenic microorganisms in atheromatous plaque. Preliminary results]. Chirurg 2002;73(6):585–91 [in German].
[29] Iwamoto Y, Nishimura F, Soga Y, et al. Antimicrobial periodontal treatment decreases serum C-reactive protein, tumor necrosis factor-alpha, but not adiponectin levels in patients with chronic periodontitis. J Periodontol 2003;74(8):1231–6.
[30] D'Aiuto F, Nibali L, Parkar M, et al. Short-term effects of intensive periodontal therapy on serum inflammatory markers and cholesterol. J Dent Res 2005;84(3):269–73.
[31] Montebugnoli L, Servidio D, Miaton RA, et al. Periodontal health improves systemic inflammatory and haemostatic status in subjects with coronary heart disease. J Clin Periodontol 2005;32(2):188–92.
[32] Mattila KJ, Asikainen S, Wolf J, et al. Age, dental infections, and coronary heart disease. J Dent Res 2000;79(2):756–60.
[33] Hung HC, Joshipura KJ, Colditz G, et al. The association between tooth loss and coronary heart disease in men and women. J Public Health Dent 2004;64(4):209–15.
[34] Hildebrandt GH, Dominguez BL, Schork MA, et al. Functional units, chewing, swallowing, and food avoidance among the elderly. J Prosthet Dent 1997;77(6):588–95.
[35] Loesche WJ. Chemotherapy of dental plaque infections. Oral Sci Rev 1976;9:65–107.
[36] Loesche WJ, Kazor C. Microbiology and treatment of halitosis. Periodontol 2000 2002;28: 256–79.
[37] Loesche WJ, Straffon LH. Longitudinal investigation of the role of Streptococcus mutans in human fissure decay. Infect Immun 1979;26(2):498–507.
[38] Florio FM, Klein MI, Pereira AC, et al. Time of initial acquisition of mutans streptococci by human infants. J Clin Pediatr Dent 2004;28(4):303–8.
[39] Wan AK, Seow WK, Purdie DM, et al. A longitudinal study of Streptococcus mutans colonization in infants after tooth eruption. J Dent Res 2003;82(7):504–8.
[40] Berkowitz RJ, Jones P. Mouth-to-mouth transmission of the bacterium Streptococcus mutans between mother and child. Arch Oral Biol 1985;30(4):377–9.
[41] Brailsford SR, Sheehy EC, Gilbert SC, et al. The microflora of the erupting first permanent molar. Caries Res 2005;39(1):78–84.
[42] Van Houte J, Sansone C, Joshipura K, et al. Mutans streptococci and non-mutans streptococci acidogenic at low pH, and in vitro acidogenic potential of dental plaque in two different areas of the human dentition. J Dent Res 1991;70(12):1503–7.
[43] Milgrom P, Riedy CA, Weinstein P, et al. Dental caries and its relationship to bacterial infection, hypoplasia, diet, and oral hygiene in 6- to 36-month-old children. Community Dent Oral Epidemiol 2000;28(4):295–306.
[44] Boyar RM, Bowden GH. The microflora associated with the progression of incipient carious lesions of children living in a water-fluoridated area. Caries Res 1985;19(4):298–306.
[45] Gustafsson BE, Quensel CE, Lanke LS, et al. The Vipeholm dental caries study; the effect of different levels of carbohydrate intake on caries activity in 436 individuals observed for five years. Acta Odontol Scand 1954;11(3–4):232–64.
[46] Fitzgerald DB, Stevens R, Fitzgerald RJ, et al. Comparative cariogenicity of streptococcus mutans strains isolated from caries active and caries resistant adults. J Dent Res 1977;56(8): 894.
[47] Gibbons RJ, Fitzgerald RJ. Dextran-induced agglutination of Streptococcus mutans, and its potential role in the formation of microbial dental plaques. J Bacteriol 1969;98(2):341–6.

[48] Guggenheim B. Enzymatic hydrolysis and structure of water-insoluble glucan produced by glucosyltransferases from a strain of streptococcus mutans. Helv Odontol Acta 1970; 14(Suppl 5):89–94.
[49] Johnson MC, Bozzola JJ, Shechmeister IL. Morphological study of Streptococcus mutans and two extracellular polysaccharide mutants. J Bacteriol 1974;118(1):304–11.
[50] Tanzer JM, Freedman ML, Fitzgerald RJ, et al. Diminished virulence of glucan synthesis-defective mutants of Streptococcus mutans. Infect Immun 1974;10(1):197–203.
[51] Johnson MC, Bozzola JJ, Shechmeister IL, et al. Biochemical study of the relationship of extracellular glucan to adherence and cariogenicity in Streptococcus mutans and an extracellular polysaccharide mutant. J Bacteriol 1977;129(1):351–7.
[52] de Stoppelaar JD, Konig KG, Plasschaert AJ, et al. Decreased cariogenicity of a mutant of Streptococcus mutans. Arch Oral Biol 1971;16(8):971–5.
[53] Loesche WJ, Kornman KS. Production of mannitol by Streptococcus mutans. Arch Oral Biol 1976;21(9):551–3.
[54] Bratthall D, Hoszek A, Zhao X. Evaluation of a simplified method for site-specific determination of mutans streptococci levels. Swed Dent J 1996;20(6):215–20.
[55] Jensen B, Bratthall D. A new method for the estimation of mutans streptococci in human saliva. J Dent Res 1989;68(3):468–71.
[56] Krasse B. Biological factors as indicators of future caries. Int Dent J 1988;38(4):219–25.
[57] Dreizen S, Brown LR. Xerostomia and dental caries. Presented at the Microbial Aspects Of Dental Caries. St Simon Island (GA), June 21–24, 1976.
[58] Loesche WJ. The rationale for caries prevention through the use of sugar substitutes. Int Dent J 1985;35(1):1–8.
[59] Scheinin A. Dental caries, sugars and xylitol. Ann Med 1993;25(6):519–21.
[60] Loesche WJ, Grossman NS, Earnest R, et al. The effect of chewing xylitol gum on the plaque and saliva levels of Streptococcus mutans. J Am Dent Assoc 1984;108(4): 587–92.
[61] Burt BA. The use of sorbitol- and xylitol-sweetened chewing gum in caries control. J Am Dent Asso 2006;137(2):190–6.
[62] Uhari M, Tapiainen T, Kontiokari T. Xylitol in preventing acute otitis media. Vaccine 2000;19(Suppl 1):S144–7.
[63] Caufield PW, Cutter GR, Dasanayake AP. Initial acquisition of mutans streptococci by infants: evidence for a discrete window of infectivity. J Dent Res 1993;72(1):37–45.
[64] Kohler B, Andreen I, Jonsson B. The effect of caries-preventive measures in mothers on dental caries and the oral presence of the bacteria Streptococcus mutans and lactobacilli in their children. Arch Oral Biol 1984;29(11):879–83.
[65] Kohler B, Andreen I. Influence of caries-preventive measures in mothers on cariogenic bacteria and caries experience in their children. Arch Oral Biol 1994;39(10):907–11.
[66] Soderling E, Isokangas P, Pienihakkinen K, et al. Influence of maternal xylitol consumption on acquisition of mutans streptococci by infants. J Dent Res 2000;79(3):882–7.
[67] Soderling E, Isokangas P, Pienihakkinen K, et al. Influence of maternal xylitol consumption on mother-child transmission of mutans streptococci: 6-year follow-up. Caries Res 2001;35(3):173–7.
[68] Thorild I, Lindau B, Twetman S. Caries in 4-year-old children after maternal chewing of gums containing combinations of xylitol, sorbitol, chlorhexidine and fluoride. Eur Arch Paediatr Dent 2006;7(4):241–5.
[69] Oliver RC, Brown LJ, Loe H. Periodontal diseases in the United States population. J Periodontol 1998;69(2):269–78.
[70] Papapanou PN. Periodontal diseases: epidemiology. Ann Periodontol 1996;1(1):1–36.
[71] Winkler JR, Murray PA, Grassi M, et al. Diagnosis and management of HIV-associated periodontal lesions. J Am Dent Assoc 1989;110(Suppl):25S–34S.
[72] Loe H, Theilade E, Jensen HB. Experimental gingivitis in man. J Periodontol 1965;36: 177–81.

[73] Loesche WJ, Syed SA. Bacteriology of human experimental gingivitis: effect of plaque and gingivitis score. Infect Immun 1978;21(3):830–9.
[74] Syed SA, Loesche WJ. Bacteriology of human experimental gingivitis: effect of plaque age. Infect Immun 1978;21(3):821–9.
[75] Kenny EB, Ash MM. Oxidation reduction potential of developing plaque, periodontal pockets and gingival sulci. J. Periodontol 1969;40:630–3.
[76] Armitage GC. Development of a classification system for periodontal diseases and conditions. Ann Periodontol 1999;4:1–6.
[77] Alaluusua S, Asikainen S, Lai CH. Intrafamilial transmission of Actinobacillus actinomycetemcomitans. J Periodontol 1991;62(3):207–10.
[78] Tuite-McDonnell M, Griffen AL, Moeschberger ML, et al. Concordance of Porphyromonas gingivalis colonization in families. J Clin Microbiol 1997;35(2):455–61.
[79] Umeda M, Miwa Z, Takeuchi Y, et al. The distribution of periodontopathic bacteria among Japanese children and their parents. J Periodontal Res 2004;39(6):398–404.
[80] Newman MG, Socransky SS. Predominant cultivable microbiota in periodontosis. J Periodontal Res 1977;12(2):120–8.
[81] Tanner AC, Visconti RA, Socransky SS, et al. Classification and identification of Actinobacillus actinomycetemcomitans and Haemophilus aphrophilus by cluster analysis and deoxyribonucleic acid hybridizations. J Periodontal Res 1982;17(6):585–96.
[82] Zambon JJ. Actinobacillus actinomycetemcomitans in human periodontal disease. J Clin Periodontol 1985;12(1):1–20.
[83] Slots J. Selective medium for isolation of Actinobacillus actinomycetemcomitans. J Clin Microbiol 1982;15(4):606–9.
[84] Slots J, Reynolds HS, Genco RJ. Actinobacillus actinomycetemcomitans in human periodontal disease: a cross-sectional microbiological investigation. Infect Immun 1980; 29(3):1013–20.
[85] Albandar JM, Brown LJ, Loe H. Putative periodontal pathogens in subgingival plaque of young adults with and without early-onset periodontitis. J Periodontol 1997;68(10):973–81.
[86] Saxen L, Asikainen S. Metronidazole in the treatment of localized juvenile periodontitis. J Clin Periodontol 1993;20(3):166–71.
[87] Brown LJ, Loe H. Prevalence, extent, severity and progression of periodontal disease. Periodontol 2000;2:57–71.
[88] Ellen RP, Galimanas VB. Spirochetes at the forefront of periodontal infections. Periodontol 2000 2005;38:13–32.
[89] Loesche WJ, Syed SA, Schmidt E, et al. Bacterial profiles of subgingival plaques in periodontitis. J Periodontol 1985;56(8):447–56.
[90] Loesche WJ, Lopatin DE, Stoll J, et al. Comparison of various detection methods for periodontopathic bacteria: can culture be considered the primary reference standard? J Clin Microbiol 1992;30(2):418–26.
[91] Grossi SG, Zambon JJ, Ho AW, et al. Assessment of risk for periodontal disease. I. Risk indicators for attachment loss. J Periodontol 1994;65(3):260–7.
[92] Grossi SG, Genco RJ, Machtei EE, et al. Assessment of risk for periodontal disease. II. Risk indicators for alveolar bone loss. J Periodontol 1995;66(1):23–9.
[93] Machtei EE, Hausmann E, Dunford R, et al. Longitudinal study of predictive factors for periodontal disease and tooth loss. J Clin Periodontol 1999;26(6):374–80.
[94] Machtei EE, Dunford R, Hausmann E, et al. Longitudinal study of prognostic factors in established periodontitis patients. J Clin Periodontol 1997;24(2):102–9.
[95] Socransky SS, Haffajee AD, Cugini MA, et al. Microbial complexes in subgingival plaque. J Clin Periodontol 1998;25(2):134–44.
[96] Papapanou PN, Baelum V, Luan WM, et al. Subgingival microbiota in adult Chinese: prevalence and relation to periodontal disease progression. J Periodontol 1997;68(7):651–66.
[97] Ximenez-Fyvie LA, Haffajee AD, Socransky SS. Comparison of the microbiota of supra- and subgingival plaque in health and periodontitis. J Clin Periodontol 2000;27(9):648–57.

[98] Avila-Campos MJ, Velasquez-Melendez G. Prevalence of putative periodontopathogens from periodontal patients and healthy subjects in Sao Paulo, SP, Brazil. Rev Inst Med Trop Sao Paulo 2002;44(1):1–5.
[99] Loesche WJ, Bretz WA, Kerschensteiner D, et al. Development of a diagnostic test for anaerobic periodontal infections based on plaque hydrolysis of benzoyl-DL-arginine-naphthylamide. J Clin Microbiol 1990;28(7):1551–9.
[100] Apsey DJ, Kaciroti N, Loesche WJ. The diagnosis of periodontal disease in private practice. J Periodontol 2006;77(9):1572–81.
[101] Slots J, Ashimoto A, Flynn MJ, et al. Detection of putative periodontal pathogens in subgingival specimens by 16S ribosomal DNA amplification with the polymerase chain reaction. Clin Infect Dis 1995;20(Suppl 2):S304–7.
[102] Loesche WJ, Bretz WA, Lopatin D, et al. Multi-center clinical evaluation of a chairside method for detecting certain periodontopathic bacteria in periodontal disease. J Periodontol 1990;61(3):189–96.
[103] Loesche WJ, Lopatin DE, Giordano J, et al. Comparison of the benzoyl-DL-arginine-naphthylamide (BANA) test, DNA probes, and immunological reagents for ability to detect anaerobic periodontal infections due to Porphyromonas gingivalis, Treponema denticola, and Bacteroides forsythus. J Clin Microbiol 1992;30(2):427–33.
[104] Shinn DL. Vincent's disease and its treatment. In: Finegold SM, editor. Metronidazole. Excerpta Medica. 1977;307–8.
[105] Tally FP, Goldin BR, Sullivan N, et al. Antimicrobial activity of metronidazole in anaerobic bacteria. Antimicrob Agents Chemother 1978;13(3):460–5.
[106] Loesche WJ, Syed SA, Laughon BE, et al. The bacteriology of acute necrotizing ulcerative gingivitis. J Periodontol 1982;53(4):223–30.
[107] Hirschfeld L, Wasserman B. A long-term survey of tooth loss in 600 treated periodontal patients. J Periodontol 1978;49(5):225–37.
[108] McFall WT Jr. Tooth loss in 100 treated patients with periodontal disease. A long- term study. J Periodontol 1982;53(9):539–49.
[109] Loesche WJ. The antimicrobial treatment of periodontal disease: changing the treatment paradigm. Crit Rev Oral Biol Med 1999;10(3):245–75.
[110] Loesche WJ, Giordano JR. Metronidazole in periodontitis V: debridement should precede medication. Compendium 1994;15(10):1198, 1201, 1203 passim; [quiz: 1218].
[111] Loesche WJ, Giordano J, Soehren S, et al. Nonsurgical treatment of patients with periodontal disease. Oral Surg Oral Med Oral Pathol Oral Radiol Endod 1996;81(5):533–43.
[112] Loesche WJ, Giordano JR, Soehren S, et al. The nonsurgical treatment of patients with periodontal disease: results after 6.4 years. Gen Dent 2005;53(4):298–306 [quiz: 307].
[113] Miyamoto T, Kumagai T, Jones JA, et al. Compliance as a prognostic indicator: retrospective study of 505 patients treated and maintained for 15 years. J Periodontol 2006;77(2): 223–32.
[114] Kamma JJ, Baehni PC. Five-year maintenance follow-up of early-onset periodontitis patients. J Clin Periodontol 2003;30(6):562–72.
[115] Haffajee AD, Cugini MA, Dibart S, et al. Clinical and microbiological features of subjects with adult periodontitis who responded poorly to scaling and root planing. J Clin Periodontol 1997;24(10):767–76.
[116] Loesche WJ, Giordano J, Hujoel PP. The utility of the BANA test for monitoring anaerobic infections due to spirochetes (Treponema denticola) in periodontal disease. J Dent Res 1990;69(10):1696–702.

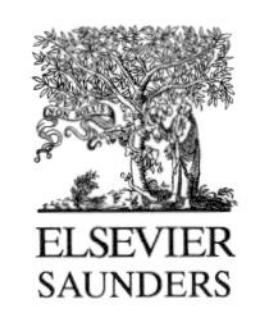

ELSEVIER
SAUNDERS

INFECTIOUS
DISEASE CLINICS
OF NORTH AMERICA

Infect Dis Clin N Am 21 (2007) 503–522

Mucositis in the Cancer Patient and Immunosuppressed Host

Joel B. Epstein, DMD, MSD, FRCD(C)[a,b,*]

[a] *Department of Oral Medicine and Diagnostic Sciences, College of Dentistry, 801 South Paulina St., Chicago, IL 60612, USA*

[b] *Oral Cancer Biology, Detection and Treatment, Chicago Cancer Center, University of Illinois at Chicago, 801 South Paulina St., Chicago, IL 60612, USA*

Oropharyngeal mucositis (OM) is the most common, distressing, and disabling complication of chemotherapy and radiotherapy in patients who have cancer and in other severely immunosuppressed hosts [1–8]. OM may develop in 10% to 75% of patients undergoing chemotherapy and in up to 75% of patients receiving hematopoietic cell transplantation (HCT). Virtually all patients who receive combined radiation and chemotherapy for head and neck cancer develop OM with enhanced severity and duration [9–14]. Standard chemotherapy regimens for non-Hodgkin's lymphoma result in clinically significant OM in 3% to 10% of patients, and similar rates are seen with doxorubicin- and taxane-based regimens for breast cancer. Severe oromucositis and esophagitis are seen during radiotherapy and concurrent platinum therapy in more than 15% of patients who have lung cancer [10]. Increased severity and duration of mucositis is seen in patients receiving hyperfractionated radiotherapy [11], and the severity of mucositis in intensity-modulated radiation therapy seems similar to that seen in conventional radiotherapy protocols with or without chemotherapy [15].

Pathogenesis

Development of oral mucositis is thought to include several phases: (1) initiation, characterized by changes in the epithelium and connective tissue; (2) primary response to tissue injury with signal amplification; (3) ulceration with barrier loss; and (4) healing [16]. Earliest changes occur in the

* Interdisciplinary Program in Oral Cancer, College of Medicine, Chicago Cancer Center, 801 South Paulina St., Chicago, IL 60612.

E-mail address: jepstein@uic.edu

doi:10.1016/j.idc.2007.03.003 **id.theclinics.com**

connective tissue in response to DNA and non-DNA damage from chemotherapy and radiation. This damage leads to the production of reactive oxygen species and proinflammatory cytokines such as interleukin (IL)-2 and IL-6, and tumor necrosis factor alpha. Reactive oxygen species cause molecular damage, activation of nuclear factor kappa B with further increased expression of genes involved in inflammation and cell death (apoptosis), and activation of the sphingomyelin pathway. Early changes occur in cell surface molecules, with an increase in integral membrane proteins such as RM3-1, and intercellular adhesion molecules [16,17]. These processes result in vascular dilation, increased cellular extravasation, apoptosis, and inflammation. Increased levels of epidermal growth factor are detected in the oral secretions of patients receiving radiation therapy [18]. In the epithelium, apoptosis and necrosis (probably related to events in the submucosa) accompany ongoing cellular proliferation. Ulceration develops when destruction of the basal cells of the epithelium exceeds proliferation of new cells. The oral microflora, which normally reside on intact mucosa, may invade deeper tissues in the submucosa when ulceration develops and further stimulate the release of inflammatory cytokines. The outcomes of infection associated with mucosal damage are conditioned by the impact of systemic therapy on the hematopoietic system and immune function. Resolution of mucositis involves interaction between the epithelial and connective tissue compartments and depends on the production of growth factors, angiogenesis, and epithelial cell regeneration/migration, which in turn may be enhanced after the return of white blood cell function [16–21].

Risk factors

Underlying systemic disease, toxic or immunosuppressive therapy, and concurrent oropharyngeal infection may all contribute to the development of oral mucositis. Other risk factors include poor oral hygiene, tobacco use, hyposalivation, lower baseline neutrophil counts, elevated serum urea nitrogen and serum creatinine levels, and older age [22–25]. The elderly may be at increased risk of mucosal toxicity because of reduced metabolic reserve and altered metabolism of chemotherapeutic agents [25]. In patients receiving HCT and intensive chemotherapy, associated myelosuppression can trigger reactivation of herpes simplex virus (HSV) and predispose the patient to the development of oropharyngeal candidiasis.

Host factors

Mucosal defenses of the healthy oral cavity include integrity of the epithelial barrier, exfoliation of mucosal epithelial cells, antimicrobial salivary constituents, salivary flow and clearance, and protective effects of the resident oral microflora [26–31]. These defenses are compromised by cancer therapy. The precise role of the oral flora and microbial end products in the genesis of oral mucositis is not clear, although high levels of dental plaque caused by poor oral hygiene have been shown to worsen the severity of mucositis [22–25,32–34]. Conversely, intensive oral hygiene has been shown to reduce both the severity and duration of oral mucositis in patients receiving HCT [32]. Cell-mediated immunity plays an important role in oral defense against intracellular pathogens, and in immunocompromised patients the risk of reactivation of viral infection occurs both regionally and systemically. Children may have fewer complications with mucositis, possibly because of fewer problems associated with pre-existing chronic dental infections and latent micro-organisms [35].

Underlying systemic disease

Underlying disease is a critical factor in determining the severity of mucositis and risk for infection. In patients receiving chemotherapy for solid tumors, approximately 10% may develop oral infection, more than two thirds of which are of fungal origin [10,36]. In immunocompromised patients who have blood dyscrasias, the frequency and severity of infection increases with the severity and duration of myelosuppression, particularly in those who have damage to the oral mucosa [37–41]. Patients who have AIDS have many of the infections and risks of complication described for patients who have cancer treated with radiation and chemotherapy. Oropharyngeal candidiasis is the most common oral presentation in HIV infection. Labial and oral HSV infections are common also.

Medical interventions

In addition to mucosal damage and immunosuppression, medical management associated with cancer therapy and hospitalization impacts the oral environment. Reduced epithelial cell turnover resulting from cancer therapy allows retention of adherent organisms and enhance the risk of infection. The oral flora is impacted by the use of prophylactic and therapeutic antibiotics, antivirals, antifungals, and steroids. A shift in the oral flora may occur with overgrowth of organisms not indigenous to the oral cavity, including nosocomial pathogens. Both radiation and chemotherapy lead to xerostomia. Immunoglobulins, reduced saliva volume, and changes in salivary constituents have major effects on the oral microenvironment. Salivary lysozyme, lactoferrin, lactoperoxidase, histidine-rich polypeptides, protegrins, and defensins inhibit both bacteria and fungi [28,29,42–44]. Salivary glycoproteins inhibit microbial attachment to the oral epithelium through competition with cellular receptor sites and by clumping of micro-organisms [27,30]. Salivary antibodies may affect the oral flora by aggregation of organisms and preventing adherence to the mucosal epithelium [27,45,46]. In patients who have dry mouth, the oral flora shifts from a predominantly gram-positive flora to a predominantly gram-negative and fungal flora

[32,47–51]. The decrease in epidermal growth factor and antimicrobial proteins in the saliva after conditioning for HCT may lead to increased risk of mucositis and mucosal infection. Reduced salivary IgA in patients treated with methotrexate has been correlated with mucositis.

Clinical manifestations of oral mucositis and oral infections

Oropharyngeal mucositis

OM is characterized by mucosal erythema, ulceration, and oropharyngeal pain (Fig. 1). OM typically develops 7 to 14 days after the initiation of chemotherapy or radiotherapy. Chemotherapy-associated OM arises on the nonkeratinized mucosa (the soft palate, ventral tongue, and floor of the mouth) and the buccal and labial mucosa. Typically, there is bilateral involvement with ulceration, foul odor, and necrotic debris. OM associated with radiation therapy involves the nonkeratinized mucosa, primarily in the high-dose fields. Healing typically occurs 2 to 4 weeks after completion of cancer chemotherapy, although with more aggressive cancer treatment protocols mucositis may persist more than 4 weeks after therapy.

Pain associated with OM is the most common and debilitating complaint by patients undergoing cancer therapy (Box 1) [8,52–54]. Pain associated with mucositis is dependent on the degree of tissue damage [21], sensitization of pain receptors, and the elaboration of inflammatory and pain mediators. There is considerable individual variation.

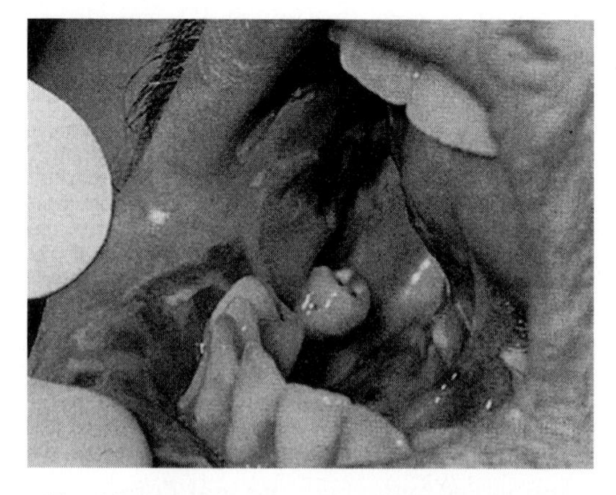

Fig. 1. Severe mucositis with marked erythema, loss of epithelial barrier, and extensive ulceration of the labial and buccal mucosa in a patient receiving radiation therapy. (*From* Epstein JB, Chow AW. Oral complications associated with immunosuppression and cancer therapies. Infect Dis Clin N Am 1999;13:915; with permission.)

Box 1. Impact of oral mucositis on quality of life

Pain, often requiring opioid analgesics
Possible oral bleeding
Impact on communication, speech, and expression
Difficulty with speech, denture use, oral hygiene, dysguesia, bad breath, and dysphagia
Inability to take nutrition or hydration by mouth, requiring tube feeding or parenteral nutrition
Inability to take medication by mouth
Portal for systemic infection (primarily n neutropenic patients) with potential mortality
Need for or prolongation of hospitalization
Increased cost of care

Oropharyngeal infections

Bacterial infections

Bacteremia and septicemia arising from oral sources have been well documented in immunosuppressed patients. Whereas gram-negative bacteria predominated in the past, more recent studies have reported an increased rate of gram-positive infections (staphylococci, streptococci, enterococci) (Fig. 2) [26,55]. Bacteremia caused by oral viridans streptococci has become more prevalent in patients who have acute leukemia and correlates with the presence of mucosal barrier injury. In such patients, elevations in serum IL-8

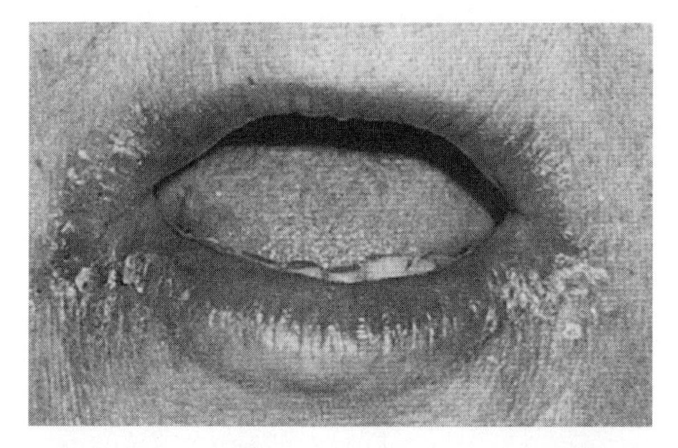

Fig. 2. Severe cheilitis producing pain and discomfort in a patient undergoing chemotherapy for breast carcinoma. Laboratory testing demonstrated a pure culture of *Staphylococcus aureus*. The intensely red, ulcerated, and crusted lesion did not improve until an antibacterial cream was applied. (*From* Epstein JB, Chow AW. Oral complications associated with immunosuppression and cancer therapies. Infect Dis Clin N Am 1999;13:915; with permission.)

and C-reactive protein often can be documented before onset of clinical infection and fever [38,39]. The change in the organisms identified in bacteremia among patients who have leukemia may be related to the use of prophylactic antibiotics such as the fluoroquinolones. Greenberg and colleagues [56] identified an oral source of septicemia in 25% of patients who had acute leukemia and who received dental care and scaling before chemotherapy. This finding contrasts with a rate of 77% among patients without such dental care before chemotherapy. The primary sources of bacteremia in these patients were pre-existing periodontal infections and infections associated with partially erupted wisdom teeth. Gingivitis and periodontitis caused by mixed bacterial infection also are common in patients who have acute nonlymphocytic leukemia and have been reported in up to 25% of all infections (Fig. 3) [57]. The clinical findings are bleeding of the gums and gingival inflammation. When the inflammation is acute, symptoms include pain, tenderness, and bad taste. Other signs of inflammation may be minimal in the immunocompromised host, however.

Fungal infections

Oropharyngeal candidiasis is the most common oropharyngeal mucosal infection after radiation therapy in patients who have cancer [47,58], in neutropenic patients [47,55,58–64], and in patients receiving myelosuppressive chemotherapy [37–40,47,53,58,65]. Oropharyngeal colonization by *Candida* species is present commonly before clinical infection and before systemic infection in myelosuppressed patients. Candidiasis may present as white and red intraoral mucosal lesions and cracking at the corners of the mouth. Pseudomembranous candidiasis (thrush) presents as adherent white plaques

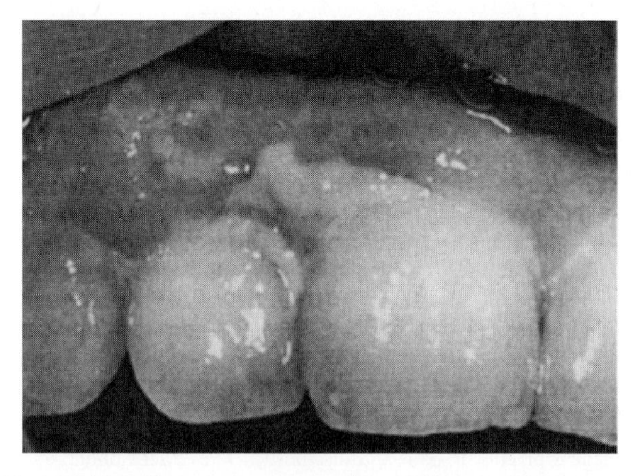

Fig. 3. Mixed bacterial infection of the periodontium leading to ulceration of the interdental papillae in a patient who has leukemia. The infection was not associated with marked erythema and was only mildly tender. (*From* Epstein JB, Chow AW. Oral complications associated with immunosuppression and cancer therapies. Infect Dis Clin N Am 1999;13:915; with permission.)

that can be wiped off the mucosa (Fig. 4). Hyperplastic candidiasis may present as white lesions that cannot be removed from the surface and requires a biopsy and special stains for diagnosis. Red lesions may represent an inflammatory lesion resulting from infection, trauma, immune-mediated reactions, or a vascular or hematologic disorder. Erythematous candidiasis may involve the dorsal surface of the tongue, typically with loss of papillae and erythema in the midline of the dorsum of the tongue. Patients who have positive cultures for Candida from multiple sites are considered at high risk of systemic infection. Disseminated candidiasis is potentially fatal and can be difficult to diagnose unless blood cultures are positive (Fig. 5).

Aspergillus species also may cause infection in neutropenic patients and is increasingly common, with the most common site of infection in the upper respiratory tract. Aspergillus infection may present as masses, ulceration, and bone loss when alveolar bone is involved [37–39,60]. Histoplasmosis, coccidiomycosis, mucormycosis, and other fungal pathogens may have a similar clinical presentation but are less common.

Viral infections

Viral reactivation occurs commonly in adults who have leukemia and is common in immunosuppressed patients. Viral infections associated with defects in cell-mediated immunity include the herpes family of viruses (HSV, varicella zoster virus, cytomegalovirus, Epstein-Barr virus, human herpesvirus-8). Herpetic lesions have a propensity to occur on keratinized or attached oral mucosa, such as gingiva and palate (Fig. 6), and on the tongue. In severely immunosuppressed patients, infection may extend

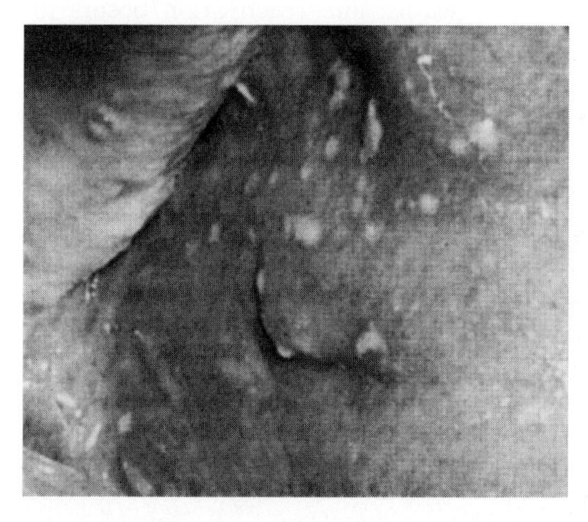

Fig. 4. Pseudomembranous candidiasis presenting with white plaques that can be wiped off, leaving an erythematous or bleeding area. The patient was immunosuppressed because of HIV infection and had symptoms of burning sensitivity in the mouth. (*From* Epstein JB, Chow AW. Oral complications associated with immunosuppression and cancer therapies. Infect Dis Clin N Am 1999;13:915; with permission.)

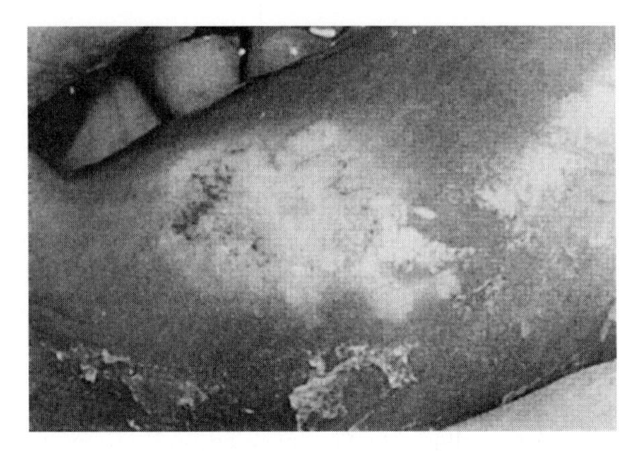

Fig. 5. This patient who had acute myelomonocytic leukemia (M4) developed an invasive candidal ulcer of the lower lip. Diagnosis required a biopsy. Systemic candidiasis was confirmed in the blood and later at postmortem. (*From* Epstein JB, Chow AW. Oral complications associated with immunosuppression and cancer therapies. Infect Dis Clin N Am 1999;13:915; with permission.)

regionally to involve nonkeratinized tissue, resulting in esophagitis, tracheitis, and disseminated infection. Varicella-zoster reactivation also is common in immunocompromised patients, with lesions initially confined to the dermatome of the involved nerve (Fig. 7) and with potential for dissemination with hematogenous spread to other organs. Epstein-Barr virus is present in the oral secretions in up to 60% of patients during HCT and has been associated with hairy leukoplakia changes in patients who have AIDS and in HCT recipients [66,67]. Cytomegalovirus causes up to 20% of posttransplantation deaths, and reactivation occurs in up to 70% of

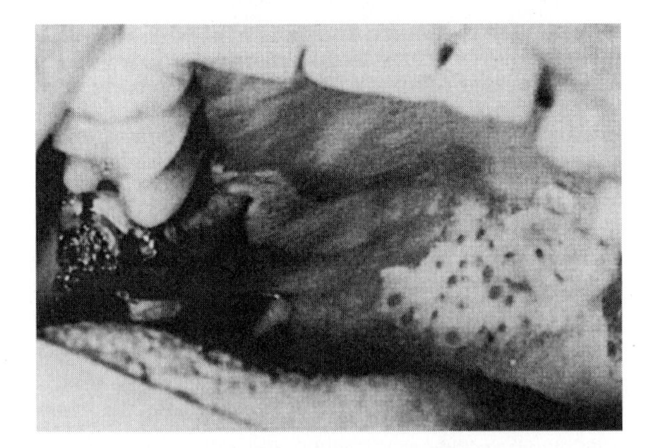

Fig. 6. Extensive palatal ulcer extending from the gingival margin to involve the hard and soft palate. This confluent, extensive ulcer was caused by HSV infection in a patient receiving bone marrow transplantation for leukemia. (*From* Epstein JB, Chow AW. Oral complications associated with immunosuppression and cancer therapies. Infect Dis Clin N Am 1999;13:915; with permission.)

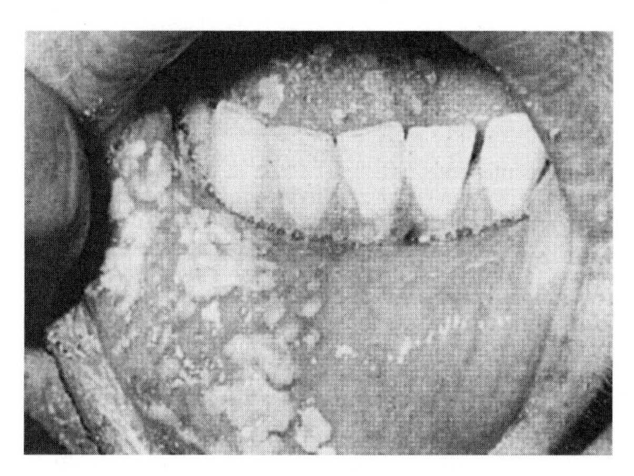

Fig. 7. Unilateral viral vesicles and ulcerations confined to the mandibular division of the trigeminal nerve, affecting the skin and oral mucosa. The diagnosis of herpes zoster virus was made in this patient who had completed chemotherapy for non-Hodgkin's lymphoma. (*From* Epstein JB, Chow AW. Oral complications associated with immunosuppression and cancer therapies. Infect Dis Clin N Am 1999;13:915; with permission.)

seropositive patients [68]. Cytomegalovirus can present as oropharyngeal mucosal ulcers involving keratinized and nonkeratinized tissues and has been associated with gingival hyperplasia [67,69].

Management of oral mucositis

The increasing understanding of the biologic basis of mucosal injury and repair in cancer therapy is leading to the development of more rational approaches to therapy. Guidelines for the management of mucositis have been published recently (Boxes 2 and 3) [9,70].

Basic oral care and good clinical practice

Good clinical practices should focus on maintaining a clean oral cavity, reducing the oral microbial load, and promoting comfort. Oral care should be directed to the individual needs of the patient, and education should include patient, staff, family, and significant others. Regular assessment of oral hygiene, mucosal condition, and oral pain is essential. Good oral hygiene reduces the density of the oral flora, which in turn reduces the likelihood of gingivitis and oral mucositis in high-risk patients [32,71–73]. It has been suggested that good oral hygiene may reduce the development and severity of oral mucositis following chemotherapy or irradiation [32,56,74–76]. Maintaining good oral hygiene has been documented to reduce the risk of bacteremia or fever in patients who have cancer treated with high-dose chemotherapy and in HCT recipients [32].

Box 2. Evidence-based clinical practice guidelines for care of patients who have oromucositis

I. Basic oral care and good clinical practices for oral mucositis
  1. Oral care protocol that includes patient and provider education
  2. Oral care protocol that includes use of a soft toothbrush
  3. Oral condition, oral pain, and impact of oral care assessed on a regular basis using validated tools

II. Patient-controlled analgesia with morphine for oral mucositis pain in patients undergoing HCT

III. Prevention of oral mucositis in radiotherapy
  1. Midline radiation blocks and three-dimensional radiation treatment to reduce mucosal injury
  2. Benzydamine for prevention in patients who have head and neck cancer, standard fractionation radiation therapy

III. Prevention of oral mucositis in standard-dose chemotherapy
  1. Cryotherapy to prevent oral mucositis with bolus 5-fluorouracil and bolus edatrexate

IV. Prevention of oral mucositis in high-dose chemotherapy with or without total body irradiation/HCT
  1. Keratinocyte growth factor-1 (palifermin) for patients undergoing autologous stem cell transplantation
  2. Cryotherapy to prevent oral mucositis with high-dose melphalan

---

Data from Rubenstein E, Peterson DE, Schubert M, et al, Clinical practice guidelines for the prevention and treatment of cancer therapy-induced oral and gastrointestinal mucositis. Cancer 2004;100:2026–46; and Keefe DM, Schubert MM, Elting KS, et al. Updated clinical practice guidelines for the prevention and treatment of mucositis. Cancer 2007;109(5):820–31.

A preventive oral care regimen should include systematic oral hygiene with a soft toothbrush, flossing, bland rinses, and lip moisturizers (Box 3). Dental assessment and dental treatment are important before the start of cancer therapy for all patients and especially for patients expected to become neutropenic and patients who have head and neck cancer receiving treatment protocols in which oral mucositis is anticipated. Pain management should include topical anesthetics or analgesics as supportive care before the use of systemic analgesics. Nonsteroidal anti-inflammatory analgesics with or without codeine should be used if pain arises, and powerful opioids may be required if pain progresses. Analgesics should be used on a time-contingent basis when topical agents are inadequate for pain control.

Box 3. Supportive care for prevention of oral mucositis

1. Manage pre-existing conditions
   Treat acute, symptomatic infection
   Control chronic, asymptomatic infection
   Eliminate sources of physical irritation
2. Suppress colonizing organisms
   Good oral hygiene, saline or bicarbonate rinses
3. Use antiseptics (chlorhexidine, povidone iodine)
   Topical antibiotics
   Topical antifungals
   Systemic antibiotics
4. Prevent reactivating HSV infection
   Systemic antivirals (acyclovir or analogues)
5. Manage xerostomia
   High fluid intake, saline or bicarbonate rinses, ice chips
   Sialogogues (pilocarpine, anetholetrithione, bethanechol, civemiline)

Prevention of mucositis

Oral rinsing with saline or a bicarbonate solution often is suggested to reduce the severity of mucositis, although there are no studies demonstrating effectiveness (Box 4) [77]. Mouthwashes that contain alcohol and phenol and intense flavoring should be avoided because they may dehydrate the mucosa and increase irritation. Coating agents such as milk of magnesia, kaopectate, aluminum hydroxide, and sucralfate have been used for symptomatic relief and prevention of mucositis, but supportive studies are lacking, although sucralfate may reduce pain report in patients who have ulcerative mucositis [78,79]. Cryotherapy is recommended to prevent oral mucositis in patients receiving drugs with short half-lives, including bolus 5-fluorouracil, high-dose melphalan (conditioning in HCT), and possibly etidronate. Compliance may be limited by the discomfort some patients experience when holding ice in the mouth for an extended period.

Benzydamine rinse is recommended for the prevention of radiation-induced oral mucositis in patients receiving standard daily-fractionated radiation therapy. Palifermin (Kepivance, Amgen Inc, Thousand Oaks, California; keratinocyte growth factor-1) is recommended for patients who have hematologic malignancies receiving high-dose chemotherapy and total body irradiation before autologous stem cell transplant. Continuing studies have shown reduced mucositis in allogeneic transplantation and in patients receiving 5-fluorouracil for colon cancer [80,81]. Additional studies are being conducted to assess its efficacy in head and neck cancer. Tissue protection conferred by palifermin has been attributed to its mitogenic effect, resulting

Box 4. Symptomatic management of oral discomfort

1. General measures: bland diet, nonirritating foods, frequent 0.9% saline or bicarbonate rinses, use of ice chips, good oral hygiene
2. Topical anesthetic rinses: Benzydamine Hcl (3M Canada, London, Ontario), dyclonine HCl, diphenhydramine HCl, viscous lidocaine
3. Topical anesthetic creams or gels: lidocaine, benzocaine, cocaine
4. Topical analgesics: doxepin, morphine
5. Coating agents: milk of magnesia, kaopectate, Amphogel (alone or mixed with anesthetics), sucralfate
6. Systemic analgesics: nonsteroidal analgesics, opioids; adjuvant pain medications (eg: tricyclics, gabapentin)

in increased thickness of the mucosal epithelium. Other mechanisms of action may include increased expression of transcription factor Nrf2 in keratinocytes and of genes that encode a series of reactive oxygen species–scavenging enzymes [82]. Palifermin increases the anti-inflammatory cytokine IL-13, which in turn suppresses tumor necrosis factor alpha, a proinflammatory cytokine that may play a key role in mucositis. Palifermin also has antiapoptotic effects and promotes angiogenesis [16]. In addition to reducing mucositis, use of palifermin has been associated with a reduced incidence of blood-borne infections and with diminished use of parental opioids. Fibroblast growth factor 10 (Velafermin, CuraGen, Corp., Branford, Connecticut), a recombinant member of the fibroblast growth factor family, is currently under study in the transplant setting.

A number of other agents are currently in development. These include topical and systemic EN-2535 (Endo Pharmaceuticals, Chaddsford, Pennsylvania), a reactive oxygen species scavenger currently being studied as a topical rinse during radiation therapy. Serenex 1012, a tetracycline derivative, is in clinical trial as a topical rinse for chemotherapy-induced mucositis. Continuing study of topical glutamine (Saforis, MGI Pharma, Minneapolis, Minnesota) is planned. Low-level laser therapy has been shown to be effective in reducing mucositis in a small number of trials; more studies are required to validate these early results.

Approaches not recommended for the prevention of mucositis include the systemic administration of glutamine for the prevention of gastrointestinal mucositis, sucralfate rinses, and topical antimicrobials for radiation-induced mucositis. Topical antimicrobials have not been shown to be effective in the prophylaxis of mucositis but may be valuable in reducing secondary bacterial and fungal infection and pseudomembrane formation when tissue damage has occurred. Granulocyte macrophage colony-stimulating factor mouthwashes also are not recommended for preventing mucositis in transplant patients. In patients who are expected to develop xerostomia, stimulation of saliva flow with sialogogues may reduce the severity of subsequent mucositis, but evidence is lacking.

Suppression of the oropharyngeal flora

Topical antibacterials, antifungals, and antiseptics are used for the prevention and treatment of local infections, particularly in reducing oral candidiasis and the risk for dental caries and gingivitis [83–85]. Chlorhexidine reduces plaque formation and disperses established plaque [57,86] and has been found effective in treating oral candidiasis and other periodontal infections in immunocompromised patients [87].

Topical amphotericin B has shown encouraging results; in cases where it was ineffective, limited compliance with its use was reported [40,88]. Troche forms of these agents are not used easily in patients who have dry mouth, and a rinse may be a better choice.

A patient who is seropositive for HSV has an approximately 80% chance of viral reactivation during induction chemotherapy for leukemia or HCT, and prophylaxis with acyclovir and analogues has become standard for seropositive patients [89–92]. Viral reactivation is not prevented in all cases, however, so vigilance and recognition of signs and symptoms of reactivation are needed. The emergence of acyclovir-resistant HSV during prolonged acyclovir treatment has been reported and may be overcome by increasing the dosage or the use of foscarnet [89,93–98].

Specific antimicrobial therapy of oropharyngeal infections

Severely immunocompromised patients are particularly at risk for unchecked and spreading orofacial infections, and in these patients empiric broad-spectrum antimicrobial therapy is warranted. The antibiotic regimen must be broad spectrum, bactericidal, and given in an appropriate dose and schedule. In patients who have leukemia and severe neutropenia after chemotherapy, it is prudent to cover for facultative gram-negative bacilli as well as oral anaerobes and streptococci. Agents with broad-spectrum activity against both aerobes and anaerobes, such as a third-generation cephalosporin, piperacillin-tazobactam, a carbapenem (eg, imipenem, meropenem, or ertapenem), or a newer fluoroquinolone with enhanced activity against gram-positive bacteria and anaerobes (eg, moxifloxacin or gemifloxacin), are desirable (Box 5). In addition, coverage for methicillin-resistant *Staphylococcus aureus* (eg, vancomycin, linezolid, daptomycin) may be required. Ciprofloxacin is active against gram-negative bacteria but lacks activity against gram-positive organisms and oral anaerobes and is not recommended as monotherapy for oromucosal infections. The addition of clindamycin or metronidazole is advised.

Box 5. Antimicrobial agents useful for odontogenic and oromucosal infections

Systemic antibacterials for dental or periodontal Infections

Penicillin G, 1–4 MU intravenously every 4–6 hours; or ampicillin-sulbactam, 1.5–3 g intravenously every 6 hours
Clindamycin, 450 mg by mouth or 600 mg intravenously every 6–8 hours
Metronidazole, 500 mg by mouth or intravenously every 8 hours
Levofloxacin, 400 mg by mouth or intravenously every 24 hours; gemifloxacin, 320 mg by mouth every 24 hours; or moxifloxacin 400 mg by mouth or intravenously every 24 hours
Cefoxitin, 1–2 g intravenously every 6 hours; cefotetan, 2 g intravenously every 12 hours; or ceftizoxime, 1–2 g intravenously every 8–12 hours
Compromised host (one of the following ± an aminoglycoside)
Ceftizoxime, 4 g intravenously every 8 hours
Cefotaxime, 2 g intravenously every 6 hours
Piperacillin-tazobactam, 3 g intravenously every 4 hours
Imipenem/cilastatin, 500 mg intravenously every 6 hours; meropenem, 1 g intravenously every 8 hours; ertapenem, 1 g intravenously every 24 hours
Moxifloxacin 400 mg intravenously every 24 hours

Systemic antifungals: fluconazole, itraconazole, caspofungin, micafungin, amphotericin B

Systemic antivirals: acyclovir, valacyclovir, famciclovir, ganciclovir, foscarnet
Topical medications
Antiseptics: chlorhexidine, povidone iodine
Antibiotics: tetracycline, vancomycin, bacitracin, polymyxin B, tobramycin lozenge, and others.
Antifungals: nystatin, amphotericin B, clotrimazole, miconazole, ketoconazole, itraconazole suspension, fluconazole suspension

Ambulatory patients who have less serious oral infections may be treated with an aminopenicillin with a β-lactamase inhibitor (eg, amoxicillin-clavulanic acid), or penicillin in combination with metronidazole. Penicillin-allergic patients may be treated with clindamycin, cefoxitin, cefotetan, cefotaxime, or ceftizoxime. Erythromycin and tetracycline are not recommended because of increasing resistance among some strains of streptococci. Newer macrolides such as clarithromycin and azithromycin may be an alternative. Metronidazole, although highly active against anaerobic gram-negative bacilli and spirochetes, is only moderately active against anaerobic cocci and is not active against aerobes, including streptococci.

Patients who have acute leukemia and HCT recipients presenting with fever and neutropenia despite broad-spectrum antibiotics are treated empirically with systemic antifungals (fluconazole, itraconazole, caspofungin, micafungin, or amphotericin) because of the risk of undiagnosed systemic fungal infection. Patients who have severe HSV or varicella zoster virus infections should be treated with acyclovir or one of the new analogues (valacyclovir or famciclovir). Cytomegalovirus infection can be treated with ganciclovir or foscarnet.

Summary

The oral manifestations of oropharyngeal infection in immunocompromised patients present a particular challenge for both medical and dental professionals because clinical signs and symptoms may be minimal, and accurate diagnosis and appropriate treatment may be difficult. Both effective control of infection and management of oral symptoms are important and may be achieved by the judicious use of topical and systemic agents and by maintaining good oral hygiene. Prevention of mucosal breakdown, suppression of microbial colonization, control of viral reactivation, and effective management of severe xerostomia are all critical steps to reduce the overall morbidity and mortality of oromucosal infections in the severely immunocompromised patient. It is anticipated that multiple and possibly timed interventions may become the standard of care for prevention and management of oropharyngeal mucositis, based on current understanding of the molecular mechanisms underlying its pathogenesis. These interventions may include topical (rinse) applications of products and systemic agents that limit tissue injury and promote healing. Although prophylactic antimicrobials have not been shown to reduce the incidence or severity of mucositis, appropriate antimicrobial therapy clearly is important for the treatment of secondary oropharyngeal infections that contribute to oral mucositis.

References

[1] Bellm LA, Epstein JB, Rose-Ped A, et al. Patient reports of complications of bone marrow transplantation. Support Care Cancer 2000;8:33–9.
[2] Rose-Ped AM, Bellm LA, Epstein JB, et al. Complications of radiation therapy for head and neck cancers: the patient's perspective. Cancer Nursing 2002;25:461–7.
[3] McGuire DB, Yaeger KA, Dudley WN, et al. Acute oral pain and mucositis in bone marrow transplant and leukemia patients: data from a pilot study. Cancer Nursing 1998;21:385–93.
[4] Dunbar PJ, Buckley P, Gavrin JR, et al. Use of patient-controlled analgesia for pain control for children receiving bone marrow transplant. J Pain Symptom Manage 1995;604–11.
[5] Perch SJ, Machtay M, Markiewicz DA, et al. Decreased acute toxicity by using midline mucosa-sparing blocks during radiation therapy for carcinoma of the oral cavity, oropharynx, and nasopharynx. Radiology 1995;197:863–6.

[6] Syrjala KL, Chapko ME. Evidence for a biopsychosocial model of cancer treatment-related pain. Pain 1995;61:69–79.
[7] Epstein JB, Stewart KH. Radiation therapy and pain in patients with head and neck cancer. Eur J Cancer B Oral Oncol 1993;29:191–9.
[8] Stiff PJ. Mucositis associated with stem cell transplantation: current status and innovative approaches to management. Bone Marrow Transplant 2001;27(Suppl 2):S3–11.
[9] Rubenstein E, Peterson DE, Schubert M, et al. Clinical practice guidelines for the prevention and treatment of cancer therapy-induced oral and gastrointestinal mucositis. Cancer 2004; 100:2026–46.
[10] Jones JA, Avritscher EBC, Cooksley CD, et al. Epidemiology of treatment-associated mucosal injury after treatment with newer regimens for lymphoma, breast, lung, or colorectal cancer. Support Care Cancer 2006;14:505–15.
[11] Modi BJ, Knab B, Feldman LE, et al. Review of current treatment practices for carcinoma of the head and neck. Expert Opin Pharmacother 2005;6:1143–55.
[12] Trotti A, Bellm LA, Epstein JB, et al. Mucositis incidence, severity and associated outcomes in patients with head and neck cancer receiving radiotherapy with or without chemotherapy: a systematic literature review. Radiother Oncol 2003;66:253–62.
[13] Peterman A, Cella D, Gandon G, et al. Mucositis in head and neck cancer: economic and quality of life outcomes. J Natl Cancer Inst 2001;29:45–51.
[14] Dodd M, Dibble S, Miakowski C, et al. A comparison of the affective state and quality of life of chemotherapy patients who do and do not develop chemotherapy-oral mucositis. J Pain Symptom Manage 2001;21:498–505.
[15] Elting L, Isitt J, Murphy BA, et al, and the OM Study Group (Brizel DM, Bellm LA, Beaumont JL, Wells N, Cella D). Retrospective and prospective studies of the severity of oral mucositis (OM) in intensity modulated radiation therapy (IMRT) compared to conventional radiation therapy in head and neck cancer (HNC) patients [abstract 2428]. Philadelphia: American Society for Therapeutic Radiation and Oncology (ASTRO); 2006.
[16] Sonis ST. The pathobiology of mucositis. Nat Rev Cancer 2004;4:277–84.
[17] Handschel J, Prott FJ, Meyer U, et al. Prospective study of the pathology of radiation-induced mucositis [in German]. Mund Kiefer Gesichtschir 1998;2:131–5.
[18] Epstein JB, Emerton S, Guglietta A, et al. Assessment of epidermal growth factor in oral secretions of patients receiving radiation therapy for cancer. Oral Oncol 1997;33:359–63.
[19] Gordon B, Spadinger A, Hodges E, et al. Effect of granulocyte-macrophage colony stimulating factor on oral mucositis after hematopoietic stem-cell transplantation. J Clin Oncol 1994;12:1917–22.
[20] Reynoso EE, Calderon E, Miranda E. GM-CSF mouthwashes to attenuate severe mucositis after high dose chemotherapy and allogeneic bone marrow transplantation (BMT) or autologous peripheral blood stem cell transplantation (APBSCT). Ann Oncol 1994;5(Suppl 8): 1062.
[21] Sonis ST, Eilers JP, Epstein JB, et al. Validation of a new scoring system for the assessment of clinical trial research of oral mucositis induced by radiation or chemotherapy. Cancer 1999; 85:2103–13.
[22] Rapoport AP, Miller-Watelet LF, Linder T, et al. Analysis of factors that correlate with mucositis in recipients of autologous and allogeneic stem-cell transplants. J Clin Oncol 1999;17: 2446–53.
[23] McCarthy GM, Awde JD, Ghandi H, et al. Risk factors associated with mucositis in cancer patients receiving 5-fluorouracil. Oral Oncol 1998;34:484–90.
[24] Dodd MJ, Miaskowski C, Shiba GH, et al. Risk factors for chemotherapy-induced oral mucositis: dental appliances, oral hygiene, previous oral lesions and history of smoking. Cancer Invest 1999;17:278–84.
[25] Epstein JB, Wigdor H. Oropharyngeal cancer and oral complications of cancer therapy: considerations in older patients. Geriatrics & Aging 2004;7:59–64.

[26] Donnelly JP, Muus P, Horrevorts AM, et al. Failure of clindamycin to influence the course of severe oromucositis associated with streptococcal bacteraemia in allogeneic bone marrow transplant recipients. Scand J Infect Dis 1993;25:43–50.

[27] Epstein JB, Truelove EL, Izutzu KT. Oral candidiasis: pathogenesis and host defense. Rev Infect Dis 1984;6:96–106.

[28] MacKay BJ, Denepitiya L, Iacono VJ, et al. Growth-inhibitory and bactericidal effects of human parotid salivary histidine-rich polypeptides on Streptococcus mutans. Infect Immun 1984;44:695–701.

[29] Pollock JJ, Denepitiya L, MacKay BJ, et al. Fungistatic and fungicidal activity of human parotid salivary histidine-rich polypeptides on Candida albicans. Infect Immun 1984;44: 702–12.

[30] Williams RC, Gibbons RJ. Inhibition of streptococcal attachment to receptors on human buccal epithelial cells by antigenically similar salivary glycoproteins. Infect Immun 1975; 11:711–8.

[31] Woo SB, Lee SJ, Schubert MM. Graft-vs-host disease. Crit Rev Oral Biol Med 1997;8: 201–16.

[32] Borowski B, Benhamou E, Pico JL, et al. Prevention of oral mucositis in patients treated with high dose chemotherapy and bone marrow transplantation: a randomized controlled trial comparing two protocols of dental care. Eur J Cancer B Oral Oncol 1994;30:93–7.

[33] Wahlin YB, Granstrom S, Persson S, et al. Multivariate study of enterobacteria and Pseudomonas in saliva of patients with acute leukemia. Oral Surg Oral Med Oral Pathol 1991;72: 300–8.

[34] Dodd MJ, Larson PJ, Dibble SL, et al. Randomized clinical trial of chlorhexidine versus placebo for prevention of oral mucositis in patients receiving chemotherapy. Oncol Nurs Forum 1996;23:921–7.

[35] Scully C, Epstein J, Porter S, et al. Viruses and chronic disorders involving the human oral mucosa. Oral Surg Oral Med Oral Pathol 1991;72 547–44.

[36] Sonis ST, Elting LS, Keefe D, et al. Perspectives on cancer therapy-induced mucosal injury: pathogenesis, measurement, epidemiology, and consequences for patients. Cancer 2004; 100(Suppl):1995–2025.

[37] Blijlevens NMA, Donnelly JP, de Pau BE. Microbiologic consequences of new approaches to managing hematologic malignancies. Rev Clin Exp Hematol 2005;9:E2.

[38] Blijlevens NMA, Donnelly JP, de Pau BE. Inflammatory response to mucosal barrier injury after myeloablative therapy in allogeneic stem cell transplant recipients. Bone Marrow Transplant 2005;36:70–7.

[39] Blijlevens NMA, Donnelly JP, de Pauw BE. Empirical therapy of febrile neutropenic patients with mucositis: challenge of risk-based therapy. Clin Microbiol Infect 2001;7(Suppl 4):47–52.

[40] Epstein JB, Truelove EL, Hanson-Huggins K, et al. Topical polyene antifungals in hematopoietic cell transplant patients: tolerability and efficacy. Support Care Cancer 2004;12: 517–25.

[41] Navari RM, Buckner CD, Clift RA, et al. Prophylaxis of infection in patients with aplastic anemia receiving allogeneic marrow transplants. Am J Med 1984;76:564–72.

[42] Diamond DL, Kimball JR, Krisanaprakornkit S, et al. Detection of β-defensins secreted by human oral epithelial cells. J Immunol Methods 2001;256:65–76.

[43] Dale BA, Fredericks LP. Antimicrobial peptides in the oral environment: expression and function in health and disease. Curr Issues Mol Biol 2005;7:119–33.

[44] Tjabringa GS, Vos JB, Olthuus P, et al. Host defense effector molecules in mucosal secretions. FEMS Immunol Med Microbiol 2005;45:151–8.

[45] Epstein JB, Pearsall NN, Truelove EL. Oral candidiasis: effects of antifungal therapy upon clinical signs and symptoms, salivary antibody and mucosal adherence of Candida albicans. Oral Surg Oral Med Oral Pathol 1981;51:32–6.

[46] Epstein JB, Kimura LH, Menard TW, et al. Effects of specific antibodies on the interaction between the fungus Candida albicans and human oral mucosa. Arch Oral Biol 1982;27: 469–74.
[47] Epstein JB, Freilich M, Le N. Risk factors for oropharyngeal candidiasis in patients who receive radiation therapy for malignant conditions of the head and neck. Oral Surg Oral Med Oral Pathol 1993;76:169–74.
[48] Epstein JB, Chin EA, Jacobson JJ, et al. The relationship among fluoride, cariogenic oral flora, and salivary flow rate during radiation therapy. Oral Surg Oral Med Oral Pathol Oral Radiol Endod 1998;86:286–92.
[49] Lockhart PB, Sonis ST. Alterations in the oral mucosa caused by chemotherapeutic agents. J Dermatol Surg Oncol 1981;7:1019–25.
[50] Silverman S Jr. Radiation effects. In: Silverman S Jr, editor. Oral cancer. 5th edition. New York: American Cancer Society, Decker (BC); 2003. p. 70–8.
[51] National Cancer Institute. Oral complications of chemotherapy and head/neck radiation (PDQ). Available at: http://cancer.gov.cancerinfo/pdq/supportivecare/oralcomplications/health-professional. Accessed August 30, 2004
[52] Spielberger R, Stiff P, Bensinger W, et al. Palifermin for oral mucositis after intensive therapy for hematologic cancers. N Engl J Med 2004;351:2590–8.
[53] Sonis ST, Oster G, Fuchs H, et al. Oral mucositis and the clinical and economic outcomes of hematopoietic stem-cell transplantation. J Clin Oncol 2001;19:2201–5.
[54] Epstein J, Emerton S, Kolbinson D, et al. Quality of life and oral function following therapy for head and neck cancer. Head Neck 1999;21:1–11.
[55] Ruescher T, Sodeifi A, Scrivani SJ, et al. The impact of mucositis on alpha haemolytic streptococcal infection in pateitns undergoing autologous bone marrow transplantation for hematoloigical malignancies. Cancer 1998;82:2275–81.
[56] Greenberg MA, Cohen SG, McKitrick JC, et al. The oral flora as a source of septicemia in patients with acuate leukemia. Oral Surg Oral Med Oral Pathol 1982;53:32–6.
[57] Overholser CD, Peterson DE, Williams LT, et al. Periodontal infection in patients with acute nonlymphocytic leukemia: prevalence of acute exacerbations. Arch Intern Med 1982;142: 551–4.
[58] Epstein JB, Ransier A, Lunn R, et al. Prophylaxis of candidiasis in leukemia and bone marrow transplant patients. Oral Surg Oral Med Oral Pathol Oral Radiol Endod 1996;81: 291–6.
[59] Khan SA, Wingard JR. Infection and mucosal injury in cancer treatment. J Natl Cancer Inst 2001;29:31–6.
[60] Newman KA, Schimpf SC, Young VM, et al. Lessons learned from surveillance cultures from patients with acute nonlymphocytic leukemia: usefulness for epidemiologic, preventive and therapeutic research. Am J Med 1981;70:423–31.
[61] Epstein JB, van der Meij EH, Lunn R, et al. Effects of compliance with fluoride gel application on caries and caries risk in patients after radiation therapy for head and neck cancer. Oral Surg Oral Med Oral Pathol Oral Radiol Endod 1996;82:268–75.
[62] Donnelly JP. Bacterial complications of transplantation: diagnosis and treatment. J Antimicrob Chemother 1995;36(B):59–72.
[63] Main BE, Calman KC, Ferguson MM, et al. The effect of cytotoxic therapy on saliva and oral flora. Oral Surg Oral Med Oral Pathol 1984;58:545–8.
[64] Johnson WG, Pierce AK, Sanford JP. Changing pharyngeal bacterial flora of hospitalized patients: emergence of gram-negative bacilli. N Engl J Med 1969;281:1137–40.
[65] Ramirez-Amador V, Silverman S Jr, Mayer P, et al. Candidal colonization and oral candidiasis in patients undergoing oral and pharyngeal radiation therapy. Oral Surg Oral Med Oral Pathol Oral Radiol Endod 1997;84:149–53.
[66] Epstein JB, Sherlock CH, Wolber RA. Hairy leukoplakia after bone marrow transplantation. Oral Surg Oral Med Oral Pathol 1993;75:690–5.

[67] Epstein JB, Page JL, Anderson GH, et al. The role of an immunoperoxidase technique in the diagnosis of oral herpes simplex virus infection in patients with leukemia. Diagn Cytopathol 1987;3:205–9.
[68] Burns JC. Diagnostic methods of herpes simplex infection: a review. Oral Surg Oral Med Oral Pathol 1980;50:346–9.
[69] Schubert MM, Epstein JB, Lloid ME, et al. Oral infections due to cytomegalovirus in immunocompromised patients. J Oral Pathol Med 1993;22:268–73.
[70] Keefe DM, Schubert MM, Elting KS, et al. Updated clinical practice guidelines for the prevention and treatment of mucositis. Cancer 2007;109(5):820–31.
[71] Epstein JB, Vickers L, Spinelli J, et al. Efficacy of chlorhexidine and nystatin rinses in prevention of oral complications in leukemia and bone marrow transplantation. Oral Surg Oral Med Oral Pathol 1992;73:682–9.
[72] Spiers AS, Dias SF, Lopez JA. Infection prevention in patients with cancer: microbiological evaluation of laminar air flow isolation, topical chlorhexidine and non-absorbable antibiotics. J Hyg (Lond) 1980;84:457–65.
[73] Foote RL, Loprinzi CL, Frank AR, et al. Randomized trial of a chlorhexidine mouthwash for the alleviation of radiation induced mucositis. J Clin Oncol 1994;12:2630–3.
[74] Beck S. Impact of a systematic oral care protocol on stomatitis after chemotherapy. Cancer Nurs 1979;2:185–99.
[75] Lindquist SF, Hickey AJ, Drane JB. Effect of oral hygiene on stomatitis in patients receiving cancer chemotherapy. J Prosthet Dent 1978;40:312–4.
[76] Peterson DE, Overholser CD, Schimpff SC, et al. Relationship of intensive oral hygiene to systemic complications in acute nonlymphocytic leukemia. Proc Am Fed Clin Res 1981; 29:440A.
[77] Schubert MM, Sullivan KM, Truelove ET. Head and neck complications of bone marrow transplantation. In: Peterson DE, Elias EG, Sonis ST, editors. Head and neck management of the cancer patient. Boston: Martinus Nijhoff; 1986. p. 401–27.
[78] Adams S, Toth B, Dudley BS. Evaluation of sucralfate as a compounded oral suspension for the treatment of stomatitis. Clin Pharmacol Ther 1985;2:178.
[79] Epstein JB, Wong FLW. The efficacy of sucralfate suspension in the prevention of oral mucositis due to radiation therapy. Int J Radiat Oncol Biol Phys 1994;28:693–8.
[80] Blazar BR, Weisdorf DJ, deFor T, et al. Phase 1/2 randomized, placebo-control trial of palifermin to prevent graft-versus-host disease (GVHD) after allogeneic hematopoietic stem cell transplantation (HSCT). Blood 2006;108:3216–9.
[81] Rosen LS, Abdi E, Davis ID, et al. Palifermin reduces the incidence of oral mucositis in patients with metastatic colorectal cancer treated with fluorouracil-based chemotherapy. J Clin Oncol 2006;24:5194–200.
[82] Braun S, Hanselmann C, Gassmann MG, et al. Nrf2 transcription factor, a novel target of keratinocyte growth factor action which regulates gene expression and inflammation in the healing skin wound. Mol Cell Biol 2002;22:5492–505.
[83] Spijkervet FKL, van Saene HKF, van Saene JJM, et al. Mucositis prevented by selective elimination of oral flora in irradiated head and neck cancer patients. J Oral Pathol Med 1991;19:480–9.
[84] Symonds RP, McIlroy P, Khorrami J, et al. The reduction of radiation mucositis by selective decontamination antibiotic pastilles: a placebo controlled double blind trial. Br J Cancer 1996;74:312–7.
[85] Okuno SH, Foote RL, Loprinzi CL, et al. A randomized trial of a nonabsorbable antibiotic lozenge given to alleviate radiation-induced mucositis. Cancer 1997;79:2193–9.
[86] Fardal O, Turnbull RS. A review of the literature on use of chlorhexidine in dentistry. J Am Dent Assoc 1986;112:863–9.
[87] Langslet A, Olsen I, Lie SO, et al. Chlorhexidine treatment of oral candidiasis in seriously diseased children. Acta Paediatr Scand 1974;63:809–11.

[88] Barrett AP. A long-term prospective clinical study of oral complications during conventional chemotherapy for acute leukemia. Oral Surg Oral Med Oral Pathol 1987;63:313–6.
[89] Epstein JB, Sherlock C, Page JL, et al. Clinical study of herpes virus infection in leukemia. Oral Surg Oral Med Oral Pathol 1990;70:38–43.
[90] Epstein JB, Scully C. Herpes simplex virus in immunocompromised patients: growing evidence of drug resistance. Oral Surg Oral Med Oral Pathol 1991;72:47–50.
[91] Epstein JB, Ransier A, Sherlock CH, et al. Acyclovir prophylaxis of oral herpes virus during bone marrow transplantation. Eur J Cancer B Oral Oncol 1996;32:158–62.
[92] Oakley C, Epstein JB, Sherlock CH. Reactivation of oral herpes simplex virus. Implications for clinical management of herpes simplex virus recurrence during radiotherapy. Oral Surg Oral Med Oral Pathol 1997;84:272–8.
[93] Cassady KA, Whitley RJ. New therapeutic approaches to alpha herpesvirus infections. J Antimicrob Chemother 1997;39:119–28.
[94] Warkentin DI, Epstein JB, Campbell LM, et al. Valacyclovir versus acyclovir for HSV prophylaxis in neutropenic patients. Ann Pharmacother 2002;36:1525–31.
[95] Burns WH, Santos GW, Saral R, et al. Isolation and characterization of resistant herpes simplex virus after acyclovir therapy. Lancet 1982;1:421–3.
[96] Crumpacker CS, Schnipper LE, Marlowe SI, et al. Resistance to anti-viral drugs of herpes simplex virus isolated from a patient treated with acyclovir. N Engl J Med 1982;306:343–6.
[97] de Clerq E. In search of a selective antiviral chemotherapy. Clin Microbial Rev 1997;10: 674–93.
[98] Wagstaff AJ, Bryson HM, Foscarnet. A reappraisal of its antiviral activity, pharmacokinetic properties and therapeutic use in immunocompromised patients with viral infections. Drugs 1994;48:199–226.

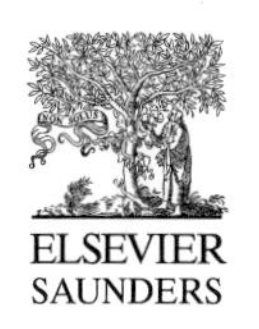

ELSEVIER
SAUNDERS

INFECTIOUS
DISEASE CLINICS
OF NORTH AMERICA

Infect Dis Clin N Am 21 (2007) 523–541

Cervical Lymphadenitis, Suppurative Parotitis, Thyroiditis, and Infected Cysts

Nawaf Al-Dajani, MD, Susan H. Wootton, MD*

Division of Infectious and Immunological Diseases, Department of Pediatrics, BC Children's Hospital, 4480 Oak Street, University of British Columbia, Vancouver, BC V6H 3N1, Canada

Neck masses are common and have a variety of infectious and noninfectious causes. A directed history and thorough physical examination are the cornerstones on which a diagnosis is made. In particular, the age of the patient is critical in formulating an appropriate differential diagnosis for neck masses. Unlike adults, neck masses in children seldom represent ominous disease. This article reviews the more common infectious causes of neck swelling—cervical lymphadenitis, suppurative parotitis, thyroiditis, and infected cysts. Noninfectious causes of neck masses include tumors, congenital anomalies, and skin and salivary gland disease.

Cervical lymphadenitis

The cervical lymphatic system involves a great array of superficial and deep lymph nodes that protect the head, neck, nasopharynx, and oropharynx against infection. Cervical lymphadenitis is characterized by inflammation of one or more of these lymph nodes. Most cases of cervical lymphadenitis, especially in children, are caused by an infectious agent; some immunologic processes and malignancies result in a similar presentation. The following section reviews the differential diagnosis and therapy of cervical lymphadenitis caused by infectious processes.

* Corresponding author. Vaccine Evaluation Center, Rm L-427, 4500 Oak Street, Vancouver, BC V6H 3N1.

E-mail address: swootton@cw.bc.ca (S.H. Wootton).

0891-5520/07/$ - see front matter
doi:10.1016/j.idc.2007.03.004

id.theclinics.com

Pathophysiology

The lymphatic system of the cervical region serves as the initial line of defense against infections for all structures within the head, neck, and upper respiratory tract. Micro-organisms of the skin, oropharynx, or respiratory tract can invade local cervical lymph nodes, resulting in localized infection [1,2]. If this initial defense fails, micro-organisms can disseminate, resulting in systemic disease. There are three groups of cervical lymph nodes: (1) Waldeyer's ring (including the adenoids and tonsils); (2) the nodes that surround Waldeyer's ring (occipital, postauricular, preauricular, parotid, and facial nodes); and (3) the submaxillary, submental, and deep and superficial jugular nodes [3]. Most cervical lymphatics drain to the submaxillary and deep cervical lymph nodes. Consequently, these nodes are often involved in cervical lymphadenitis.

Etiology

Infectious causes of cervical lymphadenitis are multiple (Table 1). The most common bacterial organisms causing acute unilateral infection are *Staphylococcus aureus* and *Streptococcus pyogenes*. In newborns adenitis may be caused by group B streptococci, whereas viruses are more common in children [4]. The presence of dental or periodontal disease suggests anaerobic bacteria [2]. In the past, anaerobic infections were uncommon; an observation that probably represented inadequate anaerobic-culturing techniques at the time.

The epidemiology of methicillin-resistant *S aureus* (MRSA) infections is changing. In the past, MRSA infections typically occurred in a hospital setting. More recently, the incidence of infections in adults and children who do not have traditional risk factors (prolonged hospitalization, surgical procedure, indwelling catheters) has increased [5]. The recent description of MRSA infection in healthy newborns is of particular concern [6]. MRSA, a common cause of skin and soft tissue infections, should be considered in patients presenting with cervical lymph node swelling.

The cause of cervical mycobacterial adenitis varies by age [7]. Adults more commonly present with *Mycobacterium tuberculosis*, whereas children, especially those age 2 to 5 years, tend to present with nontuberculous mycobacteria. In a report by Starke and colleagues [8], only 11 (10%) of 110 children who had active tuberculosis presented with cervical or supraclavicular lymphadenopathy. Species of nontuberculous mycobacteria that commonly cause infection in children include *Mycobacterium avium-intracellulare*, *Mycobacterium scrofulaceum*, and *Mycobacterium kansasii* [9].

Cat-scratch disease (CSD) is also a common cause of lymphadenitis in young children and adults and generally is self-limited. CSD was first described in 1931, but it was not until 1983 that Wear and colleagues [10] described *Bartonella henselae*, a small, gram-negative, silver-stained bacillus, as the causative agent of CSD.

Table 1
Infectious agents associated with cervical lymphadenitis

Type of organism	Common	Rare
Bacteria	*Staphylococcus* aureus	Non-group A streptococci
	Streptococcus pyogenes	Enterobacteriaceae
	Peptostreptococcus spp	*Escherichia coli*
	Peptococcus spp	*Klebsiella* spp
	Bacteroides spp	*Pseudomonas* spp
	Bartonella henselae	*Haemophilus influenzae*
		Actinomyces Israeli
		Fusobacterium spp
		Francisella tularensis
		Yersinia spp
		Corynebacterium spp
		Brucella spp
		Listeria monocytogenes
		Bacillus anthracis
Viruses	Epstein-Barr virus	
	Herpes simplex virus 1 and 2	
	Cytomegalovirus	
	Adenovirus	
	Enterovirus	
	Rubella virus	
	Roseola virus	
	Varicella-zoster virus	
	Influenza virus	
	Parainfluenza virus	
	Respiratory syncytial virus	
Mycobacteria	*Mycobacterium tuberculosis*	
	Mycobacterium avium-intracellulare	
	Mycobacterium scrofulaceum	
Fungi		*Sporothrix schenckii*
		Histoplasma capsulatum
		Aspergillus fumigatus
		Candida albicans
		Cryptococcus neoformans
		Coccidioidomycosis
Parasites		*Toxoplasma gondii*
		Leishmania spp
		Trypanosoma spp
		Filaria spp

Adapted from Brook I. The swollen neck. Cervical lymphadenitis, parotitis, thyroiditis, and infected cysts. Infect Dis Clin North Am 1988;2(1):223; with permission.

HIV is another cause of chronic cervical lymphadenitis, but patients typically develop more generalized lymphadenopathy. Early manifestations of maternally derived HIV infection can include lymphadenopathy associated with splenomegaly [11]. In adolescents (age $>$ 13 years) and adults, lymphadenopathy is recognized as a diagnostic criterion for HIV [12]. Human T-cell lymphotropic virus (HTLV), a retrovirus linked to adult T-cell leukemia/lymphoma and HTLV-1–associated myelopathy/tropical spastic paraparesis, also can present with more generalized lymphadenopathy [13].

Clinical manifestations

The presentation of cervical lymphadenitis can be classified into three broad groups: (1) acute unilateral cervical lymphadenitis; (2) acute bilateral cervical lymphadenitis; and (3) subacute or chronic cervical lymphadenitis. *S aureus* and *S pyogenes* are the most common causes of acute unilateral cervical lymphadenitis [2,3,14,15]. Lymph nodes infected with *S aureus* tend to be fluctuant, quite tender, and vary in size (2–6 cm). Often the skin overlying the infected lymph node is warm and erythematous. Systemic symptoms tend to be mild. In neonates, acute unilateral cervical lymphadenitis is generally caused by *S aureus*; however, a "cellulitis-adenitis syndrome" caused by group B streptococci has been described [4]. These infants often are male and typically present with fever, facial or submandibular cellulitis, and ipsilateral otitis media.

Acute bilateral cervical lymphadenitis often is caused by viral pathogens; however, it also may represent pharyngitis caused by *S pyogenes* as well as *Mycoplasma pneumoniae* (see Table 1). In general, the lymph nodes are small and rubbery with little redness or warmth. Additional clinical features such as gingivostomatitis (herpes simplex), herpangina (coxsackie virus or enterocytopathogenic [ECHO] virus), or rash (cytomegalovirus) may help identify the causative virus. Posterior acute bilateral cervical lymphadenitis often is associated with rubella or infectious mononucleosis. Typically, viral infections resolve within 1 to 2 weeks without complication.

Chronic unilateral cervical lymphadenitis is often caused by *B henselae,* atypical mycobacteria, or *Toxoplasma gondii.* The highest incidence of *B henselae* infection (CSD) occurs in children younger than 10 years. Patients develop lymphadenopathy, usually preceded by an erythematous papule or pustule at the inoculation site. Some children (25%) progress to more severe disease [16,17]. Atypical mycobacterial infections generally are localized to a single tonsillar or submandibular node (<3 cm), but deeper nodes may be involved. The overlying skin becomes very thin and changes from red to distinctive lilac. Some nodes (10%) drain spontaneously, resulting in sinus tract formation. Chest radiographs are normal, and Mantoux skin tests usually result in less than 15 mm of induration (usually 5–9 mm) [2].

Differential diagnosis

Differentiating between infectious and noninfectious causes of cervical lymphadenitis is of paramount importance. A detailed medical history including the presence of skin lesions, exposure to animals or feeding insects, dentition, constitutional symptoms, history of recurrent infections or lymphadenopathy, immunization status, contact with tuberculosis, place of residence, and recent travel may provide essential clues. The duration of swelling and its location also serve as diagnostic aids. For example, tumors and congenital anomalies generally are present for weeks and are often in the midline. A history of cat contact may suggest CSD, whereas coexisting dental or periodontal infection may suggest anaerobic bacteria [2,16].

Physical examination should include a thorough evaluation of the liver, spleen, and lymphatic system as well as the oropharynx, dentition, conjunctiva, and skin. Palpation of the mass to determine its location, consistency (solid or fluctuant, smooth or nodular), and motility (fixed or movable) is helpful in differentiating structures within the neck.

The extent of the diagnostic evaluation depends on the history and physical examination. For most uncomplicated cases of cervical lymphadenitis, determining the precise cause often is not necessary. For patients who do not respond to initial medical management or are acutely ill, a search for a cause should be pursued. Cultures of the blood, a complete blood cell count, liver function studies, and amylase as well as serologic tests for viruses may be indicated. Culture of material collected directly from the lymph node by fine needle aspiration (FNA) is especially valuable. The aspirate should be sent for routine Gram stain, aerobic and anaerobic bacterial culture, acid-fast stain, and mycobacterial culture. For chronic cervical lymphadenitis, methenamine-silver stain, fungal cultures, and polymerase chain reaction for *B henselae* should be done. An intradermal skin test for tuberculosis and atypical mycobacteria should be applied. In addition, high-resolution and color Doppler ultrasonography offers clues into the cause and the degree of suppuration [18]. If the diagnosis remains in doubt, an excision biopsy should be performed for both histology and cultures.

Therapy and prevention

Most cases of acute cervical lymphadenitis require no specific therapy because they are the sequelae of viral pharyngitis or stomatitis. Empiric therapy should provide adequate coverage for *S aureus* and *S pyogenes*. Oral therapy should include cephalexin, oxacillin, or clindamycin, or the combination of amoxicillin and a beta-lactamase inhibitor (clavulanic acid). Therapy given for 10 to 14 days generally is sufficient. Parenteral therapy (cefazolin, nafcillin, oxacillin, or clindamycin) may be required for toxic patients.

Lack of clinical improvement after 36 to 48 hours should indicate a need for reassessment of therapy. Culture results may guide the selection of appropriate therapeutic agents. When fluctuation or pointing is present, the abscess should be incised and drained because antibiotic therapy alone is insufficient. Surgical evacuation of the abscess is helpful in promoting resolution.

If CSD or mycobacterial infection is suspected, incision and drainage should be avoided because cutaneous fistulae often develop. Treatment for CSD depends on the severity of disease and may include gentamicin, rifampin, or trimethoprim-sulfamethoxazole; most cases do not require antibiotic therapy. Azithromycin also has been shown to be effective [19]. Total surgical removal is the most effective therapy for nontuberculous mycobacterial cervical lymphadenitis [20]. After excision, antimycobacterial agents (isoniazid and rifampin) are given until organisms are identified. If *M tuberculosis* is identified, these agents are continued for 9 to 12 months. Streptomycin and pyrazinamide arc added if isoniazid-resistant *M tuberculosis* is documented.

Conditions predisposing to cervical lymphadenitis should be managed and treated appropriately. Examples of such conditions include dental caries or abscesses, oropharyngeal or otitic infections, and skin infections involving the face or scalp. Avoiding exposure to highly contagious pathogens (*M tuberculosis*) and animals known to transmit infection (toxoplasmosis and CSD) may reduce the risk of cervical lymphadenitis further.

Suppurative parotitis

Inflammation of the parotid gland is caused by a variety of infectious agents and noninfectious systemic illnesses. Depending on the clinical presentation and cause, parotitis can be classified into several types: suppurative, viral, granulomatous, recurrent, or chronic. Determining the type of parotitis has important treatment implications.

Pathophysiology

Inflammation of the parotid gland is caused by local infection, systemic infection (eg, mumps), or hematogenous seeding. Factors that decrease or interrupt the flow of saliva increase the risk for parotitis. Risk factors include dehydration, poor oral hygiene, oral trauma, xerostomia, ductal obstruction, certain drugs (anticholinergics or antihistamines), certain chronic diseases (Sjögren's syndrome or diabetes mellitus), malnutrition, neoplasms of the oral cavity, tracheostomy, immunosuppression, and sialolithiasis [21,22].

Etiology

Infectious parotitis is caused by a wide variety of organisms (Table 2). *S aureus* is by far the most common pathogen; however, streptococci and gram-negative bacilli also have been reported [21–24]. Gram-negative organisms often are seen in neonates and in hospitalized, debilitated patients. Anaerobic infections of the parotid gland are rare; only a few cases have been reported [24]. In cases of recurrent parotitis in children, *Streptococcus* spp are the most commonly isolated organisms [25].

M tuberculosis and atypical mycobacteria, such as *M avium-intracellulare*, are rare causes of granulomatous parotitis [26]. Other causes of granulomatous parotitis include *Actinomyces* spp and gram-negative intracellular organisms such as *Francisella tularensis* and *Brucella* spp [27].

Table 2
Infectious pathogens associated with suppurative parotitis

Type of organism	Common	Rare
Bacteria	*Staphylococcus aureus*	*Streptococci pneumoniae*
	Streptococcus pyogenes	Viridans streptococci
	Alpha-hemolytic streptococci	*Haemophilus influenzae*
		Moraxella catarrhalis
		Pseudomonas aeruginosa
		Escherichia coli
		Proteus spp
		Salmonella spp
		Klebsiella spp
		Peptostreptococcus spp
		Prevotella spp
		Fusobacterium spp
		Actinobacillus spp
Mycobacteria	*Mycobacterium tuberculosis*	
	Mycobacterium avium-intracellulare	
	Other mycobacteria	
Fungi	*Candida albicans*	
Viruses	Mumps virus	
	Coxsackieviruses A and B	
	Echoviruses	
	Epstein-Barr virus	
	Influenza A virus	
	Parainfluenza viruses 1 and 3	
	Cytomegalovirus	
	Herpes simplex virus 1	
	Lymphocytic-choriomeningitis	
	Human immunodeficiency virus	

Adapted from Brook I. The swollen neck. Cervical lymphadenitis, parotitis, thyroiditis, and infected cysts. Infect Dis Clin North Am 1988;2(1):228; with permission.

Even in the postvaccine era, epidemic mumps caused by paramyxovirus is the most common viral cause of parotitis in childhood [28]. Other viral agents associated with parotid infection are coxsackie viruses, Epstein-Barr virus, influenza A virus, lymphocytic-choriomeningitis virus, parainfluenza viruses, herpes simplex virus, and cytomegalovirus [29].

Clinical manifestations

A detailed history and physical examination help to determine the cause of parotitis. Acute suppurative parotitis is characterized by the sudden onset of unilateral induration and erythema that extends from the cheek to the angle of the jaw. The parotid gland becomes swollen and extremely tender. Purulent discharge may be expressed from the orifice of the parotid duct with gentle pressure. The infection can extend locally into surrounding tissue, the face, ear, or through the fascial plane to the mediastinum resulting in severe complications such as thrombophlebitis of the jugular vein (Lemierre syndrome) or septicemia.

Mumps, the most common form of viral parotitis, is characterized by a prodrome of fever, malaise, anorexia, and headache followed by unilateral or bilateral earache and parotid tenderness. Drainage from the parotid duct is clear even though the duct is erythematous and swollen. Other viral agents may cause similar symptoms. Rarely, mumps is complicated by meningoencephalitis, pancreatitis, orchitis, myocarditis, pericarditis, arthritis, and nephritis.

Granulomatous parotitis is rare and presents as a painless enlarging mass without surrounding inflammation. Often, evidence of systemic tuberculous disease is absent. Actinomycosis of the parotid gland also causes painless nodular swelling and often is associated with oral (dental caries) or cervicofacial infection. Fistulas draining yellow or white material with sulfur granules are common [27].

Recurrent parotitis of childhood, a unique disease characterized by acute and subacute parotid gland swelling, is quite rare with a peak incidence around 6 years of age [25,30]. Children have repeated episodes of fever, pain, and unilateral parotid swelling that last up to 2 weeks, resolving spontaneously. Culture of drainage from the parotid duct often yields streptococcal organisms. The disease tends to become less frequent with age, stopping by early adulthood.

Bilateral parotid enlargement is a common finding in children who have HIV infection (20%–50%) and often is the first manifestation of HIV infection in an otherwise healthy older child [31]. Pre-existing xerostomia and secondary infections caused by immunosuppression may increase the risk for parotitis in these patients.

Differential diagnosis

Acute suppurative parotitis should be differentiated from other types of parotitis. Typically, suppurative parotitis is characterized by the expression of purulent material from the parotid duct with gentle pressure over the gland. A Gram stain of the purulent material may support bacterial infection; however, cultures may simply represent oropharyngeal contamination. In contrast, FNA of the parotid gland may yield the causative organism. Aerobic, anaerobic, fungal, and mycobacterial cultures should be performed. Surgical exploration and drainage may be indicated for diagnosis as well as for therapy.

In contrast, viral parotitis does not produce purulent discharge from the parotid duct. Mumps and other viral infections can be diagnosed using a variety of methodologies including culture, serology, and nucleic acid tests (polymerase chain reaction).

Multiple imaging techniques are available that can assist with the diagnosis of parotitis including ultrasound, CT scan, and X-ray sialography (the criterion). Unlike X-ray sialography, MR sialography is not contraindicated during acute infection and does not require the injection of contrast material. This technology may offer a promising alternative for diagnosis [32].

If infection is not found, noninfectious causes should be pursued. Such disorders include collagen vascular diseases, cystic fibrosis, alcoholism, diabetes, gout, uremia, sarcoidosis, ectodermal dysplasia syndromes, familial dysautonomia, sialolithiasis, benign and malignant tumors, metal poisoning, and drug-related disorders. Nonparotid swelling that may simulate parotitis includes lymphoma, lymphangitis, cervical adenitis, external otitis, dental abscess, actinomycosis not involving the parotid, anaerobic infection of the buccal space, and infected cysts.

Therapy and prevention

Maintenance of adequate hydration, parotid massage, sialagogues (eg, lemon drops, hard candy), and administration of parenteral antimicrobial therapy are essential. The choice of antibiotics depends on the agent responsible. Most cases respond to antimicrobial therapy, but some inflamed glands may reach a stage of abscess formation that requires surgical drainage. Broad antimicrobial therapy is indicated to cover all possible aerobic and anaerobic pathogens, including adequate coverage for *S aureus*, hemolytic streptococci, and anaerobic bacteria.

A penicillinase-resistant penicillin or a first-generation cephalosporin plus clindamycin in combination with an aminoglycoside is generally adequate [33], but vancomycin for MRSA or ceftazidime for broader gram-negative coverage may be required. If the patient does not respond to medical therapy, or if fluctuance increases, surgical incision and drainage are indicated. Treatment of viral parotitis includes antipyretics, analgesia, and hydration. For mycobacterial infection, excision of the gland and specific antimicrobial therapy may be required [26]. Patients who have actinomycosis should be managed with penicillin G [27]. Children who have recurrent parotitis should be treated with appropriate antibiotics, but chronic suppressive therapy is not recommended.

Active immunization against the mumps virus has reduced the occurrence of mumps significantly. Unfortunately, outbreaks continue to occur within unvaccinated populations [34]. Maintenance of good oral hygiene, adequate hydration, and early and proper therapy of bacterial infection of the oropharynx may reduce the occurrence of suppurative parotitis.

Thyroiditis

The thyroid gland is remarkably resistant to infection, and infectious thyroiditis is quite rare. Infectious thyroiditis can be classified into three groups: (1) acute suppurative (AST); (2) subacute (ST); and (3) chronic thyroiditis. The incidence of infectious thyroiditis is unknown, but AST is estimated to account for 0.1% to 0.7% of all thyroid pathology [35,36]. AST, first described by Bauchet in 1857, carries substantial risk and should be treated as a medical emergency. In the preantimicrobial era, the case-fatality rate of AST was 22% [37]. Early recognition of AST is crucial for preventing devastating complications.

Pathogenesis and risk factors

The rarity of thyroid infections has been attributed to several factors of the thyroid gland: its high content of iodine, hydrogen peroxide production, rich blood supply with anastomotic arterial network, abundant lymphatic drainage, and unique encapsulated location [2,38,39]. Most cases of AST involve the left thyroid lobe because of the persistence of piriform sinus fistula, but the right lobe or both lobes may be involved [40,41]. Other routes of infection include hematogenous spread, additional congenital defects, direct spread from adjacent infected tissue, or lymphatic spread [2,38]. In ST, both lobes often are involved. Predisposing factors for infection include previous thyroid disease (goiter or adenoma), preceding infection in a distant site, trauma, postpartum or postabortal status, advanced age, diabetes mellitus, smoking, immunocompromising conditions, and chemotherapy [2,39].

Pathogens and infecting agents

In the largest review of infectious thyroiditis to date, bacteria were isolated in the majority of patients [42]. Gram-positive cocci are the most common organisms and include *S aureus*, *S pyogenes*, *Streptococcus viridans*, *Streptococcus pneumoniae*, and *Staphylococcus epidermidis* (Table 3). Gram-negative aerobic organisms such as *Klebsiella* spp, *Salmonella typhi*, and *Escherichia coli*, as well as anaerobic bacteria such as *Bacteroides* spp and *Peptostreptococcus* spp, have been reported. Anaerobic infections are commonly polymicrobial [43,44]. In ST, measles virus, influenza virus, adenovirus, echovirus, mumps virus, and Epstein-Barr virus are common [45–47]. Mycobacterial species have also been reported but usually are associated with miliary or disseminated disease. Other rare causes include parasites (*Echinococcus*, *Taenia solium*, and *Strongyloides stercoralis*) and *Treponema pallidum* [42]. Fungal etiologies include *Aspergillus* spp and *Coccidioides immitis* [48]. In patients who have HIV infection, *Pneumocystis jiroveci* is the most common organism in autopsy specimens [38].

Clinical manifestations

The most frequent symptoms of infectious thyroiditis are pain (which may refer to the ear or occiput), fever, dysphagia, dysphonia, hoarseness, chills, and preceding sore throat. In AST, clinical manifestations are similar in children and adults (Table 4) [40,49]. Stridor or dyspnea may develop because of tracheal narrowing (Fig. 1). Expectoration of purulent sputum should raise the suspicion of anatomic abnormalities. Death may occur because of tracheal obstruction, tracheal perforation, mediastinitis, or thyroid

Table 3
Pathogens associated with infectious thyroiditis

Type of organism		
Bacterial	Gram-positive aerobes	Gram-positive anaerobes
	Staphylococcus aureus	Peptostreptococci
	Group A streptococci	*Clostridium septicum*
	Streptococcus viridans	*Actinomyces* spp
	Streptococcus pneumoniae	Gram-negative anaerobes
	Staphylococcus epidermidis	*Bacteroides* spp
	Group B streptococci	*Prevotella* spp
	Enterococci	*Fusobacterium* spp
	Corynebacterium spp	Spirochete
	Nocardia asteroids	*Treponema pallidum*
	Rhodococcus equi	
	Gram-negative aerobes	
	Enterobacteriaceae	
	Escherichia coli	
	Salmonella spp	
	Klebsiella pneumoniae	
	Acinetobacter spp	
	Enterobacter cloacae	
	Others	
	Pseudomonas aeruginosa	
	Brucella spp	
	Haemophilus spp	
	Eikenella corrodens	
	Bartonella spp	
	Coxiella burnetii	
	Mycobacterium	
	Mycobacterium tuberculosis	
	Mycobacterium chelonia	
	Mycobacterium avium-intracellulare	
Fungal	*Pneumocystis jiroveci*	
	Aspergillus spp	
	Candida spp	
	Coccidioides immitis	
	Pseudoallescheria boydii	
	Cryptococcus spp	
	Histoplasma capsulatum	
Parasitic	*Echinococcus* spp	
	Trypanosome spp	
	Falciparum spp	
	Strongyloides stercoralis	
	Taenia solium	
Viral	Measles virus	Mumps virus
	Influenza virus	Epstein-Barr virus
	Adenovirus	Cytomegalovirus
	Echovirus	St. Louis encephalitis virus
	Human foamy virus	Herpes Simplex virus
	Rubella virus	Human T-cell Lymphotropic virus

Table 4
Manifestations of acute suppurative thyroiditis in children

Symptom	Children (%)	Adult (%)
Neck mass	100	100
Pain/tenderness	93	100
Left lobe involvement	87	85
Fever	80	100
Dysphagia/sore throat	40	90
Antecedent upper respiratory tract infection	33	88

Adapted from Chi H, Lee YJ, Chiu NC, et al. Acute suppurative thyroiditis in children. Pediatr Infect Dis J 2002;21(5):385; with permission; and Szabo SM, Allan DB. Thyroiditis. Differentiation of acute suppurative and subacute. Case report and review of the literature. Clin Pediatr (Phila) 1989; 28(4):173; with permission.

abscess rupture. Other complications include pneumonia, sepsis, vocal cord paralysis, regional sympathetic nerve disruption, and thyroid dysfunction [2,42]. Occasionally, patients may show symptoms of thyroid dysfunction, nervousness, gastrointestinal disturbance, or tremor. In patients who have mycobacterial, fungal, or parasitic infections resulting in chronic thyroiditis, specific symptoms usually are lacking. Diagnosis often is made intraoperatively or postmortem in autopsies [2]. The symptoms of ST generally are milder than those of AST and are more common in women (Table 5) [42,50].

Diagnosis

Thyroiditis should be suspected in patients presenting with anterior neck swelling associated with fever, dysphagia, and hoarseness. Leukocytosis and

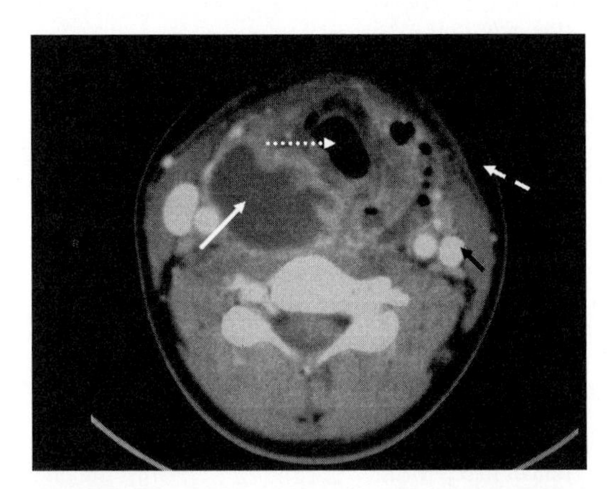

Fig. 1. CT scan of thyroid gland showing (*A*) thyroid abscess (*white solid arrow*), (*B*) mass effect on trachea (*white dotted arrow*), (*C*) air bubble (*white dashed arrow*) suggesting fistula/communication with posterior pharynx, and (*D*) vascular structure, left internal jugular vein (*black arrow*). "(*Courtesy of* Nawaf Al-Dajani, MD, Vancouver, British Columbia, Canada, 2006.)"

Table 5
Clinical features differentiating acute suppurative thyroiditis from subacute thyroiditis

Characteristic	Acute suppurative thyroiditis	Subacute thyroiditis
Preceding upper respiratory tract infection	88%	17%
Fever	100%	54%
Thyrotoxicosis	Uncommon	Common
Sore throat	90%	36%
Painful thyroid gland	100%	77%
Left side affected	85%	Not specific
Migrating tenderness	Possible	27%

Adapted from Szabo SM, Allan DB. Thyroiditis. Differentiation of acute suppurative and subacute. Case report and review of the literature. Clin Pediatr (Phila) 1989;28(4):173; with permission.

elevated sedimentation rate as well as C-reactive protein are observed frequently. Fewer than 6% of patients have coexisting bacteremia or fungemia. Thyroid function tests generally are normal (83%) [38,40]. In AST, the T4 level can be high during the acute stages because of the abundant release of T4 from the inflamed lobe. In prolonged ST or chronic thyroiditis, T4 can be low as hypothyroidism evolves. In mycobacterial thyroiditis, 50% of patients tend to be hyperthyroid; the opposite occurs in fungal thyroiditis [42].

Multiple imaging studies can assist with the diagnosis of infectious thyroiditis. Ultrasonography can identify lobe involvement and abscess formation [51]. In AST, thyroid radionuclide scans show focal reduced uptake or a cold nodule (90%–95%), whereas diffuse reduced uptake is seen in ST. Thyroid CT or MRI scans can delineate abscess extension and identify anatomic abnormalities [52,53]. Upper gastrointestinal contrast studies may show a fistula after successful treatment with antibiotics. Upper airway endoscopies can identify the piriform sinus and assess vocal cords and airways status. The criterion for diagnosis is FNA (ultrasound- or CT-guided) or biopsy for culture. Specimens should be sent for aerobic, anaerobic, fungal, and mycobacterial culture.

Management

Because AST can be fatal, initial therapy includes establishing an airway and intravenous access. Antibiotics tailored toward common pathogens, oral flora, and anaerobes (penicillin, cefazolin or cloxacillin in combination with clindamycin) are initiated. Broad-spectrum antibiotics such as cefotaxime and meropenem can be used in severe cases as well as vancomycin (if MRSA is suspected) and metronidazole. Fungal infection can be treated with amphotericin B, fluconazole, voriconazole, or caspofungin [48].

In the case of airway obstruction, failure of medical therapy, or clinical deterioration, prompt surgical intervention is indicated. Surgery also is indicated for patients who have persistent piriform sinus fistula or thyroglossal cyst after successful medical management. Recently, endoscopic fibrin glue has also been used with success [54]. Thyroid function tests should be followed because hypothyroidism may develop. Most patients who have AST and who are appropriately treated recover completely, but disease will recur in 16%. Treatment for ST is symptomatic; initial therapy includes nonsteroidal anti-inflammatory drugs. Some patients may require steroids. Again, thyroid function tests must be followed in patients who have ST because hypothyroidism develops in approximately 10% of these patients. ST generally is self limited, with most patients recovering within several weeks [50].

Infected cysts

Thyroglossal duct cyst

Thyroglossal duct cysts (TDC) account for 70% of congenital neck anomalies. TDC arise from the embryonic remnant of the thyroglossal duct that connects the foramen cecum (at the base of the tongue) with the thyroid gland. Most patients remain asymptomatic for years. A midline neck mass developing during late childhood, adolescence, or even adulthood is the most common presentation. There is a slight male predominance [55].

Dermoid and epidermoid cysts

Dermoid cysts and epidermoid cysts are the second most common congenital neck cysts. They typically occur in the midline of the neck anywhere from the hyoid bone to the mouth floor. Depending on their location, such cysts can interfere with breathing and swallowing. In contrast to epidermoid cysts, dermoid cysts contain skin appendages (eg, sebaceous glands, hair follicles) [56]. Surgical removal is almost always necessary to prevent infection or recurrence.

Branchial cleft cyst

Branchial cleft cysts arise from the incomplete obliteration of the branchial clefts during embryogenesis. Almost all branchial cleft anomalies arise from the second cleft (95%). Branchial cleft cysts usually are located in the anterior triangle of the neck at the junction of the middle and upper third of the sternocleidomastoid muscle. Often presenting at birth, branchial cleft cysts may become evident later in infancy or childhood. Branchial cleft cysts often become infected with sinus tract or abscess formation. Occasionally, internal drainage into the pharynx or external auditory meatus can occur. Interference with swallowing and breathing also may occur [57,58].

Laryngocele

A laryngocele is a cystic dilation of the laryngeal saccule. The congenital form is a remnant of air sac, whereas the acquired form develops from increased intraglottic pressure, excessive coughing, or glass blowing. Laryngoceles are rarely bilateral. The size can vary, increasing with Valsalva's maneuver. Most patients present with dysphonia, neck mass, or airway obstruction. Laryngoceles can become infected, especially if the saccule orifice becomes blocked [56,59].

Cystic hygroma

Cystic hygromas are lymphangiomas, a benign developmental condition of unknown origin. Cystic hygromas develop when communication between lymphatic sac and internal jugular vein or thoracic duct fails to develop, resulting in the accumulation of lymph and cystic formation [60]. Most present during the neonatal or childhood period (1 in 6000 births) and generally are located in the posterior triangle of the neck. Cystic hygromas can be single or multicystic. They are soft and fluctuant and transilluminate. Cystic hygromas can grow rapidly within the first few weeks, extending to internal structures of the neck, pharynx, larynx, and epiglottis. Airway compromise is common and can be challenging during delivery and neonatal resuscitation.

Pathogenesis and causative agents

In patients who have TDC, secretions of the thyroglossal duct epithelial cells accumulate, leading to dilation of the duct and gradual development of a cystic structure. This development, in combination with inadequate drainage and low oxygen tension, contributes to bacterial overgrowth and abscess formation. Connection to the mouth floor facilitates oral flora migration to the cyst cavity. TDC frequently become infected (40%–60%) [61]. *S aureus* and *S pyogenes* are the predominant pathogens. Alpha hemolytic *streptococci*, *Peptostreptococcus* spp, and gram-negative anaerobes (*Prevotella*, *Porphyromonas*, and *Bacteroides* spp) are common also [59]. Other types of congenital cysts become infected by the same mechanism (blocking of cyst orifice) with similar pathogens [59].

Clinical presentation

Most patients who have infected TDC present with a painful midline neck mass that is erythematous and warm. Hoarseness, dysphagia, or odynophagia are associated symptoms. Fever, chills, and other constitutional symptoms are uncommon [62]. In addition, the mass moves upward with swallowing. Fluctuation suggests abscess formation. In rare cases, airway compromise and suffocation may develop, especially if the TDC developed at the base if the tongue. This presentation can be fatal. Other forms of congenital neck cyst present in a similar fashion (Table 6). Purulent discharge may develop if a sinus tract has formed. Enlarged regional lymph node also may occur. Occasionally mass effect on surrounding organs, trachea, or pharynx may occur.

Table 6
Common congenital neck cysts by location, signs, and age range of onset

Type	Location	Signs	Age
Thyroglossal duct	Midline	Cyst moves with swallowing	Birth–elderly
Dermoid/epidermoid	Midline	Cyst may move with swallowing	Birth–adult
Branchial	Anterior neck triangle Lateral	Associated with draining sinus	Childhood–adult
Laryngocele	Lateral neck	Size fluctuates Transilluminates	Infancy–adult
Cystic hygroma	Posterior neck triangle	Soft, enlarges in first few weeks of life	Birth–infancy

Diagnosis

The diagnosis of infected neck cysts is based on clinical presentation (see Table 6). Most infected TDC present with a midline neck mass that moves with swallowing, whereas others, such as branchial cleft cyst or laryngocele, are lateral. Ultrasound scans can differentiate cystic from solid structures, detect abscesses, and guide FNA. CT and MRI scans detect suppuration and identify anatomic structure before surgical intervention. Fistulography can delineate the course of the fistula and identify the level of brachial cleft involvement. Pharyngoscopy and laryngoscopy identify internal orifices and mass effects. FNA or intraoperative cultures and histopathology are the criterion for identifying infectious agents and confirming developmental anomalies or malignant transformation [2,59]. Cultures should be processed for aerobes, anaerobes, fungi, and mycobacteria.

Management

Antibiotics (penicillin or cefazolin in addition to clindamycin) are targeted toward oral flora. Antibiotic regimens should be adjusted based on culture and sensitivity results. Oral antibiotics such as first-generation cephalosporins, amoxicillin/clavulanate, or clindamycin may be adequate for mild cases. Broad-spectrum antibiotics should be reserved for severe cases. Incision and drainage are indicated for abscesses and if medical therapy is unsuccessful. To prevent recurrences, surgical intervention ("Sistrunk procedure" for TDC) is required ultimately [59]. Such surgery is delayed until an acutely inflamed cyst has resolved [54].

References

[1] Barton LL, Feigin RD. Childhood cervical lymphadenitis: a reappraisal. J Pediatr 1974;84(6):846–52.

[2] Brook I. The swollen neck. Cervical lymphadenitis, parotitis, thyroiditis, and infected cysts. Infect Dis Clin North Am 1988;2(1):221–36.

[3] Scobie WG. Acute suppurative adenitis in children: a review of 964 cases. Scott Med J 1969; 14(10):352–4.
[4] Baker CJ. Group B streptococcal cellulitis-adenitis in infants. Am J Dis Child 1982;136(7): 631–3.
[5] Herold BC, Immergluck LC, Maranan MC, et al. Community-acquired methicillin-resistant *Staphylococcus aureus* in children with no identified predisposing risk. JAMA 1998;279(8): 593–8.
[6] CDC. Community-associated methicillin-resistant Staphylococcus aureus infection among healthy newborns— Chicago and Los Angeles county, 2004. MMWR Morb Mortal Wkly Rep 2006;55(12):329–32.
[7] Lai KK, Stottmeier KD, Sherman IH, et al. Mycobacterial cervical lymphadenopathy: relation of etiologic agents to age. JAMA 1984;251(10):1286–8.
[8] Starke JR, Taylor-Watts KT. Tuberculosis in the pediatric population of Houston, Texas. Pediatrics 1989;84(1):28–35.
[9] Wolinsky E. Mycobacterial lymphadenitis in children: a prospective study of 105 nontuberculous cases with long-term follow-up. Clin Infect Dis 1995;20(4):954–63.
[10] Wear DJ, Margileth AM, Hadfield TL, et al. Cat-Scratch disease: a bacterial infection. Science 1983;21(4618):1403–5.
[11] Scott GB, Hutto C, Makuch RW, et al. Survival in children with perinatally acquired human immunodeficiency virus type 1 infection. N Engl J Med 1989;321(26):1791–6.
[12] Centers for Disease Control and Prevention. 1993 Revised classification system for HIV infection and expanded surveillance case definition for AIDS among adolescents and adults. MMWR Morb Mortal Wkly Rep 1992;41(RR-17):1–19.
[13] Edlich RF, Arnette JA, Williams FM. Global epidemic of human T-cell lymphotropic virus type-1 (HTLV-1). J Emerg Med 2000;18(1):109–19.
[14] Dajani AS, Garcia RE, Wolinsky E. Etiology of cervical lymphadenitis in children. N Engl J Med 1963;268(24):1329–33.
[15] Yamauchi T, Ferrieri P, Anthony BF. The aetiology of acute cervical adenitis in children: serological and bacteriological studies. J Med Microbiol 1980;13(1):37–43.
[16] Bass JW, Vincent JM, Person DA. The expanding spectrum of Bartonella infection. II. Cat-scratch disease. Pediatr Infect Dis J 1997;16(2):163–79.
[17] Arisoy ES, Correa AG, Wagner ML, et al. Hepatosplenic cat-scratch disease in children: selected clinical features and treatment. Clin Infect Dis 1999;28(4):778–84.
[18] Papakonstantinou O, Bakantaki A, Paspalaki P, et al. High-resolution and color Doppler ultrasonography of cervical lymphadenopathy in children. Acta Radiol 2001;42(5): 470–6.
[19] Bass JW, Freitas BC, Freitas AD, et al. Prospective randomized double blind placebo-controlled evaluation of azithromycin for treatment of cat-scratch disease. Pediatr Infect Dis J 1998;17(6):447–52.
[20] American Thoracic Society. Diagnosis and treatment of disease caused by nontuberculosis mycobacteria. Am J Respir Crit Care Med 1997;156(2 Pt 2):S1–25.
[21] Petersdorf RG, Forsyth BR, Bernanke D. Staphylococcal parotitis. N Engl J Med 1958; 259(26):1250–4.
[22] Krippaehne WW, Hunt TK, Dunphy JE. Acute suppurative parotitis: a study of 161 cases. Ann Surg 1962;156(2):251–7.
[23] Leake DL, Krakowiak FJ, Leake RC. Suppurative parotitis in children. Oral Surg Oral Med Oral Pathol 1971;31(2):174–9.
[24] Brook I, Frazier EH, Thompson DH. Aerobic and anaerobic microbiology of acute suppurative parotitis. Laryngoscope 1991;101:170–2.
[25] Giglio MS, Landaeta M, Pinto ME. Microbiology of recurrent parotitis. Pediatr Infect Dis J 1997;16(4):386–90.
[26] O'Connell JE, George MK, Speculand B, et al. Mycobacterial infection of the parotid gland: an unusual case of parotid swelling. J Laryngol Otol 1993;107(6):561–4.

[27] Hensher R, Bowerman J. Actinomycosis of the parotid gland. Br J Oral Maxillofac Surg 1995;23(2):128–34.
[28] Cherry JD, Jahn CL. Exanthem and enanthem associated with mumps virus infection. Arch Environ Health 1966;12(4):518–21.
[29] Clark JR, Campbell JR. Parotitis. In: Feigin RD, Cherry JD, Demmler GJ, Kaplan SL, editors. Textbook of pediatric infectious diseases, 5th edition. Philadelphia: Saunders; 2004. p. 197–201.
[30] Ericson S, Zetterlund B, Ohman J. Recurrent parotitis and sialectasis in childhood: clinical, radiologic, immunologic, bacteriologic, and histologic study. Ann Otol Rhinol Laryngol 1991;100(7):527–35.
[31] Sperling NM, Lin P. Parotid disease associated with human immunodeficiency virus infection. Ear Nose Throat J 1990;69(7):475–7.
[32] Varghese JC, Thornton F, Lucey BC, et al. A prospective comparative study of MR sialography and conventional sialography of salivary disease. AJR Am J Roentgenol 1999;173(6): 1497–503.
[33] Brook I. Diagnosis and management of parotitis. Arch Otolaryngol Head Neck Surg 1992; 118(5):469–71.
[34] Centers for Disease Control and Prevention. Update: multistate outbreak of mumps—United States, Jan 1–May 2, 2006. MMWR Morb Mortal Wkly Rep 2006;55(20): 559–63.
[35] Henderson J. Abscess of the thyroid. A discussion and report of four cases. Am J Surg 1935; 29:36–41.
[36] Hendrick JW. Diagnosis and management of thyroiditis. JAMA 1957;164:127–33.
[37] Robertson WS. Acute inflammation of the thyroid gland. Lancet 1911;1:930–1.
[38] Farwell AP. Infectious thyroiditis. In: Braverman LE, Utiger RD, editors. Werner & Ingbar's the thyroids: a fundamental and clinical text. 8th edition. Philadelphia: Lippincott Williams and Wilkins; 2000. p. 1044–50.
[39] Pearce EN, Farwell AP, Braverman LE. Thyroiditis. N Engl J Med 2003;348(26):2646–55.
[40] Chi H, Lee YJ, Chiu NC, et al. Acute suppurative thyroiditis in children. Pediatr Infect Dis J 2002;21(5):384–7.
[41] Pereira KD, Davies JN. Piriform sinus tracts in children. Arch Otolaryngol Head Neck Surg 2006;132(10):1119–21.
[42] Berger SA, Zonszein J, Villamena P, et al. Infectious diseases of thyroid gland. Rev Infect Dis 1983;5(1):108–22.
[43] Yu EH, Ko WC, Chuang YC, et al. Suppurative Acinetobacter baumanii thyroiditis with bacteremic pneumonia: case report and review. Clin Infect Dis 1998;27(5):1286–90.
[44] Jacobs A, Gros DA, Gradon JD. Thyroid abscess due to Acinetobacter calcoaceticus: case report and review of the causes of and current management strategies for thyroid abscesses. South Med J 2003;96(3):300–7.
[45] Volpe R. The management of subacute (de Quervain's) thyroiditis. Thyroid 1993;5:253–5.
[46] Parmar RC, Bavdekar SB, Sahu DR, et al. Thyroiditis as a presenting feature of mumps. Pediatr Infect Dis J 2001;20(6):637–8.
[47] Volta C, Carano N, Street ME, et al. Atypical subacute thyroiditis caused by Epstein-Barr virus infection a three year old girl. Thyroid 2005;15(10):1189–91.
[48] Goldani LZ, Zavascki AP, Maia AL. Fungal thyroiditis: an overview. Mycopathologia 2006;161(3):129–39.
[49] Szabo SM, Allan DB. Thyroiditis. Differentiation of acute suppurative and subacute. Case report and review of the literature. Clin Pediatr (Phila) 1989;28(4):171–4.
[50] Sniezek JC, Francis TB. Inflammatory thyroid disorders. Otolaryngol Clin North Am 2003; 36(1):55–71.
[51] Ahuja AT, Griffithes JF, Roebuck DJ, et al. The role of ultrasound and oesophagography in the management of acute suppurative thyroiditis in children associated with congenital pyriform fossa sinus. Clin Radiol 1998;53(3):209–11.

[52] Weber Al. CT and MR imaging evaluation of neck infections with clinical correlations. Radiol Clin North Am 2000;38(5):941–68.
[53] Stone ME. A new role for computed tomography in the diagnosis and treatment of pyriform sinus fistula. Am J Otolaryngol 2000;21(5):323–5.
[54] Cigliano B, Cipolletta L, Baltogliannis N, et al. Endoscopic fibrin sealing of congenital pyriform sinus fistula. Surg Endosc 2004;18(3):554–6.
[55] Ostlie DJ, Burjonrappa SC, Snyder CL, et al. Thyroglossal duct infections and surgical outcomes. J Pediatr Surg 2004;39(3):396–9.
[56] Koeller KK, Alamo L, Adair C, et al. Congenital cystic masses of the neck: radiologic-pathologic correlation. Radiographics 1999;19(1):121–46.
[57] Waldhausen JH. Branchial cleft and arch anomalies in children. Semin Pediatr Surg 2006; 15(2):64–9.
[58] Mandell DL. Head and neck anomalies related to the branchial apparatus. Otolaryngol Clin North Am 2000;33(60):1309–32.
[59] Brook I. Microbiology and management of infected neck cysts. J Oral Maxillofac Surg 2005; 63(3):392–5.
[60] Velez I, Mintz S. Cystic hygroma. N Y State Dent J 2006;72(5):51–2.
[61] Brousseau V, Solares C, Xu M, et al. Thyroglossal duct cyst: presentation and management in children versus adult. Int J Pediatr Otorhinolaryngol 2003;67(12):1285–90.
[62] Mohan P, Chokshi R, Moser R, et al. Thyroglossal duct cysts: a consideration in adults. Am Surg 2005;71(6):508–11.

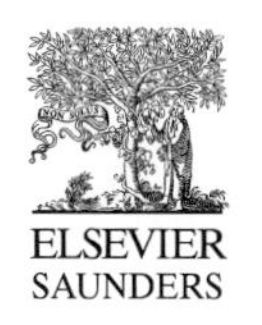

ELSEVIER
SAUNDERS

INFECTIOUS
DISEASE CLINICS
OF NORTH AMERICA

Infect Dis Clin N Am 21 (2007) 543–556

Cervicofacial Actinomycosis and Mandibular Osteomyelitis

Abdu A. Sharkawy, BMSc, MD, FRCPC

Department of Medicine, Division of Infectious Diseases,
University of Toronto and Toronto Western Hospital,
8-East Wing Room 418, 399 Bathurst Street, Toronto, ON M5T 2S8, Canada

Cervicofacial actinomycosis

Actinomycosis is a chronic disease characterized by abscess formation, draining sinus tracts, fistulae, and tissue fibrosis. Cervicofacial infection is the most common manifestation of the disease, accounting for nearly 50% of presentations [1–4]. Other forms of actinomycosis involving the central nervous system, lung and thoracic wall, and abdominal and pelvic organs are less common.

Microbiology

Cervicofacial actinomycosis is caused by organisms belonging to the order Actinomycetales, family Actinomycetaceae, genus *Actinomyces* [1]. Of note, both *Mycobacteria* and *Nocardia* species are classified in the same order and may be difficult to distinguish clinically or histologically from *Actinomyces* species [1]. At least 14 *Actinomyces* species have been described. Disease in humans is primarily caused by *A israelii*. *A bovis* is known to cause "lumpy jaw" disease in cattle but has never been cultured in humans [5]. Less common causes of human disease include *A odontolyticus, A naeslundii, A meyeri, A viscosus, A gerencseriae, A pyogenes, A georgiae*, and *A graevenitzii* [6–8]. Other implicated organisms include *Propionibacterium propionicus* (formerly *Arachnia propionicus*) and the coryneform bacteria *A neuii, A radingae*, and *A turicensis* [8,9].

Actinomyces are slow growing, non–spore-forming, gram-positive rods which are either strict or facultative anaerobes. Their morphology by Gram stain is variable, ranging from diphtheroidal to mycelial (Fig. 1). The name "actinomycosis" literally translates to "ray fungus" and reflects

E-mail address: abdu.sharkawy@uhn.on.ca

0891-5520/07/$ - see front matter
doi:10.1016/j.idc.2007.03.007

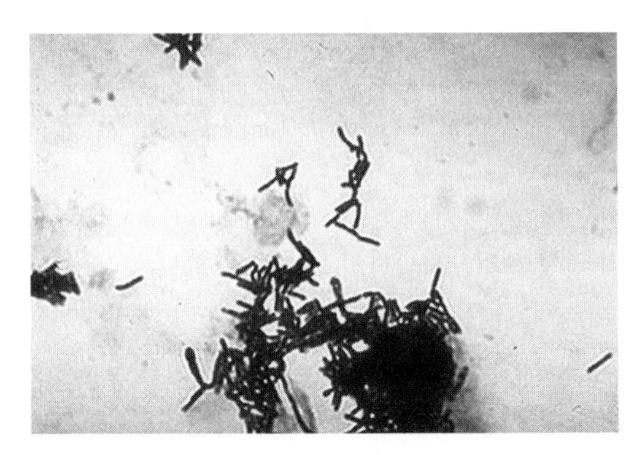

Fig. 1. Gram stain of a broth culture of *Actinomyces israelii*. Variable morphologies of these gram-positive organisms are visible, ranging from diphtheroidal to coccoid filaments. (*Courtesy of* Diane L. Roscoe, MD, Vancouver, British Columbia, Canada.)

its filamentous, fungal-like appearance [10]. Actinomyces, however, are true bacteria with filaments much narrower than fungal hyphae. Although actinomycotic filaments readily fragment into bacillary forms, tubular hyphae of molds never fragment and exhibit distinct branching patterns. Another distinguishing feature is reproduction, which occurs by bacterial fission and never by spores or budding [1].

Actinomyces are fastidious organisms that require culturing in enriched brain-heart infusion media. Incubation at 37°C with 6% to 10% carbon dioxide provides optimal growth conditions. Given their slow-growing nature, it is recommended that cultures be observed for at least 14 to 21 days to allow adequate detection [8].

Actinomyces almost invariably is isolated as part of polymicrobial flora, which commonly includes *Actinobacillus actinomycetemcomitans, Eikenella corrodens*, and species of *Fusobacterium, Bacteroides, Capnocytophaga, Staphylococcus, Streptococcus*, and *Enterococcus* [4,8,11,12]. In one study of more than 650 cases of actinomycosis, no *Actinomyces* species was isolated in pure culture in any single case. *A actinomycetemcomitans* and *Haemophilus aphrophilus* were most commonly identified with Actinomyces in this study [7].

Epidemiology

Actinomycosis was originally described in 1878 by Israel and Wolfe [13,14], who initially isolated the organism in culture and defined its anaerobic nature [8]. Actinomyces are not found in nature, and humans are, in fact, the only natural reservoir for the species causative of cervicofacial disease [8]. It is a rare condition, with most major medical centers reporting an average of one case per year [5]. Actinomycosis has a worldwide distribution with no predilection for age, race, season, or occupation [7]. For reasons that are unclear, a male predominance of 1.5 to 3:1 is reported in many series [2]. Predisposing factors include dental extractions, caries, gingivitis, gingival trauma, and infection in erupting secondary teeth [15]. Adult men who have poor oral hygiene seem to be at greatest risk. Other predisposing conditions include diabetes, immunosuppression, malnutrition, and local tissue damage by neoplastic disease or radiation [15,16]. Although not characterized as an opportunistic infection per se, its diagnosis in children should arouse suspicion of an underlying immunodeficiency state, particularly chronic granulomatous disease [7].

Pathogenesis

Actinomyces are normal constituents of the oral flora and are commensals of the periodontal pockets, carious teeth, dental plaque and calculus, gingival crevices, and tonsillar crypts [1]. Although not characteristically described as opportunistic pathogens, *Actinomyces* species capitalize on tissue injury or mucosal breach to invade adjacent structures in the head and neck regions. As a result, dental infections, manipulations, and oromaxillofacial trauma are common antecedent events [5]. Disease occurs almost exclusively by direct invasion, rarely by metastatic or hematogenous spread. A hallmark of cervicofacial actinomycosis is the tendency to spread without regard for anatomic barriers, including fascial planes or networks of lymphatic drainage.

The presence of other oral commensals, including gram-negative and anaerobic species intimately associated with Actinomyces, has led some to suggest that these organisms have an important role as facilitators of actinomycotic disease. Specifically, these organisms can reduce local oxygen tension, enabling Actinomyces to survive in abscess cavities or within the relatively avascular milieu of chronic fibrosis and inflammatory tissue. In addition, it is strongly believed that the presence of dense fibrosis, particularly in chronic disease states, provides a mechanism of resistance to both host phagocytosis and antibiotic penetration [17,18]. All these factors may explain the tendency of Actinomyces to pursue a chronic, often relapsing, disease course, particularly if not recognized early with initiation of appropriate therapy.

Pathology

Actinomyces are noted for forming characteristic sulfur granules in infected tissue but not in vitro. The term "sulfur granule" is a misnomer, reflecting only the yellow color of the granules in pus, because the granules contain no sulfur at all. The granules actually are discreet, macroscopic grains of hard consistency, 100 to 1000 μm in diameter, often visible to the naked eye or on low (× 10) magnification by microscopy (Fig. 2). They are composed of an internal tangle of mycelial fragments and a rosette of peripheral clubs. The complex is stabilized by a protein–polysaccharide complex and mineralized by host calcium phosphate [1]. Some authors

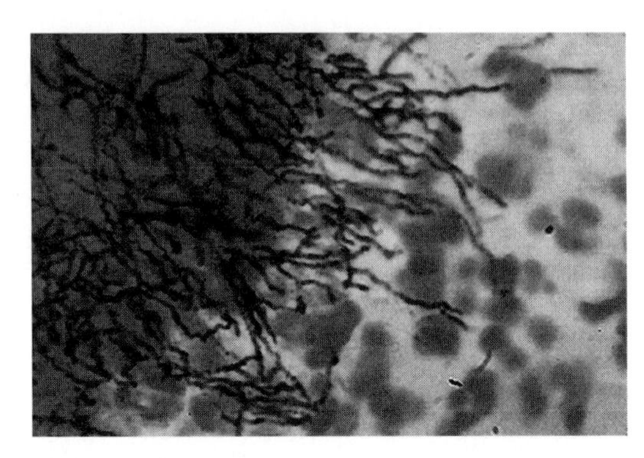

Fig. 2. Sulfur granules of actinomycosis. Gram stain of aspirate from oral abscess (original magnification × 1000). Actinomyces frequently grows in aggregates, termed "sulfur granules." Note the branching, gram-positive filaments on the edge of this granule. Actinomyces is a fastidious obligate anaerobe requiring anaerobic culture. (*Courtesy of* Harriet Provine, Boston, MA.)

suggest that the protein–polysaccharide complex provides a mechanism of resistance to host phagocytic activity among other defenses. Normal filaments within a granule are often seen with Gram's stain or silver methenamine stain, although more calcified granules may be difficult to identify [1,19].

Similar granules are formed by other organisms, notably *Nocardia* species, and in particular, *N brasiliensis* (mycetoma). Numerous other species, including fungi, *Streptomyces madurae* (mycetoma), and *Staphylococcus aureus* (botryomycosis), also produce granules, but these are best distinguished by an absence of peripheral clubs, which seem to be specific to *Actinomyces* species. Finally, it should be noted that not all Actinomyces species form sulfur granules (eg, *A odontolyticus*), and a peripheral fringe of clubs may be absent in certain instances, such as in tonsillar crypt infection, where minimal surrounding tissue reaction is provoked [1,3,20].

Sections of biopsy material typically reveal acute or chronic inflammatory granulation tissue with neutrophilic infiltration, surrounding dense fibrosis, foamy macrophages, plasma cells, and lymphocytes. Tissue fibrosis and a relative increase in plasma cells are more evident with chronic infection. Healing lesions tend to demonstrate profound fibrosis, even avascular in nature, often in proximity to areas of acute suppuration [1,21]. Sulfur granules may comprise no more than 1% of total tissue in a given lesion and hence are easily missed. Often a series of biopsies is required to confirm a pathologic diagnosis [18].

Clinical manifestations

Cervicofacial actinomycosis may present with a wide range of clinical signs and symptoms, but it usually develops in one of two distinct patterns. Typically, it presents as a chronic, slowly progressive, nontender, indurated mass that evolves into multiple abscesses, fistulae, and draining sinus tracts. Less commonly, it may present as an acute suppurative infection with a rapidly, progressive, fluctuant mass of pyogenic nature. At this stage pain and trismus may arise that seem disproportionate to local (visible) inflammation. With infections of the perimandibular space, inflammation of the muscles of mastication also may elicit significant pain and trismus. Fistulization from the perimandibular region is the most easily recognized manifestation of cervicofacial actinomycosis [1].

In general however, pain is an uncommon feature, particularly in chronic cases, although it may be prominent as a result of compression of adjacent structures in the ororespiratory tract such as the tongue [5,16]. Dyspnea and dysphagia may occur but are similarly uncommon. Occasionally, fever and constitutional symptoms including fatigue and malaise are notable in the acute, pyogenic form of the disease. Because actinomycosis spreads by direct extension, without regard for normal tissue planes, regional lymphadenopathy is rare until quite late in the disease course and tends to be reactive in nature [18].

Characteristic lesions usually develop slowly over weeks to months with adherence to overlying skin, giving a bluish or reddish appearance. This presentation often is mistaken for cellulitis but in fact more likely represents venous congestion. Over time, sinus tracts invariably form on the skin surface or oral mucosae, eventually erupting to express a thick, yellow-serous exudate that yields the characteristic sulfur granules [1]. Inflammatory, cicatricial scarring is one of the more noticeable long-term sequelae [15].

Cervicofacial actinomycosis may involve almost any tissue or structure surrounding the upper or lower mandible, but the mandibular region itself is consistently the most commonly identified site of infection [1]. In one study of 317 patients at the University of Cologne between 1952 and 1975, the distribution of affected sites were mandible, 53.6%; cheek, 16.4%; chin, 13.3%; submaxillary ramus and angle, 10.7%; upper jaw, 5.7%; and mandibular joint, 0.3% [1,22]. Although direct bony invasion is uncommon, periostitis and posttraumatic osteomyelitis occurred in 11.7% of cases in this study. Although most cases of cervicofacial actinomycosis are of odontogenic origin, primary infections have been reported in numerous structures within the head and neck, often quite remote from any potential periodontal source. In fact, primary infections of the thyroid gland [23], of a thyroidectomy incision site, and as a complication of transtracheal aspiration have been reported [24]. Furthermore, infections of the temporal region [25], paranasal sinuses [26], palate [27], tongue [28], and posterior triangle of the neck [18] also have been documented.

Diagnosis

Cervicofacial actinomycosis has been dubbed "the great masquerader of head and neck disease" [29], highlighting both its elusive nature in microbial etiology and its relative lack of familiarity to most clinicians. As a consequence, because the index of suspicion is usually low, appropriate steps to obtain an adequate specimen for culture and histopathologic examination are often impeded. Furthermore, such infections often respond, at least in the short term, to brief courses of antibiotic therapy. This treatment creates two key problems. (1) Isolation of the causative organism from culture is exceedingly rare if a patient has received antibiotics within 7 to 10 days of the time of specimen acquisition. (2) Falsely negative culture results can delay diagnosis, leading to additional fibrosis and a more chronic disease course. The enhanced fibrosis further hinders identification of granules by histologic examination [30].

As the disease progresses with repeated courses of antibiotic therapy, the fibrotic, "woody" induration often comes to resemble a malignant process. Occasionally, the granulomatous appearance of a biopsy specimen is mistaken for tuberculous disease. Perhaps even more commonly, granules are misidentified by staining or biopsy as an indication of nocardiosis. These pitfalls can be avoided by remembering that malignant lesions should not respond at all to antimicrobial therapy and that both *Nocardia* and mycobacterial species are typically acid fast, whereas Actinomyces is not.

Diagnostic confirmation requires recovering *Actinomyces* species from an appropriately cultured specimen, typically by fine-needle aspiration of an abscess, fistula, or sinus tract or from a large biopsy specimen. Care must be taken to avoid contamination by other normal oral flora. Anaerobic or at least, microaerophilic incubation for a minimum of 14 days is recommended [1]. Ideally, empiric antimicrobial therapy should be withheld before obtaining specimens by fine-needle aspiration or biopsy of diseased tissues. Multiple sections of a biopsy specimen from different tissue levels are suggested to optimize histopathologic diagnosis [1,31].

Although at one time routine staining was considered a mainstay in diagnosing cervicofacial actinomycosis, it now is known that small colonies and single filaments are easily missed. Furthermore, filaments of *Nocardia* and *Actinomyce*s species are next to impossible to differentiate by conventional methods such as Grocott-Gomori-methenamine stain or hematoxylin and eosin [1,8]. Other methods, including p-aminosalicylic acid, MacCallen-Goodpasture, and Brown-Brenn stains, do not seem to offer additional sensitivity. As a result, specific fluorescent-conjugated monoclonal antibody stains have been popularized for their rapid and highly specific identification of various *Actinomyces* species, even in mixed infections and after fixation in formalin. An additional advantage of this technique is the ability to define single filaments in granulation tissue [8].

Although agglutinins and complement-fixing antibodies appear in the serum of some patients who have cervicofacial actinomycosis, they may represent cross-precipitating antibodies formed by other disease processes, such as tuberculosis [32]. Hence, at present, serodiagnosis does not seem to be a practical or reliable diagnostic tool. Rapid serodiagnosis by immunoelectrophoresis or monospecific antigen-antibody systems is being developed and refined [32] but is not widely available for routine use.

Treatment

Since the advent of antibiotic therapy, the principles for management of cervicofacial actinomycosis have emphasized a prolonged treatment schedule coupled with surgical management when necessary. Difficulty in penetrating areas of dense fibrosis, suppuration, and perhaps even granules in particular provides the rationale for a prolonged course of high-dose therapy. High-dose penicillin remains the treatment of choice [8,30,33,34]. For mild infections, when significant suppuration or fistulous tracts are not present, oral antibiotic therapy is reasonable; a 2-month course of oral penicillin V, 2 to 4 g/d in four divided daily doses, is generally appropriate [33]. Oral amoxicillin, 500 mg three times daily, is equally efficacious [35]. Surgical intervention may not be mandated in these cases [33], particularly if therapy is commenced early in the course of the disease. In the setting of more complicated disease, surgical excision of recalcitrant fibrotic lesions or drainage of extensive abscesses or persisting sinus tracts often is required in conjunction with ongoing antimicrobial therapy for definitive cure [36]. Surgical intervention also is recommended for excision of necrotic tissue and curettage of affected bony tissue [36]. Surgical management alone however, is rarely, if ever successful as definitive treatment [8].

In complicated cases, parenteral penicillin G, 10 to 20 million units daily divided every 6 hours for 4 to 6 weeks, followed by oral penicillin V, 2 to 4 g/d divided four times daily for 6 to 12 months, is recommended [33,35]. Duration of therapy should be guided by the severity of the disease and ongoing assessment for clinical or pathologic remission. Acceptable alternatives to penicillin include the tetracyclines, erythromycin, clindamycin, and imipenem [34,37,38]. Various other agents generally are deemed to have poor activity against *Actinomyces* species and *P propionicus,* and probably should be avoided. These agents include oral cephalexin, oxacillin and dicloxacillin, the fluoroquinolones, metronidazole, aminoglycosides, and aztreonam [37,39–41]. For patients who are allergic to penicillin, the tetracyclines probably offer the best alternative, with some studies suggesting equivalency with penicillin, especially in milder disease presentations [33,38]. Therapy need not be directed against other oral flora recovered with Actinomyces, because regimens effective against Actinomyces specifically are usually curative [33].

Prevention

There are no specifically defined measures for preventing cervicofacial actinomycosis. Maintenance of good oral hygiene and appropriate plaque removal can limit the tendency of Actinomyces to establish dense colonization and subclinical periodontal infection, an important precipitant for more extensive disease [8].

Mandibular osteomyelitis

Mandibular osteomyelitis is an infrequently reported condition; however, emerging experience suggests that it probably is more common than currently appreciated [42,43]. Because it may be difficult to distinguish from other conditions affecting the mandible – including malignancy, osteonecrosis, chronic relapsing multifocal osteomyelitis, and the synovitis, acne, hyperostosis, and osteitis syndrome, the true incidence of mandibular osteomyelitis is unknown [42].

Pathogenesis

Mandibular osteomyelitis arises primarily from odontogenic infection incited by one of two major events: extension of periapical tooth abscess or posttraumatic or postsurgical complication. Numerous other predisposing conditions have been reported, however. Prominent among these are underlying bony pathologies such as Paget's disease and osteopetrosis, compound fracture, history of local irradiation, and host-compromising conditions such as diabetes mellitus and systemic corticosteroid therapy [44].

Because of anatomic considerations, the mandible is more susceptible to osteomyelitis than are other facial bony structures, including those in the oromaxillofacial region. In particular, a relatively thin cortical plate and poor vascular supply to its medullary tissue predispose the mandible, rather than the maxilla, to bony infection [44]. Areas at greatest risk of perforation in the mandible are the lingual aspect in the region of molar teeth and anteriorly on the buccal aspect [44,45]. Considering the frequency of odontogenic infections in general, as well as the intimate association of teeth with the medullary cavity, it is surprising that mandibular osteomyelitis is not more common [44].

With initiation of infection, intramedullary pressure increases markedly, compromising the vascular supply and setting the stage for bony necrosis. Purulent material readily traverses networks of Haversian and perforating canals, eventually accumulating under the periosteum and lifting it from its bony cortex. As the accumulation of pus proceeds unabated, periosteal perforation can occur, ultimately forming abscesses and, often, fistulous tracts within mucosal or cutaneous tissues [44]. In chronic cases, granulation tissue forms as well as characteristic lesions of dead bone (sequestrum) separated from surrounding healthy tissue, and eventually, a reactive sleeve of new periosteal tissue (involucrum) forms [44].

Microbiology

The microbiologic causes of mandibular osteomyelitis comprise a wide spectrum, reflecting the polymicrobial nature of odontogenic infection in general and agents associated with suppurative infection and periapical abscesses in particular. Organisms with a tendency to colonize the tooth surface and, by extension, causative of dental caries, include those of the mutans Streptococcus group, such as *S mutans* and *S sobrinus*, along with *Actinomyces* species, namely *A naeslundii* and *A viscosus* [46].

Well-established periodontitis is associated with a more complex array of offending pathogens, including anaerobic gram-negative bacilli and motile oral spirochetes. Prominent among these are *A actinomycetemcomitans* (a HACEK organism), *Porphyromonas gingivalis, Prevotella intermedia, Bacteroides forsythus*, and *Treponema denticola* [47].

Suppurative odontogenic infection, including periapical abscess and mandibular osteomyelitis, usually is polymicrobial in nature as well, but *Fusobacterium nucleatum*, pigmented *Prevotella*, *Peptostreptococcus*, *Actinomyces*, and *Streptococcus* species are the predominant isolates [48,49]. With the exception of hosts who have serious underlying illnesses, facultative gram-negative bacilli and *S aureus* are uncommon etiologic isolates for suppurative infections predisposing to mandibular osteomyelitis [47–49].

Clinical manifestations

Mandibular osteomyelitis may present with myriad clinical features, including those that reflect a precipitating odontogenic condition, such as pulpitis, gingivitis, or periapical abscess. Regardless of the inciting event, severe localized jaw pain is a nearly universal presenting symptom. Pain may be diffuse but typically localizes to the body or ramus of the mandible [50,51]. Facial swelling, which is brawny and indurated in character, is common and raises the specter of concurrent cervicofacial actinomycosis. Sensory disturbances, including anesthesia or hypoesthesia on the affected side of the face, are variably present. In protracted cases, limitation in mouth opening and even frank trismus may occur [50,51]. Garre's chronic sclerosing osteomyelitis or proliferative periostitis is a clinical variant that presents with a hard, nontender, localized swelling over the mandible. This entity is commonly associated with actinomycosis or radiation necrosis as causes of osteomyelitis [50,51]. Various presentations of mandibular osteomyelitis progressing to frank osteonecrosis are illustrated in Fig. 3. Unless associated with an acute suppurative or necrotizing process, fever, lymphadenopathy, and constitutional symptoms are uncommon features of mandibular osteomyelitis per se, and their presence should alert the clinician to either a complicating event or an alternative diagnosis altogether [52].

Diagnosis

The diagnosis of mandibular osteomyelitis rests on appropriate specimen collection and processing for identification of microbiologic isolates and on imaging studies to determine the extent of disease. The presence of normal resident oral flora complicates the interpretation of specimens obtained for

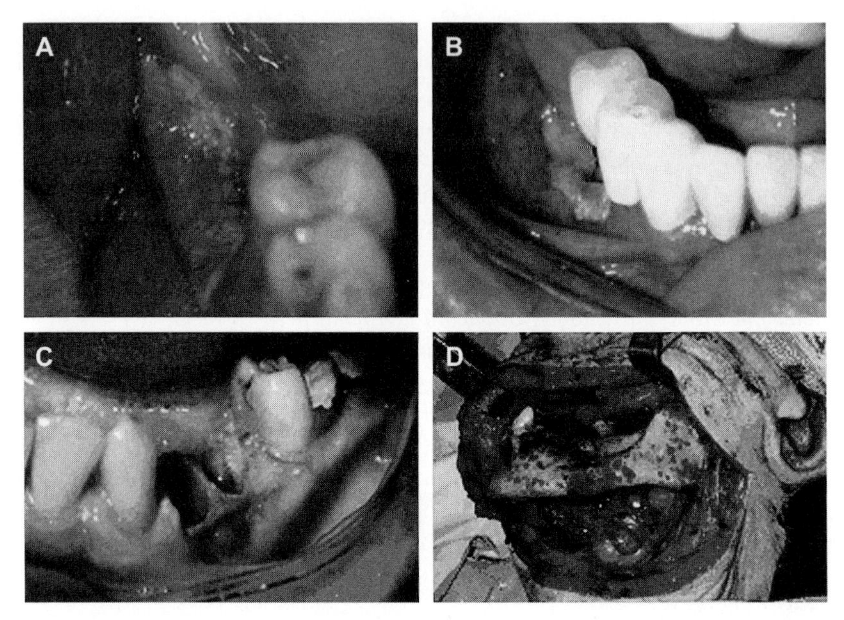

Fig. 3. Clinical presentation of osteonecrosis of the jaw. (*A*) Typical lesion of osteonecrosis of the jaw showing exposed infected bone involving the mylohyoid ridge. (*B*) Osteonecrotic bone below a dental implant. (*C*) Spontaneous exfoliated teeth with underlying exposed dead bone. (*D*) Operative picture showing well-demarcated dead bone involving the whole alveolus. (*From* Badros A, Weikel D, Salama A, et al. Osteonecrosis of the jaw in multiple myelomoa patients: clinical features and risk factors. J Clin Oncol 2006;24:948; with permission. Copyright © 2006 by American Society of Clinical Oncology.)

culture, and some degree of contamination effect is inevitable with sampling of intraoral lesions [51]. Therefore direct tissue biopsy of bony lesions is recommended whenever possible. Specimens should be examined routinely for histopathologic evidence of inflammation and/or infection. In chronic mandibular osteomyelitis, soft tissue swelling and draining fistulous tracts provide useful sources for aspiration and subsequent specimen analysis [51]. The same cannot be said for sinus tract sampling, however. Because these tracts are by definition in communication with the external environment, the microbiologic isolates obtained may reflect colonization of the tract itself rather than underlying bony infection [51]. Ultimately, bone biopsy for histopathology and culture is required to establish a definitive diagnosis.

The evolution of imaging modalities during the past 2 decades has greatly enhanced the diagnostic work-up of mandibular osteomyelitis. Nuclear medicine studies, such as technetium bone scanning, used in conjunction with gallium- or indium-labeled white blood cell scanning, are useful screening tools in the diagnosis of osteomyelitis [53,54]. Characteristic uptake patterns also can aid in differentiating acute and chronic infection from alternative diagnoses, including trauma and malignancy [51]. In acute bony infection, both bone and gallium/indium scans are likely to be positive. In chronic osteomyelitis, however, technetium scans may or may not be positive, and labeled scans often are negative [51]. Other useful imaging studies include plain-film radiographs, which can demonstrate characteristic lesions, including radiolucencies, sequestra, and even frank cortical destruction in advanced stages of disease. The earliest sign of osteomyelitis seen on plain films is periosteal reaction, which may be visible to the keen observer as early as 2 to 3 weeks after the onset of infection [53]. CT and MRI demonstrate superior sensitivity in the diagnosis of acute osteomyelitis. MRI, in particular, is an excellent modality for identifying associated soft tissue disease or deep fascial infection [53], an important consideration in the assessment of any significant infection of the head and neck region.

Treatment

A combination of appropriately targeted antimicrobial therapy and thorough surgical débridement is the cornerstone of management for most cases of mandibular osteomyelitis. Antibiotic therapy is complicated by the presence of teeth and persistent exposure to resident oral flora. With the emergence of β-lactamase–producing strains of oral anaerobes, namely pigmented *Prevotella* species and *Fusobacterium* species, empiric penicillin monotherapy has met with increasing failures and is no longer recommended [55]. Ampicillin-sulbactam (2 g intravenously every 4 hours) extends coverage against β-lactamase–producing oral anaerobes and is effective against most anaerobic gram-negative bacilli as well as *Actinomyces* species. For this reason, it is the treatment of choice for most serious odontogenic infections [51] and, by extension, is probably the best option in the empiric treatment of mandibular osteomyelitis. Penicillin G (2 to 4 MU intravenously every 4 to 6 hours) in combination with metronidazole (500 mg intravenously or by mouth every 6 hours) is an appropriate alternative [51,56]. For patients who have penicillin allergy, clindamycin (600 mg intravenously or by mouth every 6 hours) is recommended [51]. In special host-compromised populations, such as patients who have hematologic malignancy and febrile neutropenia or patients receiving immunosuppressive therapy, broad-spectrum coverage against facultative gram-negative bacilli as well as oral aerobes and anaerobes is recommended. A third-generation cephalosporin, carbapenem, and ureidopenicillin are appropriate empiric options [51]. Whenever possible, antibiotic selection should be guided by specimen culture and sensitivity results and should be modified accordingly. Regardless of the agent chosen, antibiotic therapy for mandibular osteomyelitis requires a prolonged duration, often spanning several weeks to months [44,51,57].

Hyperbaric oxygen has been proposed as adjuvant therapy to hasten the bone repair [50,51]. In one study of 33 patients who had early, chronic mandibular osteomyelitis, 79% were symptom free 10 to 34 months after combined hyperbaric oxygen therapy and surgical débridement [51,58]. The clinical utility of hyperbaric oxygen is offset by its lack of routine availability in most medical centers, however.

Surgical intervention for mandibular osteomyelitis is aimed at thorough drainage and débridement of necrotic or devitalized tissues that serve as a nidus for ongoing infection, and measures that promote tissue healing and bony remodeling. Various procedures, including sequestrectomy, saucerization, decortication, and closed-wound suction irrigation, may be necessary. In rare cases of advanced disease, radical excision of an entire segment of infected jaw may be warranted [44,51,52]. Because of the magnitude and complexity of this procedure and the risk of lasting cosmetic disfigurement, this procedure usually is a measure of last resort.

References

[1] Lerner PI. The lumpy jaw. Cervicofacial actinomycosis. Infect Dis Clin North Am 1988;2(1): 203–20.
[2] Kwartler JA, Limaye A. Pathologic quiz case 1. Cervicofacial actinomycosis. Arch Otolaryngol Head Neck Surg 1989;115(4):524–6.
[3] Brown JR. Human actinomycosis. A study of 181 subjects. Hum Pathol 1973;4:319–30.
[4] Weese WC, Smith IM. A study of 57 cases of actinomycosis over a 36 year period. Arch Intern Med 1975;135:1562–5.
[5] Belmont MJ, Behar PM, Wax MK. Atypical presentations of actinomycosis. Head Neck 1999;21(3):264–8.
[6] Schaal KP, Lee HJ. Actinomycete infections in humans—a review. Gene 1992;115: 201–11.
[7] Jacobs RF, Schutze GE. Actinomycosis. In: Berhman RE, editor. Nelson textbook of pediatrics. 16th edition. Philadelphia: WB Saunders; 2000. p. 823–5.
[8] Smego RA Jr, Foglia G. Actinomycosis. Clin Infect Dis 1998;26:1255–63.
[9] Funke G, von Graevenitz A. Infections due to Actinomyces neuii (former "CDC coryneform group 1" bacteria. Infection 1995;23:73–5.
[10] Rippon JW. Medical mycology. Philadelphia: WB Saunders; 1974. p. 13–28.
[11] Holm P. Studies on aetiology of actinomycosis. I. The "other" microbes of actinomycosis and their importance. Acta Pathol Microbiol Scand 1950;27:736–43.
[12] Holm P. Studies on aetiology of human actinomycosis. II. Do the "other" microbes of actinomycosis possess virulence? Acta Pathol Microbiol Scand 1951;28:391.
[13] Israel J. Neve Beobactungen anf dem Bebiete der Mykosen des Menshen. Virchows Arch Pathol Anat Physiol Klin Med 1878;74:15–53 [in German].
[14] Wolfe M, Israel J. Ueber Reincultur des Actinomyces and seine Uebertragbarkeit auf Thiere. Virchows Arch Pathol Anat Physiol Klin Med 1891;126:11–59 [in German].
[15] Feder HM Jr. Actinomycosis manifesting as an acute painless lump of the jaw. Pediatrics 1990;85(5):858–64.
[16] Mitchell TG. Actinomycetes. In: Joklik WK, Wilett HP, Amos BD, editors. Zinsser microbiology. 18th edition. Norwalk (CT): Appleton-Centery-Crofts Press; 1982. p. 583–94.
[17] Ermis I, Topalan M, Aydin A, et al. Actinomycosis of the frontal and parotid regions. Ann Plast Surg 2001;46(1):55–8.
[18] Burns BV, al-Ayoubi A, Ray J, et al. Actinomycosis of the posterior triangle: a case report and review of the literature. J Laryngol Otol 1997;111(11):1082–5.

[19] Pine L, Overman JR. Determination of the structure and composition of "sulphur granules" of *Actinomyces bovis*. J Gen Microbiol 1963;32:209.

[20] Hotchi M, Schwarz J. Characterization of actinomycotic granules by architecture and staining methods. Arch Pathol 1972;93:393.

[21] Emmons CW, Binfor CH, Utz JP, et al. Medical mycology. 3rd edition. Philadelphia: Lea & Febiger; 1977. p. 77.

[22] Schaal KP, Beaman BL. Clinical significance of actinomycetes. In: Goodfellow M, Mordarski M, Williams ST, editors. The biology of the actinomycetes. New York: Academic Press; 1983. p. 389–424.

[23] Dan M, Garcia A, Von Westarp C, et al. Primary actinomycosis of the thyroid mimicking carcinoma. J Otolaryngol 1984;13:109.

[24] Rothman NI, Kamholz SL, Pinsker KL. Actinomycotic cervical abscess. A complication of transtracheal aspiration. Chest 1979;76:228.

[25] Zajc I, Orihovac Z, Bagutin M. Temporal actinomycosis: report of a case. J Oral Maxillofac Surg 1999;57:1370–2.

[26] Roth M, Montone KT. Actinomycosis of the paranasal sinuses: a case report and review. Otolaryngol Head Neck Surg 1996;114:818–21.

[27] Herman WW, Whitaker SB, Williams MF, et al. Acute actinomycosis presenting as an ulcerated palatal mass. J Oral Maxillofac Surg 1998;56:1098–101.

[28] Ficarra G, Di Lollo S, Pierleoni F, et al. Actinomycosis of the tongue: a diagnostic challenge. Head Neck 1993;15:53–5.

[29] Rankow RM, Abraham DM. Actinomycosis: a masquerader in the head and neck. Ann Otolaryngol 1978;87:230–7.

[30] Peabody JW, Seabury JH. Actinomycosis and nocardiosis. A review of basic differences in therapy. Am J Med 1960;28:99–115.

[31] Pollock PG, Meyers DS, Frable WJ, et al. Rapid diagnosis of actinomycosis by thin-needle aspiration biopsy. Am J Clin Pathol 1978;70:27.

[32] Lerner PI. Serologic screening for actinomycosis. In: Balows A, editor. Anaerobic bacteria role in disease. Springfield (IL): Charles C. Thomas; 1974. p. 571.

[33] Smego RA Jr. Actinomycosis. In: Hoeprich PD, editor. Infectious diseases. New York: Lippincott Company; 1994. p. 493–7.

[34] Gilbert DN, Moellering RC Jr, Sande MA. The Sanford guide to antimicrobial therapy. 31st edition. Sperryville (VA): Antimocrobial Therapy Inc.; 2001. p. 70.

[35] Martin M. The use of oral amoxicillin for the treatment of actinomycosis. Br Dent J 1984; 156:252–4.

[36] Bennhoff D. Actinomycosis: diagnostic and therapeutic considerations and a review of 32 cases. Laryngoscope 1984;94:1198–217.

[37] Lerner PI. Susceptibility of pathogenic actinomycetes to antimicrobial compounds. Antimicrob Agents Chemother 1974;5:302–9.

[38] Martin MV. Antibiotic treatment of cervicofacial actinomycosis for patients allergic to penicillin: a clinical and in vitro study. Br J Oral Maxillofac Surg 1985;23:428–35.

[39] Fass RJ, Scholand JF, Hodges GR. Clindamycin in the treatment of serious anaerobic infections. Ann Intern Med 1973;78:853–9.

[40] Wade WG. In-vitro activity of ciprofloxacin and other agents against oral bacteria. J Antimicrob Chemother 1989;24:683–7.

[41] Tanaka-Bandoh K, Watanabe K, Kato N, et al. Susceptibilities of *Actinomyces* species and *Propionibacterium propionicus* to antimicrobial agents. Clin Infect Dis 1997;25(Suppl 2): S262–3.

[42] Robinson JL, Vaudry WL, Dobrovolsky W. Actinomycosis presenting as osteomyelitis in the pediatric population. Pediatr Infect Dis J 2005;24:365–9.

[43] Lugassy G, Shaham R, Nemets A, et al. Severe osteomyelitis of the jaw in long-term survivors of multiple myeloma: a new clinical entity. American Journal of Medicine 2004;117 (6):440–1.

[44] Chow AW. Infection of the oral cavity, neck and head. In: Mandell GL, Bennett JE, Dolin R, editors. Principles and practice of infectious diseases. 6th edition. Philadelphia: Churchill Livingstone; 2005. p. 787–98.
[45] Thadepalli H, Mandal AK. Anatomic basis of head and neck infections. Infect Dis Clin North Am 1988;2(1):21–34.
[46] Hamada S, Slade HD. Biology, immunology, and cariogenicity of Streptococcus mutans. Microbiol Rev 1980;44:331.
[47] Chow AW. Epidemiology, pathogenesis and clinical manifestations of odontogenic infections. In: Rose BD, editor. UptoDate 14.3, Wellesely (MA): UptoDate; 2006.
[48] Tanner A, Stillman N. Oral and dental infections with anaerobic bacteria: clinical features, predominant pathogens and treatment. Clin Infect Dis 1993;16(Suppl 4):S304–9.
[49] Brook I. Microbiology and management of endodontic infections in children. J Clin Pediatr Dent 2003;28(1):13–7.
[50] Topazian RG. Osteomyelitis of the jaws. In: Topazian RG, Goldberg MH, editors. Oral and maxillofacial infections. 2nd edition. Philadelphia: WB Saunders; 1987. p. 204.
[51] Chow AW. Complications, diagnosis and treatment of odontogenic infections. In: Rose BD, editor. Uptodate 14.3. Wellesely (MA): UptoDate; 2006.
[52] Harris LF. Chronic mandibular osteomyelitis. South Med J 1986;79(6):696–7.
[53] Gold RH, Hawkins RA, Katz RD. Bacterial osteomyelitis: findings on plain radiography, CT, MR, and scintigraphy. AJR Am J Roentgenol 1991;157(2):365–70.
[54] Revskin AB. Radiographic and other diagnostic imaging techniques. In: Topazian RG, Goldberg MH, editors. Oral and maxillofacial infections. 2nd edition. Philadelphia: WB Saunders; 1987. p. 105.
[55] Brook I. Antibiotic resistance of oral anaerobic bacteria and their effect on the management of upper respiratory tract and head and neck infections. Semin Respir Infect 2002;17(3): 195–203.
[56] Hood FJC. The place of metronidazole in the treatment of acute orofacial infection. Antimicrob Agents Chemother 1978;15:71.
[57] Van Merkesteyn JPR, Groot RH, van den Akker HP, et al. Treatment of chronic suppurative osteomyelitis of the mandible. Int J Oral Maxillofac Surg 1997;26:450–4.
[58] Aitosalo K, Niinikoski J, Grenman R, et al. A modified protocol for early treatment of osteomyelitis and osteoradionecrosis of the mandible. Head Neck 1998;20(5):411–7.

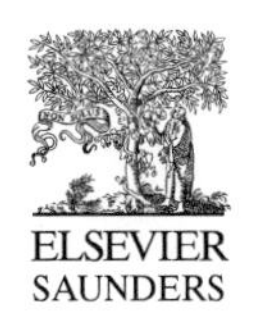

ELSEVIER
SAUNDERS

Infect Dis Clin N Am 21 (2007) 557–576

INFECTIOUS
DISEASE CLINICS
OF NORTH AMERICA

Life-Threatening Infections of the Peripharyngeal and Deep Fascial Spaces of the Head and Neck

Steven C. Reynolds, MD, FRCPC[a],
Anthony W. Chow, MD, FRCPC, FACP[b,*]

[a]*Division of Critical Care Medicine, Department of Medicine, University of British Columbia, Vancouver Hospital, ICU2, JPPN 2nd Floor, Room 2438, 855 West 12th Ave., Vancouver, BC V5Z 1M9, Canada*
[b]*Division of Infectious Diseases, Department of Medicine, University of British Columbia, Vancouver Hospital Health Sciences Centre, 2733 Heather Street, Vancouver, BC V5Z 3J5, Canada*

Life-threatening infections of the head and neck are relatively uncommon in the postantibiotic era, and many physicians are not familiar with the clinical manifestations and natural history of such infections. This was not always the case. In fact, Lemierre asserted in 1936 that the clinical manifestation of "post-anginal sepsis" were so characteristic that they could not be missed [1]. With the widespread use of effective antibiotics instituted early in the clinical course of head and neck infections, complications such as Lemierre syndrome are rarely seen and may not be recognized by many physicians. Indeed, Lemierre syndrome has often been called "a forgotten disease."

Although any infection can be life threatening in particular circumstances, infections in three potential spaces in the head and neck are considered of primary importance (Fig. 1): the submandibular, lateral pharyngeal, and the retropharyngeal-danger-prevertebral spaces. An understanding of the anatomic boundaries and connections of these potential spaces provides valuable insight into the pathophysiology, clinical manifestations, and potential complications of each of these infections. Because there are multiple synonyms for potential spaces in the head and neck, it is important to identify clearly which cervical spaces are being discussed (Table 1).

* Corresponding author.
E-mail address: tonychow@interchange.ubc.ca (A.W. Chow).

0891-5520/07/$ - see front matter
doi:10.1016/j.idc.2007.03.002

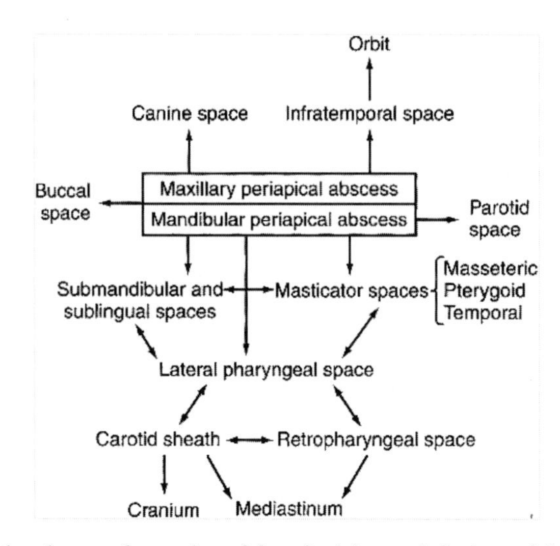

Fig. 1. Potential pathways of extension of deep fascial space infections of the head and neck. (*From* Chow AW. Infections of the oral cavity, head and neck. In: Mandell GL, Bennett JE, Dolin R, editors. Principles and practice of infectious diseases. 6th edition. Philadelphia: Elsevier Churchill Livingston; 2005, p. 791; with permission.)

Table 1
Names of cervical spaces and their synonyms

Space	Synonyms
Superficial space	Space 1 of Grodinsky and Holyoke (G&H)
Retropharyngeal space	Posterior visceral, retrovisceral, retroesophageal, posterior part of space 3 of G&H, retropharyngeal part of visceral compartment
Danger space	Space 4 of G&H
Prevertebral space	Space 5 of G&H
Submandibular space	
Sublingual	Floor of the mouth
Submylohyoid	Submaxillary (includes submental), submandibular
Lateral pharyngeal space	Parapharyngeal, peripharyngeal, pharyngomaxillary, pterygopharyngeal
Masticator spaces	Masticatory, masseter-mandibulopterygoid
Masseteric	Temporal pouches
Pterygoid	
Temporal	
Parotid	
Peritonsillar	
Anterior visceral space	Pretracheal

Data from Blomquist IK, Bayer AS. Life-threatening deep fascial space infections of the head and neck. Infect Dis Clin North Am 1988;2:238.

The anatomic location, clinical manifestation, potential complications, and therapy of these three potential space infections are discussed in this article. Vascular and parameningeal infections are discussed elsewhere in this issue. The reader is referred to the article discussing the microbial flora of the oropharynx, because it is of particular relevance to understanding effective antimicrobial therapy in severe head and neck infections.

CT and MRI scans of the head and neck are most valuable in these clinical circumstances. They allow proper disease delineation in cases with associated trismus that may limit the physical examination. Appropriate imaging also allows identification of spread between spaces that may not be clinically apparent. Clinical examination alone may underestimate the extent of disease in 70% of cases [2]. Also, appropriate imaging facilitates early recognition of complications and can expedite relevant therapeutic interventions. Finally, CT and MRI can help identify the original nidus of infection if it is not already apparent by history and physical examination [3–5]. A significant caveat is that pus may not be identified during surgical exploration of up to 25% of cases following CT scans suggestive of deep space infections [6].

Infections of the submandibular space

The most infamous of submandibular space infections is Ludwig's angina (Fig. 2). This clinical entity has been known by various names, such as "angina maligna," "morbus strangulatorius," and "garotillo," all of which refer to its historically highly lethal nature. One can only imagine the horror of slow

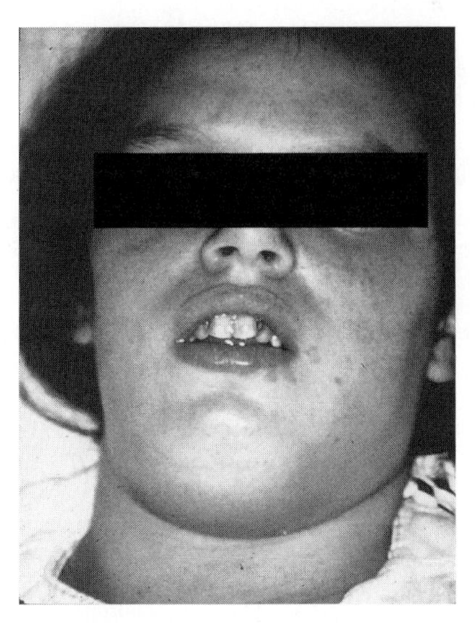

Fig. 2. Early appearance of patient who has Ludwig's angina with characteristic submandibular "woody" swelling. (*From* Megran DW, Scheifele DW, Chow AW. Odontogenic infections. Pediatr Infect Dis 1984;3:262; with permission.)

asphyxiation associated with many submandibular infections in the preantibiotic era. A series comparing mortality rates in cases of Ludwig's angina in 1940 and 1943 demonstrated a drop from 54% to 10% [7]. Mortalities now are considered very rare in Ludwig's angina because of the ubiquity of effective antibiotics and multiple supportive airway modalities [8]. The availability of effective treatment options makes this entity no less a medical emergency, however, because timely interventions are critical to patient survival.

Anatomy and pathogenesis

The submandibular potential space extends from the floor of the mouth rostrally to fascial and muscular attachments at the hyoid bone. It is bounded anteriorly and laterally by the mandible and inferiorly by the superficial layer of the deep cervical fascia (Fig. 3). The submandibular space is separated into the sublingual and submylohyoid spaces by the mylohyoid muscle. The mylohyoid muscle extends from its attachments on the mandible and forms a sling around which the submandibular and sublingual spaces can communicate freely around its posterior border. Although these spaces may be infected in isolation, their proximity and easy communication means that infections rapidly involve the whole submandibular space, and it is useful to consider them as a single unit.

Infections in the submandibular spaces typically are odontogenic in nature, although other reported etiologies include lacerations of the mouth floor, mandibular fractures, foreign bodies [9], mandibular or lingual malignancies [10], sialadenitis [11], lymphadenitis [12], and inferior alveolar nerve

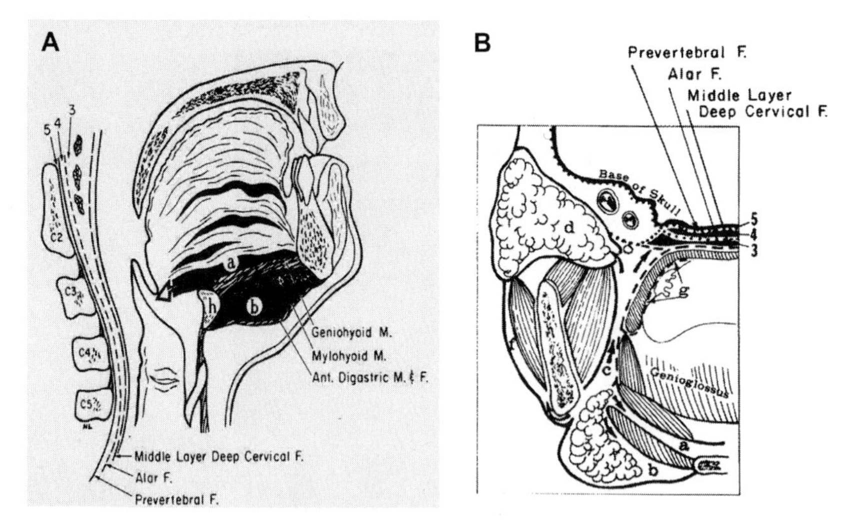

Fig. 3. Anatomic relationships in submandibular infections. (*A*) Sagittal and (*B*) oblique sections. a, sublingual space; b, submylohyoid space; c, lateral pharyngeal space; d, parotid gland; f, fascia; g, peritonsillar space; h, hyoid bone; m, muscle; 3, retropharyngeal space; 4, danger space; 5, prevertebral space. (*From* Blomquist IK, Bayer AS. Life-threatening deep fascial space infections of the head and neck. Infect Dis Clin North Am 1988;2:242; with permission.)

blocks [13]. Odontogenic infections in the submandibular space arise from the spread of periapical abscesses of the mandibular molars, most typically from the second or third molar teeth. Extensions of periapical abscesses penetrate where the bone is thinnest, that is, the lingual aspect in the case of the mandibular molars. The bone is thinnest on the buccal aspect of the premolar teeth, and periapical infections in these teeth tend to extend outwards (Fig. 4) [14].

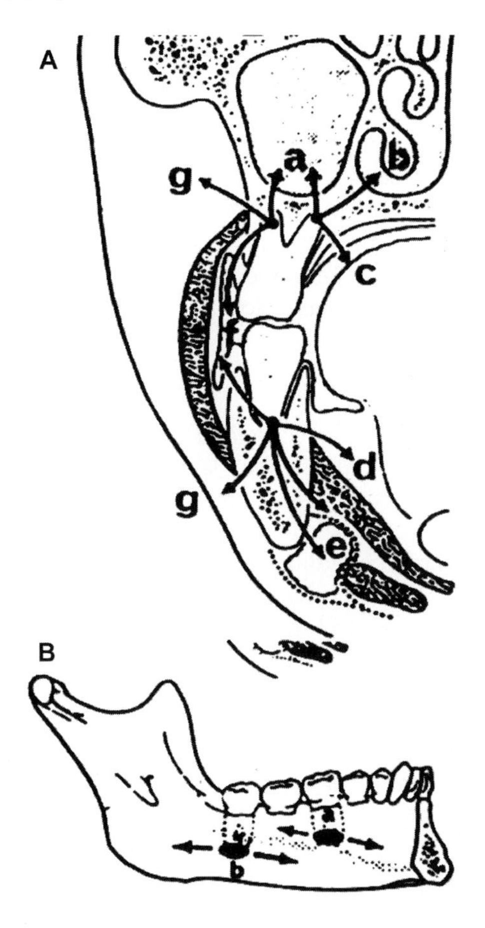

Fig. 4. Routes of spread of odontogenic orofacial infections along planes of least resistance. (*A*) Coronal section in the region of the first molar teeth. a, maxillary antrum; b, nasal cavity; c, palatal plate; d, sublingual space (above the mylohyoid muscle); e, submandibular space (below the mylohyoid muscle); f, intraoral presentation with infection spreading through the buccal plates inside the attachment of the buccinator muscle; g, extraoral presentation to buccal space with infection spreading through the buccal plates outside the attachment of the buccinator muscle. (*B*) Lingual aspect of the mandible. a, apices of the involved tooth above the mylohyoid muscle, with spread of infection to the sublingual space; b, apices of involved tooth below the mylohyoid muscle, with spread of infection into the submandibular space. (*From* Chow AW, Roser SM, Brady FA. Orofacial odontogenic infections. Ann Intern Med 1978;88:396; with permission.)

The mylohyoid muscle attaches to the mandible at an angle, leaving the first molar below its attachment and the second and third molars above its attachment. The important clinical consequence is that periapical abscesses involving the first molar initially infect the sublingual space, whereas infections originating from the second and third molars infect the submylohyoid space. As noted previously, these infections of the submandibular space can spread quickly to involve the entire submandibular space, thereby making source identification impossible based on the location of infection alone.

Another important communication between potential spaces exists at the buccopharyngeal gap, which connects the submandibular and lateral pharyngeal spaces. This connection is created by the penetration of the styloglossus muscle from its origin at the tongue, extending between the middle and superior constrictor muscles to its attachment at the styloid process. The buccopharyngeal gap allows spread of infection from the submandibular space to the lateral pharyngeal space and thence to the retropharyngeal space. This spread can yield multiple clinical manifestations and complications, depending on the infected space and its extensions.

Clinical manifestations

The predominant presenting complaint is usually mouth pain, stiff neck, drooling, and dysphagia. Patients may speak in a muffled voice if they are able to speak at all. Systemic signs of infection are present with fever, chills, and malaise.

In infections of the submandibular space, there is a characteristic lack of trismus (Table 2) [15]. Trismus develops from an irritation of the masticatory muscles, the masseter and the internal pterygoid muscles, which insert into the mandibular ramus. The submandibular space is not contiguous with these muscles, and trismus indicates a spread into the lateral pharyngeal space along the styloglossus muscle. This clinical finding has important ramifications for the location and extent of surgical débridement, if required.

Ludwig's original clinical descriptions of five patients who had a "gangrenous induration of the connective tissues that cover the small muscles between the larynx and the floor of the mouth" holds true today. Patients experience a rapidly spreading "woody" inflammation of the submandibular area that can lead to insidious or rapidly progressive asphyxiation if left untreated. There is characteristically no lymph node involvement. The firmness of the tissue is described appropriately as "woody," because it is very firm with an absence of the normal tissue compliance to palpation. There are no signs of superficial skin involvement. Once felt, this characteristic firmness is not soon forgotten by the careful clinician.

The most obvious finding on physical examination is the patient's protruding tongue, which is caused by the limitation on external swelling imposed by the strong fibers of the deep cervical fascia. Therefore, the easily distendable tissues of the mouth are forced posteriorly, superiorly, and

Table 2
Comparative clinical features of deep neck infections

Space	Pain	Trismus	Swellng	Dysphagia	Dyspnea
Submandibular	Present	Minimal	Mouth floor (tender), submylohyoid	Present if bilateral involvement	Present if bilateral involvement
Lateral pharyngeal					
Anterior	Severe	Prominent	Anterior lateral pharynx, angle of jaw	Present	Occasional
Posterior	Minimal	Minimal	Posterior lateral pharynx (hidden)	Present	Severe
Retropharyngeal (and danger)	Present	Minimal	Posterior pharynx	Present	Present
Masticator					
Masseteric and pterygoid	Present	Prominent	May not be seen	Absent	Absent
Temporal	Present	None	Face, orbit	Absent	Absent
Buccal	Minimal	Minimal	Cheek	Absent	Absent
Parotid	Severe	None	Angle of jaw	Absent	Absent

Data from Megran DW, Scheifele DW, Chow AW. Odontogenic infections. Pediatr Infect Dis 1984;3:261.

anteriorly to accommodate. The tongue is displaced, and the whole floor of the oropharynx is elevated, erythematous, and tender to palpation. Occasionally the inflammation spreads to involve the epiglottis.

Potential complications

Infections of the submandibular space can be rapidly life threatening because of airway compromise. Warning signs include any element of increased work of breathing, such as marked tachypnea with shallow respirations, use of accessory muscles, orthopnea, dyspnea, stridor, and the patient's adoption of a "sniffing position" to maximize airway patency. These findings mark a critical stage in disease progression and indicate a need to secure an appropriate artificial airway rapidly. Not all patients require intubation, but if an initial course of careful observation is decided on, it should be performed within an ICU to allow frequent airway evaluations. It also is prudent to have an emergency tracheostomy kit at the bedside and physicians who are familiar with its use readily available.

Although a detailed discussion regarding the best method of intubation of these patients is beyond the scope of this article, a few key points require emphasis [16]. As with any issue of airway control, institution of an artificial airway ideally should be made before an emergency develops and as promptly as possible when the decision to secure the airway is made. Blind endotracheal intubation is possible but is made difficult by altered airway anatomy, potential epiglottal involvement, and friability of oropharyngeal tissue and should be attempted only when other methods cannot be used. Use of paralytics may precipitate an occlusion of the airway because of loss of tone of the maximally strained pharyngeal musculature. This loss of tone can contribute to the development of the catastrophic clinical circumstance of "can't intubate, can't ventilate." Therefore, awake intubation techniques that use direct visualization, classically fiberoptic bronchoscopy modalities, usually are the most prudent approach. Consideration also needs to be given to awake tracheostomy, depending on the clinical circumstance and availability of the relevant specialty personnel. Early involvement of the anesthesia service and the critical care team is vital to ensure a positive outcome in these patients.

Other potential complications include the spread of infection beyond the submandibular space into the lateral pharyngeal space and beyond (see Fig. 1). The manifestations and complication of those infections are discussed later.

Therapeutic considerations

Antibiotic therapy in immunocompetent individuals should be directed at the typical organisms of the mouth. Infections are predominantly mixed, with an average of five pathogens identified if careful collection and culture techniques are undertaken [17]. Furthermore, the mixed nature of these infections suggests a synergistic interaction resulting in increased pathogenicity of the organisms involved [18]. Careful specimen collection and culture techniques have shown that up to two thirds of such infections involve anaerobes [19,20]. Typical recommendations for head and neck infections include penicillin G and metronidazole, although patients who are immunocompromised or recently hospitalized warrant broader antibiotic coverage to include facultative gram-negative rods and *Staphylococcus aureus* [21,22]. In particular, the Asian literature has reported an increased incidence of infections caused by *Klebsiella pneumoniae* in patients who have diabetes mellitus [20,23,24]. A recent report from New Jersey did not find any risk factors associated with the isolation of gram-negative organisms [25].

Aerobic and anaerobic beta-lactamase–producing organisms are cultured regularly from head and neck abscesses [17,26,27]. Because of the life-threatening nature of these infections, it is reasonable to initiate therapy with broader coverage until culture and sensitivity data indicate that narrower therapy is adequate [28]. Therefore, an initial regimen that is effective against beta-lactamase–producing aerobic or anaerobic gram-positive cocci and gram-negative bacilli is appropriate. Although noted only in case reports, there is the potential concern of mixed infections involving methicillin-resistant *S aureus* [25,29] and penicillin-resistant pneumococcus [30]. Community-acquired methicillin-resistant *S aureus* is being recognized increasingly as a nasal colonizer in individuals who have few or no risk factors [31,32]. Because the microbiology of retropharyngeal, lateral pharyngeal, submandibular, and danger space infections primarily reflects that of the oropharynx, and because 27% of normal individuals may be colonized nasally by methicillin-sensitive or -resistant *S aureus,* it is conceivable that these organisms also can play a role in mixed infections [33]. Although only rarely isolated, *Candida* and *Aspergillus* species have been reported consistently as compromising a small percentage of head and neck infections and should be considered if the patient has risk factors or if there is no clinical response to broad-spectrum antimicrobial agents [17,25,34].

Prudent antimicrobial choices in life-threatening infections include penicillin-derivative/beta-lactamase inhibitor combinations (ampicillin/sulbactam, ticarcillin/clavulanic acid, or piperacillin/tazobactam), carbepenems (imipenem, meropenem, ertapenem), clindamycin with initial gram-negative coverage for possible Klebsiella (some centers also add penicillin to this combination), cephalomycins (cefoxitin or cefotetan), or third- or fourth-generation cephalosporins with metronidazole. Vancomycin may be added for patients who are thought to be at particular risk for carriage of methicillin-resistant *S aureus*, who are at high risk for rapid deterioration, or who have evidence of overwhelming sepsis.

Purulent collections can be difficult to detect and tend to develop late in the clinical course, after approximately 24 to 36 hours. If collections of pus are identified, they can be drained under radiographic guidance. Patients who do not respond to initial antibiotic therapy may require surgical exploration and drainage, preferably with a cuffed tracheostomy in situ. Appropriate dental management of apical abscesses by tooth extraction is important to allow decompression of the nidus of infection.

Infections of the lateral pharyngeal space

The lateral pharyngeal space serves as an anatomic hub for deep space infections of the head and neck (see Fig. 1). Its communication with all of the major fascial planes facilitates spread of infections between these spaces. Initial clinical manifestations may be quite subtle, but missed infections can spread into other life-threatening potential spaces leading to devastating complications.

Anatomy and pathogenesis

The lateral pharyngeal space is a 2.5-cm-long inverted cone extending from the hyoid to the sphenoid bone (Fig. 5). It is bordered laterally by the parotid gland, mandible, and the attached internal pterygoid muscle. The lateral border is covered entirely by a superficial layer of deep cervical fascia except for the upper inner aspect of the parotid gland. This gap in fascial coverage allows infections from the parotid gland to penetrate rapidly into the lateral pharyngeal space, or vice versa. The medial aspect is

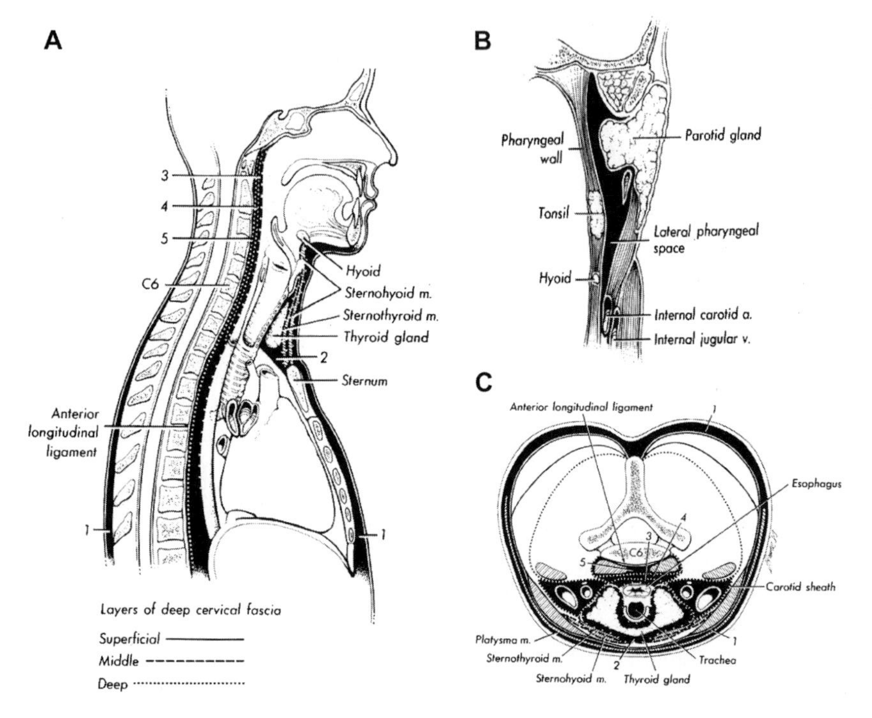

Fig. 5. Lateral pharyngeal, retropharyngeal, danger, and prevertebral spaces and their elationship with each other. (*A*) Midsagittal section of the head and neck. (*B*) Coronal section in the suprahyoid region of the neck. (*C*) Cross-section of the neck at the level of the thyroid isthmus. A, artery; m, muscle; v, vein; 1, superficial space; 2, pretracheal space; 3, retropharyngeal space; 4, danger space; 5, prevertebral space. (*From* Chow AW. Life-threatening infections of the head and neck. Clin Infect Dis 1992;14:992; with permission.)

composed of the buccopharyngeal fascia covering the lateral surface of the superior constrictor muscle. Infection may spread from the peritonsillar space through the superior constrictor and the buccopharyngeal fascia into the lateral pharyngeal space. A blind cul-de-sac is formed inferiorly at the angle of the jaw; palpable swelling in this region may be a subtle sign of lateral pharyngeal space infections. The pterygomandibular raphe, which is formed by the junction of the buccinator and the superior constrictor muscles, comprises the anterior border. The posterior aspect is delimited by the prevertebral fascia and communicates with the retropharyngeal space, allowing rapid spread of infection between these spaces.

The styloid process penetrates into the lateral pharyngeal space and separates the spaces into two communicating compartments, the anterior or muscular compartment and the posterior or neurovascular compartment. As indicated by its name, the anterior compartment contains no vital structures and is connected closely to the tonsillar fossa and the internal pterygoid muscle. On the other hand, the posterior compartment contains such key structures as the carotid sheath, the ninth to twelfth cranial nerves, and the cervical sympathetic trunk. Complications from infections in the posterior compartment can be deduced easily from the vital structures that it contains, as discussed later.

Infections involving the lateral pharyngeal space can develop from various sources throughout the neck including the pharynx, teeth, tonsils, adenoids, parotid gland, submandibular space, retropharyngeal space, masticator space, and local lymph nodes [12,35]. Peritonsillar abscesses are a particularly common cause of infections of the lateral pharyngeal space.

Clinical manifestations

The clinical manifestations of infections of the lateral pharyngeal spaces can be quite subtle and depend on whether the anterior and/or posterior compartments are involved. Infections of either compartment are associated with systemic toxicity, fevers, chills, and potentially rigors. The classic clinical signs of infection in the anterior compartment are dysphagia, trismus, and pain involving the ipsilateral side of the neck and jaw, with potential referral to the ipsilateral ear. Side flexion of the neck to the contralateral side intensifies pain by physical compression of the lateral pharyngeal space and flexion of the sternocleidomastoid muscles. Trismus develops because of the close proximity of the internal pterygoid muscle with the lateral pharyngeal space and its subsequently associated inflammation.

On physical examination, swelling and induration may be appreciated at the angle of the ipsilateral jaw caused by swelling of the blind cul-de-sac of the lateral pharyngeal space. If an adequate pharyngeal examination is possible, the lateral pharyngeal wall often is found to be distorted medially with normal overlying mucosa. There may be other physical findings associated with the portal of infection of the lateral pharyngeal space.

Often the infections causing a portal of entry into the lateral pharyngeal space do not cause prominent symptoms. An antecedent pharyngitis or tonsillitis may already have resolved by the time symptoms of lateral space infection develop. Occasionally, a patient's only antecedent complaint is of a nonspecific upper respiratory tract infection or general malaise several weeks before the patient presents with a lateral pharyngeal space infection [36].

Isolated infections of the posterior compartment lack the intense trismus associated with anterior compartment infections (see Table 2). Some patients have no specific localizing signs and may present with sepsis of occult origin. In these cases, the diagnosis may become apparent only on imaging or after the development of neurologic or vascular complications. Edema may involve the epiglottis and larynx, yielding marked dyspnea. An oropharyngeal examination may miss swelling of the pharyngeal wall because the swelling can be hidden behind the palatopharyngeal arch. The parotid gland is adjacent to the posterior compartment of the lateral pharyngeal space, and swelling of the parotid space occurs occasionally.

Potential complications

Complications arising from infections of the lateral pharyngeal space are caused predominantly by involvement of the posterior compartment space and the vital structures contained within it. Such complications include laryngeal edema and obstruction and sudden death syndromes attributed to involvement of the vagal nerve. Ipsilateral Horner's syndrome or cranial nerve nine to twelve palsies may occur and suggest carotid sheath involvement [35,37–39]. In addition, infections of the lateral pharyngeal space can lead to infection of many of the other spaces of the head and neck; therefore a high index of suspicion for their involvement must be maintained (see Fig. 1).

Suppurative jugular thrombophlebitis (Lemierre syndrome), described in detail elsewhere in the review of vascular infections of the head and neck, is the most common vascular complication of lateral pharyngeal space infections. This syndrome is characterized by an anaerobic septic thrombus occluding the internal jugular vein, often with bacteremia and metastatic foci of infection. The prototypical infecting organism is *Fusobacterium necrophorum*, and bacteremias with this organism must raise the possibility of this clinical syndrome [40,41]. Other causative organisms include anaerobic streptococci and *Prevotella* and *Bacteroides* species [42,43]. Lemierre syndrome can be difficult to detect clinically, but an indurated swelling may be appreciated behind the sternocleidomastoid muscle. Carotid artery erosion and rupture also can occur, with devastating consequences, characteristically preceded by small "herald bleeds" [44].

Therapeutic considerations

Infections of the lateral pharyngeal space have a tendency to be suppurative. If pus is present, timely surgical intervention with adequate drainage can prevent spread into other compartments of the head and neck. Antibiotic therapy follows the same general principles elaborated previously. Some limited data suggest that infections localized to the posterior lateral pharyngeal space with no clinical evidence of sepsis or airway compromise may respond to intravenous antibiotics without surgery [45–48]. In this regard, Sichel and colleagues [49] suggested that because infections of the posterior lateral pharyngeal space often arise from the lymph nodes and are contained within fibrous tissue, infections rarely spread into other spaces, and such infections may respond well to intravenous antibiotics without surgery. Conversely, because infections of the anterior lateral pharyngeal space are usually polymicrobial and odontogenic in origin, they tend to liquefy the fat in the anterior space rapidly, forming potentially large amounts of pus. Because there are no limiting boundaries, these infections are characterized by rapid spread with multiple complications and therefore are best addressed by surgical drainage plus antibiotic therapy. These two forms of lateral pharyngeal infection can be differentiated by contrast CT scans.

Suppurative jugular thrombophlebitis usually responds to antibiotic therapy, although a prolonged course of 4 to 6 weeks should be administered. Fevers may be prolonged. Surgical ligation of the internal jugular vein is needed only rarely, in cases that do not respond to adequate antibiotics. Impending carotid artery rupture requires immediate surgical intervention, which can be life saving, although at this stage the morbidity and mortality rates are exceedingly high [35,37].

Infections of the retropharyngeal, prevertebral, and danger space

The retropharyngeal, prevertebral, and danger spaces are the common pathway for caudal extension of infections from the head and neck (see Fig. 5). Although separated by fascial planes, these spaces are considered together because of their anatomic proximity and their propensity for extension of infections beyond the head and neck. Infections in the prevertebral space are primarily hematogenous in nature, and their microbiology and pathogenesis are very different from those of the other infections of the head and neck discussed in this article.

Anatomy and pathogenesis

The retropharyngeal, prevertebral, and danger spaces are situated between the posterior aspect of the pharynx-esophagus and the anterior portion of the spine. To understand the clinical relatedness of these spaces and their manifestations and complications, it is critical to appreciate the structure of the fascial planes that delineate them (see Fig. 5). The deep layer of the deep cervical fascia originates at the spinous processes and extends anteriorly, encompassing the splenius, erector spinae, and the semispinalis muscles. As this fascia continues to pass anteriorly, it fuses with the transverse processes and splits into the alar fascia anteriorly and the prevertebral fascia posteriorly. These fascial layers extend in a circle anteriorly, fuse to the contralateral transverse process, and subsequently merge en route to complete its circular route.

The existence of these two facial layers anteriorly gives rise to three separate spaces. The retropharyngeal space is the most anterior and extends from the constrictor muscles and their fascia anteriorly to the alar fascia posteriorly. The retropharyngeal space extends downwards from the base of the skull to approximately the C7/T1 region. Because of the direct extension of the fascial planes of the retropharyngeal space, mediastinal spread can occur, resulting in involvement of the superior anterior and superior posterior mediastinum. The middle layer of the deep cervical fascia also projects anteriorly, where it is called the "pretracheal" or "anterior visceral fascia," and there it fuses with the parietal pericardium and adventitia of the great vessels. Therefore, infections of the retropharyngeal space can track around the visceral space composed of the esophagus and trachea and extend into the superior anterior mediastinum. As with posterior extension of infections from the retropharyngeal space, this extension can cause purulent pleural and pericardial infections.

Two chains of lymph nodes (the deep cervical chain) extend along the retropharyngeal space on either side of the midline (Fig. 6) [50]. Suppurative adenitis of these lymph nodes may lead to the development of an infection in the retropharyngeal space. These lymph nodes tend to regress by age 4 years, thereby explaining the relatively greater frequency of retropharyngeal abscesses in young children. Other causes of retropharyngeal abscesses include trauma from esophageal instrumentation (endoscopy, nasogastric tubes, frequent suctioning, intubation attempts), foreign bodies, traumatic esophageal rupture, and spread from contiguous spaces [51].

The danger space is located posterior to the alar fascia and is bounded by the prevertebral fascia posteriorly. The danger space also is delineated superiorly by the base of the skull, but it extends inferiorly through the posterior

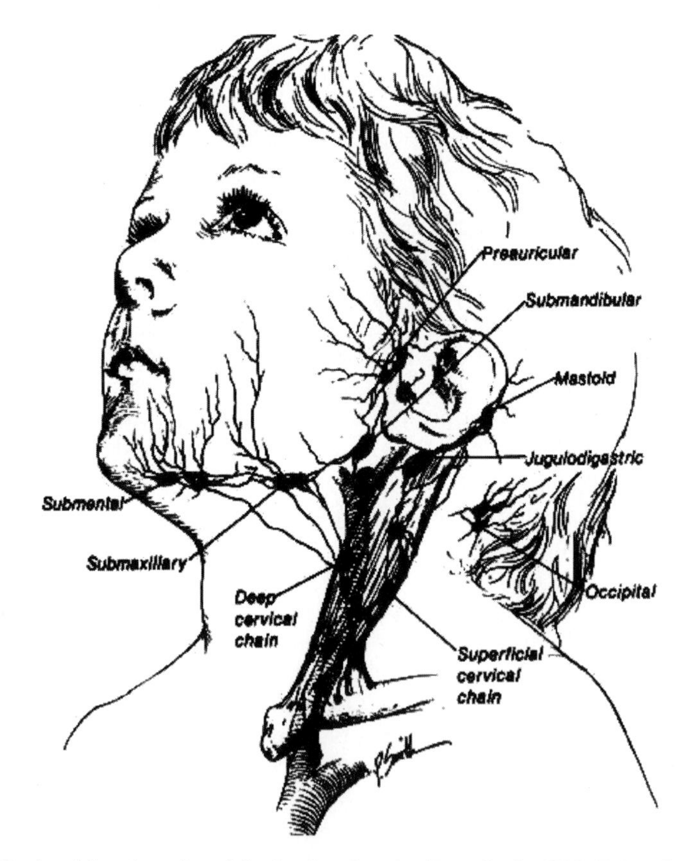

Fig. 6. Regional lymph nodes of the head and neck. (*From* Butler KM, Baker CJ. Cervical lymphadenitis. In: Fegin RD, Cheery JD, editors. Textbook of pediatric infectious diseases. 3rd edition. Philadelphia: Elsevier W.B. Saunders; 1992. p. 221; with permission.)

mediastinum to the diaphragm. Infections in the danger space develop following contiguous spread from adjacent spaces.

The prevertebral space comprises the area posterior to the prevertebral fascia to the vertebral bodies. It extends from the base of the skull down to the coccyx and is contiguous with the psoas muscle sheath, explaining the predilection for psoas muscle abscesses with prevertebral space infections. Infections of the prevertebral space usually develop from cervical spine infections that have been seeded hematogenously, by local instrumentation of the trachea or esophagus, or by contiguous spread from vertebral osteomyelitis/discitis [52]. Intravenous drug use, immunosuppression, alcoholism, and diabetes are known risk factors [53,54]. Therefore, the bacteriology of these infections is very different from that of the head and neck infections discussed previously, with a predominance of gram-positive organisms, the most common being *S aureus*. In contrast to the other infections of the head and neck, anaerobic microbes play a very minor role in infections of the prevertebral space. Less common organisms implicated in prevertebral space infections include Brucella [55] and various other gram-negative rods, Mycobacterium [56], Nocardia, fungi, and, rarely, parasites [57].

Clinical manifestations

Clinical manifestations of retropharyngeal space infections and abscesses can vary from mild retropharyngeal pain and malaise to severe respiratory distress and systemic toxicity. Patients often complain of a sore throat with dysphagia, dyspnea, and a stiff neck. Noisy breathing may be observed, and respiratory distress can develop because of the anterior displacement of the pharyngeal wall and the supraglottic structures. Patients may hold their heads rigidly tilted toward the contralateral side. Pleuritic chest pain is an ominous sign indicating extension into the mediastinum. A pharyngeal mass may be seen or palpated. On examination, bulging of the posterior oropharynx may be appreciated, although palpation of the lesion may precipitate abscess rupture with aspiration or asphyxiation.

Manifestations of infection of the prevertebral space vary depending on the degree of spinal cord compression and subsequent neurologic manifestations of descending spinal cord dysfunction. Approximately 75% of patients complain of back or neck pain, 50% present with fever, and one third have neurologic deficits ranging from nerve root pain to paralysis [57]. Bacteremia detected at the time of presentation with an epidural abscess occurs in only 60% of cases [58]. The initial diagnosis of prevertebral abscesses can be quite challenging, with approximately half of all cases being misdiagnosed initially [59].

Potential complications

Severe laryngeal inflammation may precipitate airway occlusion. Rupture of a retropharyngeal abscess into the posterior oropharynx may cause an aspiration of purulent necrotic material with asphyxia or the development of a potentially severe pneumonia.

The most lethal complication of retropharyngeal and danger space infections is descending necrotizing mediastinitis. Infections of the danger space can extend easily throughout the posterior mediastinum and may involve the retroperitoneum with widespread necrosis. Occasionally, the purulent material from the posterior mediastinum ruptures into the pleural cavity, causing a pyothorax and secondary pleural effusions [60]. Another feared consequence of mediastinal invasion is pericardial involvement with the development of a pericardial effusion and potentially tamponade. Aspiration pneumonia complicates up to 50% of cases of mediastinitis, probably because of impairment of swallowing. As such, it is imperative that oral intake in the recovering patient be delayed until a swallow assessment can be performed. Débridement and appropriate antibiotics are the foundations of treatment for mediastinitis. Even with effective therapy, mortality may be as high as 25% [61].

As noted previously, infections of the prevertebral space act in a very different manner from infections of the retropharyngeal and danger spaces. Complications commonly arise from spinal epidural collections causing potentially catastrophic cord compression. Irreversible paralysis occurs in 4% to 22% of patients [54,57]. Also, seemingly distant sites of loculation may develop in the psoas muscle sheath because of the open communication of the prevertebral space down to the psoas muscle [62]. Spread of infections to or from the vertebrae or disc may cause local destruction with mechanical instability of the spine.

Therapeutic considerations

Much of the discussion of the treatment of infections of the lateral pharyngeal and submandibular spaces also applies to infections of the retropharyngeal and danger spaces. Adequate anaerobic and oral gram-positive coverage is required and is the mainstay of therapy. Mediastinal extension requires surgical débridement of necrotizing infections and drainage of purulent material in the pleura and pericardium. If antibiotics are initiated before the development of purulent collections, surgical or drainage usually is not required, and the infections often respond to medical management alone [63–65]. There has been reported success with minimally invasive drainage and washout procedures [66].

Surgical drainage is the cornerstone of management for prevertebral space infections to control the source of infection and avoid progression of neurological deficits. There are limited reports of conservative therapy with antibiotics alone for prevertebral abscesses. The use of antibiotics alone is not ideal therapy and should be undertaken only if other factors or patient decisions limit the combined surgical and medical approach. A significant number of patients deteriorate eventually, require surgery, and may suffer greater morbidity and mortality than those receiving early surgical treatment [58]. There is still some controversy about this issue, because older reports have advocated conservative management for patients who are stable, have rapid access to MRI, and have minimal neurologic deficit [67].

Infections of the prevertebral space have a significantly different microbiology and require broad coverage until an organism is identified. Specifically, initial coverage for gram-positive organisms including methicillin-resistant *S aureus* is required. In addition, empiric coverage with an antibiotic effective against gram-negative rods, such as a third- or fourth-generation cephalosporin, ureidopenicillin/beta-lactamase inhibitor or a carbepenem, also should be considered, particularly if risk factors, such as a history of intravenous drug use or urinary tract infection, are present [54]. These recommendations must be mitigated by the local microbiological ecology, antimicrobial resistance patterns, and host factors identified. For a detailed discussion of spinal epidural abscesses, the reader is referred to the excellent recent review by Darouiche [54] and an exhaustive meta-analysis and literature review by Reihsaus and colleagues [57].

Summary

Life-threatening infections of the head and neck can be challenging in their diagnosis and management. A high index of suspicion is required, because many physicians are not familiar with these relatively uncommon infections. Because of the anatomic communication between these spaces, vigilance must be maintained for complications and extension beyond the original site of infection. With early diagnosis, adequate therapy, and appropriate airway support, morbidity and mortality from infections of the submandibular, lateral pharyngeal, retropharyngeal, danger, and prevertebral spaces can be minimized.

References

[1] Hughes CE, Spear RK, Shinabarger CE, et al. Septic pulmonary emboli complicating mastoiditis: Lemierre's syndrome revisited. Clin Infect Dis 1994;18:633–5.

[2] Crespo AN, Chone CT, Fonseca AS, et al. Clinical versus computed tomography evaluation in the diagnosis and management of deep neck infection. Sao Paulo Med J 2004;122:259–63.

[3] El-Sayed Y, Al Dousary S. Deep-neck space abscesses. J Otolaryngol 1996;25:227–33.

[4] Holt GR, McManus K, Newman RK, et al. Computed tomography in the diagnosis of deep-neck infections. Arch Otolaryngol 1982;108:693–6.

[5] Lazor JB, Cunningham MJ, Eavey RD, et al. Comparison of computed tomography and surgical findings in deep neck infections. Otolaryngol Head Neck Surg 1994;111:746–50.

[6] Smith JL 2nd, Hsu JM, Chang J. Predicting deep neck space abscess using computed tomography. Am J Otolaryngol 2006;27:244–7.

[7] Williams AC, Guralnick WC. The diagnosis and treatment of Ludwig's angina: a report of twenty cases. N Engl J Med 1943;228:443–50.

[8] Patterson HC, Kelly JH, Strome M. Ludwig's angina: an update. Laryngoscope 1982;92: 370–8.

[9] Meyers BR, Lawson W, Hirschman SZ. Ludwig's angina. Case report, with review of bacteriology and current therapy. Am J Med 1972;53:257–60.
[10] Fischmann GE, Graham BS. Ludwig's angina resulting from the infection of an oral malignancy. J Oral Maxillofac Surg 1985;43:795–6.
[11] Tsuji T, Shimono M, Yamane G, et al. Ludwig's angina as a complication of ameloblastoma of the mandible. J Oral Maxillofac Surg 1984;42:815–9.
[12] Levitt GW. Cervical fascia and deep neck infections. Laryngoscope 1970;80:409–35.
[13] Rothwell BR. Odontogenic infections. Emerg Med Clin North Am 1985;3:161–78.
[14] Chow AW, Roser SM, Brady FA. Orofacial odontogenic infections. Ann Intern Med 1978; 88:392–402.
[15] Megran DW, Scheifele DW, Chow AW. Odontogenic infections. Pediatr Infect Dis 1984;3: 257–65.
[16] Ovassapian A, Tuncbilek M, Weitzel EK, et al. Airway management in adult patients with deep neck infections: a case series and review of the literature. Anesth Analg 2005;100: 585–9.
[17] Brook I. Microbiology and management of peritonsillar, retropharyngeal, and parapharyngeal abscesses. J Oral Maxillofac Surg 2004;62:1545–50.
[18] Brook I, Hunter V, Walker RI. Synergistic effect of bacteroides, clostridium, fusobacterium, anaerobic cocci, and aerobic bacteria on mortality and induction of subcutaneous abscesses in mice. J Infect Dis 1984;149:924–8.
[19] Har-El G, Aroesty JH, Shaha A, et al. Changing trends in deep neck abscess. A retrospective study of 110 patients. Oral Surg Oral Med Oral Pathol 1994;77:446–50.
[20] Huang TT, Tseng FY, Yeh TH, et al. Factors affecting the bacteriology of deep neck infection: a retrospective study of 128 patients. Acta Otolaryngol 2006;126:396–401.
[21] Chow AW. Infections of the oral cavity, head and neck. In: Mandell GL, Bennett JE, Dolin R, editors. Principles and practice of infectious diseases. 6th edition. Philadelphia: Elsevier Churchill Livingstone; 2005. p. 787–802.
[22] Chow AW. Life-threatening infections of the head and neck. Clin Infect Dis 1992;14: 991–1002.
[23] Wang LF, Kuo WR, Tsai SM, et al. Characterizations of life-threatening deep cervical space infections: a review of one hundred ninety-six cases. Am J Otolaryngol 2003;24:111–7.
[24] Lin HT, Tsai CS, Chen YL, et al. Influence of diabetes mellitus on deep neck infection. J Laryngol Otol 2006;120:650–4.
[25] Rega AJ, Aziz SR, Ziccardi VB. Microbiology and antibiotic sensitivities of head and neck space infections of odontogenic origin. J Oral Maxillofac Surg 2006;64:1377–80.
[26] Coulthard M, Isaacs D. Retropharyngeal abscess. Arch Dis Child 1991;66:1227–30.
[27] Brook I. Beta-lactamase-producing bacteria in mixed infections. Clin Microbiol Infect 2004; 10:777–84.
[28] Kumar A, Roberts D, Wood KE, et al. Duration of hypotension before initiation of effective antimicrobial therapy is the critical determinant of survival in human septic shock. Crit Care Med 2006;34:1589–96.
[29] Sato K, Izumi T, Toshima M, et al. Retropharyngeal abscess due to methicillin-resistant Staphylococcus aureus in a case of acute myeloid leukemia. Intern Med 2005;44: 346–9.
[30] Kobayashi KI, Haruta T, Kubota M, et al. A case of retropharyngeal abscess caused by penicillin-resistant Streptococcus pneumoniae. J Infect 2002;44:267–9.
[31] Frazee BW, Lynn J, Charlebois ED, et al. High prevalence of methicillin-resistant Staphylococcus aureus in emergency department skin and soft tissue infections. Ann Emerg Med 2005;45:311–20.
[32] Zetola N, Francis JS, Nuermberger EL, et al. Community-acquired meticillin-resistant Staphylococcus aureus: an emerging threat. Lancet Infect Dis 2005;5:275–86.
[33] Wertheim HF, Melles DC, Vos MC, et al. The role of nasal carriage in Staphylococcus aureus infections. Lancet Infect Dis 2005;5:751–62.

[34] Kuriyama T, Karasawa T, Nakagawa K, et al. Antimicrobial susceptibility of major pathogens of orofacial odontogenic infections to 11 beta-lactam antibiotics. Oral Microbiol Immunol 2002;17:285–9.

[35] Blomquist IK, Bayer AS. Life-threatening deep fascial space infections of the head and neck. Infect Dis Clin North Am 1988;2:237–64.

[36] Scully RE, Galdabini JJ, McNeely BU. Case records of the Massachusetts General Hospital. Weekly clinicopathological exercises. Case 33-1975. N Engl J Med 1975;293:394–9.

[37] Blum DJ, McCaffrey TV. Septic necrosis of the internal carotid artery: a complication of peritonsillar abscess. Otolaryngol Head Neck Surg 1983;91:114–8.

[38] Wills PI, Vernon RP Jr. Complications of space infections of the head and neck. Laryngoscope 1981;91:1129–36.

[39] Ramsey PG, Weymuller EA. Complications of bacterial infection of the ears, paranasal sinuses, and oropharynx in adults. Emerg Med Clin North Am 1985;3:143–60.

[40] Chirinos JA, Lichtstein DM, Garcia J, et al. The evolution of Lemierre syndrome: report of 2 cases and review of the literature. Medicine (Baltimore) 2002;81:458–65.

[41] Dool H, Soetekouw R, van Zanten M, et al. Lemierre's syndrome: three cases and a review. Eur Arch Otorhinolaryngol 2005;262:651–4.

[42] Sinave CP, Hardy GJ, Fardy PW. The Lemierre syndrome: suppurative thrombophlebitis of the internal jugular vein secondary to oropharyngeal infection. Medicine (Baltimore) 1989; 68:85–94.

[43] Brazier JS. Human infections with Fusobacterium necrophorum. Anaerobe 2006;12:165–72.

[44] Knouse MC, Madeira RG, Celani VJ. Pseudomonas aeruginosa causing a right carotid artery mycotic aneurysm after a dental extraction procedure. Mayo Clin Proc 2002;77: 1125–30.

[45] Sichel JY, Dano I, Hocwald E, et al. Nonsurgical management of parapharyngeal space infections: a prospective study. Laryngoscope 2002;112:906–10.

[46] McClay JE, Murray AD, Booth T. Intravenous antibiotic therapy for deep neck abscesses defined by computed tomography. Arch Otolaryngol Head Neck Surg 2003; 129:1207–12.

[47] Sakaguchi M, Sato S, Ishiyama T, et al. Characterization and management of deep neck infections. Int J Oral Maxillofac Surg 1997;26:131–4.

[48] Boscolo-Rizzo P, Marchiori C, Zanetti F, et al. Conservative management of deep neck abscesses in adults: the importance of CECT findings. Otolaryngol Head Neck Surg 2006;135: 894–9.

[49] Sichel JY, Attal P, Hocwald E, et al. Redefining parapharyngeal space infections. Ann Otol Rhinol Laryngol 2006;115:117–23.

[50] Butler KM, Baker CJ. Cervical lymphadenitis. In: Fegin RD, Cheery JD, editors. Textbook of pediatric infectious diseases. 3rd edition. Philadelphia: Elsevier W.B. Saunders; 1992. p. 220–30.

[51] Barratt GE, Koopmann CF Jr, Coulthard SW. Retropharyngeal abscess–a ten-year experience. Laryngoscope 1984;94:455–63.

[52] Grewal S, Hocking G, Wildsmith JA. Epidural abscesses. Br J Anaesth 2006;96:292–302.

[53] Gordon RJ, Lowy FD. Bacterial infections in drug users. N Engl J Med 2005;353: 1945–54.

[54] Darouiche RO. Spinal epidural abscess. N Engl J Med 2006;355:2012–20.

[55] Pina MA, Modrego PJ, Uroz JJ, et al. Brucellar spinal epidural abscess of cervical location: report of four cases. Eur Neurol 2001;45:249–53.

[56] Krishnan A, Patkar D, Patankar T, et al. Craniovertebral junction tuberculosis: a review of 29 cases. J Comput Assist Tomogr 2001;25:171–6.

[57] Reihsaus E, Waldbaur H, Seeling W. Spinal epidural abscess: a meta-analysis of 915 patients. Neurosurg Rev 2000;23:175–204 [discussion: 205].

[58] Curry WT Jr, Hoh BL, Amin-Hanjani S, et al. Spinal epidural abscess: clinical presentation, management, and outcome. Surg Neurol 2005;63:364–71 [discussion: 371].

[59] Davis DP, Wold RM, Patel RJ, et al. The clinical presentation and impact of diagnostic delays on emergency department patients with spinal epidural abscess. J Emerg Med 2004; 26:285–91.
[60] Bulut M, Balci V, Akkose S, et al. Fatal descending necrotising mediastinitis. Emerg Med J 2004;21:122–3.
[61] Takao M, Ido M, Hamaguchi K, et al. Descending necrotizing mediastinitis secondary to a retropharyngeal abscess. Eur Respir J 1994;7:1716–8.
[62] Muckley T, Schutz T, Kirschner M, et al. Psoas abscess: the spine as a primary source of infection. Spine 2003;28:E106–13.
[63] Chow AW. Life-threatening infections of the head, neck and upper respiratory tract. In: Hall JB, Schmidt GA, Wood LD, editors. Principles of critical care. 3rd edition. New York: McGraw-Hill; 2005. p. 881–96.
[64] Plaza Mayor G, Martinez-San Millan J, Martinez-Vidal A. Is conservative treatment of deep neck space infections appropriate? Head Neck 2001;23:126–33.
[65] Ungkanont K, Yellon RF, Weissman JL, et al. Head and neck space infections in infants and children. Otolaryngol Head Neck Surg 1995;112:375–82.
[66] Adelson RT, Murray AD. Minimally invasive transoral catheter-assisted drainage of a danger-space infection. Ear Nose Throat J 2005;84:785–6.
[67] Hanigan WC, Asner NG, Elwood PW. Magnetic resonance imaging and the nonoperative treatment of spinal epidural abscess. Surg Neurol 1990;34:408–13.

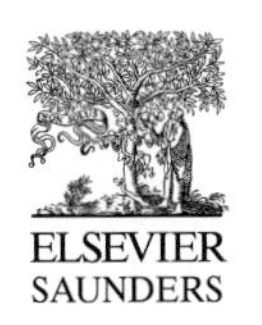

ELSEVIER
SAUNDERS

INFECTIOUS
DISEASE CLINICS
OF NORTH AMERICA

Infect Dis Clin N Am 21 (2007) 577–590

Vascular and Parameningeal Infections of the Head and Neck

Kevin B. Laupland, MD, MSc, FRCPC[a,b,c,d,*]

[a]*Department of Medicine, University of Calgary, Room 1W-415, #9, 3535 Research Road NW, Calgary, Alberta, Canada T2L 2K8*
[b]*Department of Critical Care Medicine, University of Calgary, Room 1W-415, #9, 3535 Research Road NW, Calgary, Alberta, Canada T2L 2K8*
[c]*Department of Pathology and Laboratory Medicine, University of Calgary, Room 1W-415, #9, 3535 Research Road NW, Calgary, Alberta, Canada T2L 2K8*
[d]*Department of Community Health Sciences, University of Calgary, Room 1W-415, #9, 3535 Research Road NW, Calgary, Alberta, Canada T2L 2K8*

Vascular and parameningeal infections of the head and neck are rare in populations with ready access to modern medical care, but, when they occur, they are associated with significant morbidity and mortality. Vascular infections of the head and neck include intracranial and extracranial septic venous thrombophlebitis and arterial mycotic aneurysms and erosions. Parameningeal infections include subdural empyema and epidural abscesses. These infections usually arise as complications of meningitis or odontogenic, paranasal sinus, or otogenic infections or may arise as a consequence of major trauma [1–8]. Their clinical presentations are varied and are related in part to the primary infection site and the adjacent anatomic structures involved. In many cases, more than one of these infections may coexist. Although there is a propensity for some of these infections to be associated with specific microbial agents [9,10], their microbiology largely reflects that of the primary source, as reviewed in detail elsewhere in this issue. This article focuses on a review of the clinical features, diagnosis, and management of these important infections.

Intracranial septic venous thrombosis

Septic intracranial thrombophlebitis is diagnosed when there is thrombosis of cerebral veins or dural venous sinuses in association with an infectious

* Department of Critical Care Medicine, University of Calgary, #9, 3535 Research Road NW, Room 1W-414, Calgary, Alberta, Canada T2L 2K8.
E-mail address: Kevin.laupland@calgaryhealthregion.ca

doi:10.1016/j.idc.2007.03.011

entity. Although population-based incidence rates are unknown, available data indicate that these infections are uncommon. Large observational cohort studies reported from Italy and Portugal [11,12] and one multinational study [13] have identified that only 10% to 15% of all intracranial venous thromboses are associated with infection. Aseptic intracranial thrombosis includes puerperal, marantic, and traumatic etiologies as well as congenital and acquired coagulation disorders including protein S, protein C, and antithrombin III deficiency [14]. Although intracranial aseptic thrombosis may, rarely, become secondarily infected through bloodstream infection, intracranial septic venous thrombosis usually arises from an adjacent infection [12,14–18]. Although intracranial septic thrombosis may involve any venous anatomy within the head, the vast majority involves the dural venous sinuses (either alone or concurrently with other veins), and therefore this article focuses on septic dural sinus thrombosis [19–24].

The dural sinuses may be grouped generally into the sagittal, lateral (including the transverse, sigmoid, and petrosal sinuses), and cavernous sinuses [25,26]. These dural sinuses receive blood from cerebral veins and drain primarily through the internal jugular veins. The dural sinuses also may receive blood from sphenoparietal sinuses through communicating veins in the bone, through other veins in the head such as the ophthalmic veins, and through emissary veins that connect with extracranial veins in the head and neck. The cerebral and emissary veins and dural sinuses are valveless, so infection and clot can propagate in either direction and therefore involve multiple venous structures concurrently [16].

Although superior sagittal sinus thrombosis is the most frequently observed intracranial venous thrombosis, it usually is associated with noninfectious causes [11,12,27]. When it does have an infectious cause, frontal sinusitis and meningitis are the most important underlying infections, and it generally is recognized to have a poor prognosis that, at least in part, may reflect the severity of the underlying infection [28]. In one series of pneumococcal meningitis in adults, the superior sagittal sinus was involved in three of four patients who had dural sinus thrombosis [17].

Septic lateral sinus thrombosis most commonly follows otitis media and its complications and therefore is more frequent in children and adolescents [6,7,25,29–34]. At least one half of cases are associated with chronic infections in which direct infection occurs through erosion through infected bone. Acute infection may result from spread through emissary veins without eroded bone [25]. Septic lateral sinus thrombosis frequently is associated with brain and epidural abscesses, subdural empyema, and meningitis, with one or more of these complications noted in approximately one quarter of cases in one series [32]. Increased intracranial pressure and associated symptoms may arise through sigmoid sinus obstruction [25]. In the absence of these complications, the clinical features of septic lateral sinus thrombosis often are nonspecific, are difficult to discern from the underlying middle ear process, and may not be severe. Persistent spiking fever despite appropriate antimicrobial therapy for an otogenic infection may be the only clinical feature alerting the clinician to investigate this diagnosis further.

Because of its complex neurovascular anatomic relationships, the most important intracranial septic thrombosis occurs within the cavernous sinus [16,28,35–44]. It arises most commonly as a complication of sphenoid and ethmoid and to a lesser degree frontal sinusitis, but it also may result from infections of face, orbits, middle ears, and oral cavity, especially the maxillary teeth [36,40]. The presentation typically is acute, with fever and marked toxicity, but on occasion may be subacute. The clinical findings largely arise as a result of venous obstruction and from impairment of cranial nerves that course through or within the walls of the cavernous sinus [28]. Venous obstruction may manifest as headache, proptosis, chemosis, and periorbital swelling. The oculomotor (III) nerve (with parasympathetics), trochlear (IV) nerve, and the ophthalmic and maxillary divisions of the trigeminal (V) nerve run along the lateral walls of the cavernous sinus, and the abducens (VI) nerve, along with sympathetic nerves associated with the internal carotid artery, course through its lumen. Septic thrombosis of the cavernous sinus therefore may result in external ophthalmoplegia, ptosis, and pupillary abnormalities. Because the optic (II) nerve runs outside of the cavernous sinus, visual loss is relatively uncommon, but impairment or even permanent blindness may result from retinal and optic nerve ischemia and by other mechanisms [37–39,45,46]. Although symptoms typically are unilateral initially, bilateral spread within 24 to 48 hours through anterior and posterior intercavernous sinuses is common and is highly suspicious for this diagnosis [35,36]. The internal carotid artery runs through the cavernous sinus and, rarely, may be compromised. Further symptoms may arise as a result of the direct spread to other dural sinuses and the internal jugular vein, and meningitis, subdural empyema, brain abscess, and pituitary necrosis may arise from extension into adjacent tissue [16,36,41,42].

The diagnosis of intracranial venous thrombosis is best established using MRI, but contrast-enhanced CT also performs very well (Fig. 1), may be more readily accessible in many centers, and may provide complementary information [47–49].

Although little empiric evidence exists for the management of septic intracranial thrombosis, it is widely accepted that the key management includes early intravenous antibiotics and surgical débridement of any underlying primary source of infection such as paranasal sinusitis, mastoiditis, or oral infection. Antibiotics should be chosen to cover the usual pathogens associated with the underlying source of infection, but it also is important that the agents selected and dosing achieve adequate central nervous system levels. Although treatment must be individualized, in most cases the combination of ceftriaxone and metronidazole is a reasonable empiric regimen with the addition of vancomycin if there is clinical concern for methicillin-resistant *Staphylococcus aureus* [38]. An antipseudomonal penicillin, cephalosporin, or carbapenem may need to be substituted for

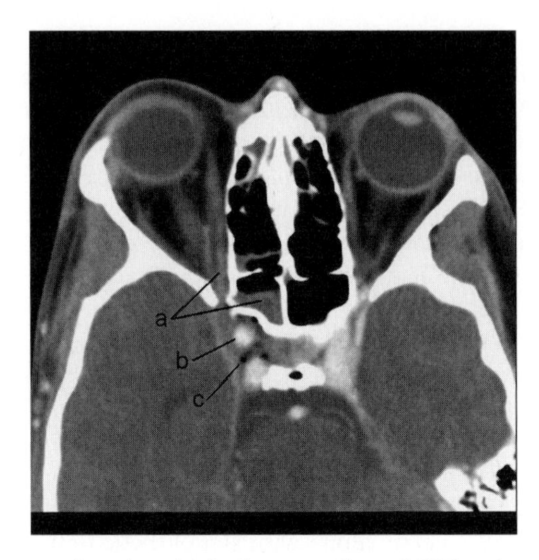

Fig. 1. Septic cavernous sinus thrombosis. Contrast-enhanced CT imaging of the orbits reveals acute right-sided ethmoid and sphenoid sinusitis with adjacent inflammatory stranding in the right orbital apex (*a*). The contrast-enhanced cavernous internal carotid artery is seen as a separate tubular structure within the cavernous sinus (*b*). The right cavernous sinus is thrombosed, with a low-density, nonenhancing appearance, several internal air blebs (*c*), and a lateral border that bowed laterally toward the middle cranial fossa. (*Courtesy of:* James N. Scott, MD, FRCPC, Calgary, Alberta, Canada.)

ceftriaxone if *Pseudomonas aeruginosa* is likely, as in chronic complicated otogenic infections [34]. Antifungal treatment directed at *Aspergillus* species and mucormycosis may be required in immune-compromised patients [50]. Often, prolonged antibiotic treatment ($\geq$ 4 weeks) is required, but duration of treatment depends on factors not limited to the rapidity of symptom resolution, resolution of thrombosis, eradication of primary infection, or immunocompetence. Supportive care in the ICU and treatment of complications such as seizures, pituitary-associated endocrinopathy, and increased intracranial pressure may be required [42,51]. Routine use of steroids is not indicated, but some authors have argued that they may provide some benefit in the setting of cranial neuropathies [35].

Given that the prevention of clot extension or resolution is of clear theoretical benefit, anticoagulants and thrombolytics have been proposed as therapies for dural venous sinus septic thrombosis, but their use is controversial [35,52,53]. A large observational cohort study and two small, randomized clinical trials have suggested the safety and potential efficacy of anticoagulants in septic and nonseptic cerebral sinus thrombosis [11,54,55]. Although a large, adequately powered study has not been conducted specifically within the septic intracranial thrombosis population, it is reasonable to give anticoagulation therapy to patients who do not have evident contraindications, especially if there is a large clot burden or progressive disease despite optimal antimicrobial therapy and surgical management of the underlying infection source [35]. No randomized trials have investigated the use of thrombolytics in intracranial venous thrombosis [56]. Canhao and colleagues [56] systematically reviewed the literature investigating the use of thrombolytics in septic and nonseptic cerebral venous or dural sinus thrombosis and identified 169 cases in the literature. They found that among these published reports the use of thrombolytics (mostly infused locally) was safe in most cases but that the efficacy could not be demonstrated clearly. At present, the use of thrombolytics in septic dural sinus septic thrombosis is experimental and should be considered only for severe refractory cases [14].

Septic internal jugular vein thrombosis

The syndrome of septic thrombophlebitis of the internal jugular vein in association with oropharyngeal infection, bacteremia, and metastatic foci is widely recognized as Lemierre syndrome [57–64]. Although a wide range of organisms may cause the syndrome, approximately 80% of cases are associated with *Fusobacterium necrophorum* bacteremia, and its presence is virtually pathognomonic of this syndrome [9,10,59,60]. Much more common in the preantibiotic era, Lemierre syndrome now is rare in developed countries. Hagelskjaer and colleagues [58] conducted a retrospective population-based study of all *F necrophorum* bacteremias during a 6-year period in Denmark and found 24 cases for an overall rate of 0.8 per million population. None of the patients died. Other large series confirm the rarity of the syndrome and suggest that it complicates 1% or less of contemporary deep neck infections [63,64]. In a review of 118 anecdotal case reports in the literature, Chirinos [59] found that this syndrome was most commonly reported in young adults, the initial site of infection was pharyngitis in 87%, and that lungs were the most frequently reported metastatic focus, followed by joints. The overall case-fatality rate in this series was 6%.

The presentation of septic internal jugular vein thrombosis typically is acute with toxicity, fever, neck pain, and tenderness and swelling along the course of the sternocleidomastoid muscle. Symptoms arising from an associated carotid artery thrombosis may, rarely, occur [65]. A thrombosed vein may be palpable, and trismus, dysarthria, dysphagia, and torticollis may be observed. Patients presenting with these symptoms should be investigated radiologically for this diagnosis, particularly if there is persistent fever or toxicity despite appropriate antibiotic therapy, severe pain, or evidence of a metastatic focus of infection or *F necrophorum* bacteremia. Doppler ultrasonography of the vessel is a highly sensitive and specific test to demonstrate clot and is readily available, inexpensive, and does not require contrast injection. Views above the level of the mandible are limited, however. Contrast-enhanced CT is sensitive for the presence of intravenous clot (Fig. 2) and has the added advantage of defining the underlying

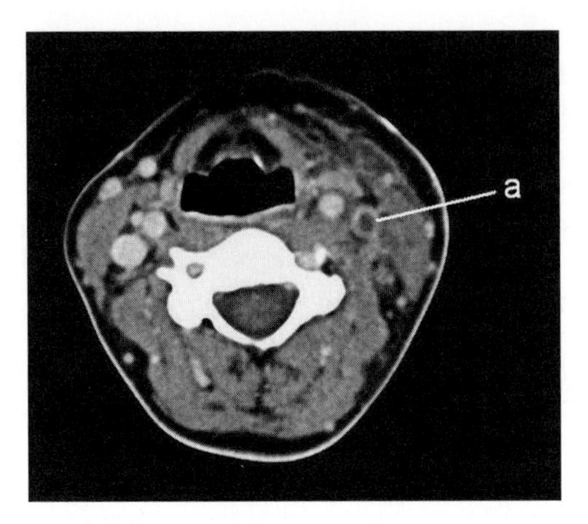

Fig. 2. Septic internal jugular vein thrombosis (Lemierre syndrome). Contrast-enhanced CT imaging reveals a thrombosed left internal jugular vein lacking normal luminal contrast (*a*) and diffuse soft tissue inflammatory stranding tracking along the left sternocleidomastoid muscle. (*Courtesy of* James N. Scott, MD, FRCPC, Calgary, Alberta, Canada.)

infection source that may assist with surgical planning. MRI probably has the highest sensitivity and specificity, but there is less published experience with this modality, and it may be less available than ultrasound or infused CT [61].

Treatment of the underlying infection with intravenous antibiotics and surgical drainage of collections or abscesses associated with the underlying oropharyngeal infection are the first principles of therapy. Empiric antimicrobial coverage for *F necrophorum*, as well as for other *Fusobacterium* species, *Bacteroides* species, *Peptostreptococcus* species, pigmented *Prevotella*, and alpha- and beta-hemolytic streptococci is required [10]. Metronidazole in combination with penicillin or a cephalosporin is appropriate empiric therapy pending cultures in most cases. Management of the underlying source of infection usually results in resolution of the thrombosis, although surgical ligation of the vein may be required in a small number of cases ($< 10\%$) refractory to medical management [59]. The use of anticoagulants and thrombolytics is controversial; there are no empiric data or expert consensus to guide their use, and a case-by-case decision is needed. Intravenous antimicrobial therapy for prolonged periods of 4 weeks and more often is required; duration depends on systemic clinical response, resolution of thrombus, and degree of local and metastatic complications.

Infection-associated arterial aneurysms and carotid erosion

Infections of the arteries of the head and neck are rare and may include aneurysms, pseudoaneurysms, and erosions [46,66–70]. Infection-associated arterial aneurysms involve dilatation of an arterial wall in association with an infection. Although collectively these aneurysms often are referred to as "mycotic aneurysms," strictly speaking, the term "mycotic aneurysm" should be reserved for a fungal origin, and the term "bacterial aneurysm" should be used to denote those caused by bacterial agents. Overall, most intracranial arterial aneurysms are have noninfectious causes; infection is the cause in approximately only 5% [68]. Most (80%) intracranial infection-associated aneurysms are secondary to embolization from endocarditis, although syphilis and extension from adjacent meningitis, cavernous sinus thrombosis, sinusitis, and skull osteomyelitis may occur [46,66,71]. Knouse and colleagues [72] summarized 74 cases of infection-associated carotid aneurysms reported in the literature and found that bacteremia with seeding was most common cause, followed by postoperative infection, endocarditis, and cervical adenopathy or neck abscess. Erosions into the internal carotid artery are rare, but when they occur they usually are extracranial and arise from infection of the lateral pharyngeal space [10]. Ludwig's angina, infection of the deep cervical lymph nodes, and Lemierre syndrome may result in carotid erosions [59,72,73]. Arterial infections and pseudoaneurysms also may be associated with patch angioplasty after carotid endarterectomy, and this risk has been noted particularly with the use of Dacron patches [70].

The clinical presentation of arterial infections of the head and neck depends on the anatomic location. Symptoms may arise from compression of adjacent vessels and nerves, and rupture, thrombosis, distal embolus, or stenosis of the affected vessel will manifest according to neurovascular territory. Carotid pseudoaneurysms usually present as an asymptomatic, pulsatile, neck mass, whereas erosions may present as fever in association with minor hemorrhages from nose, mouth, or ear [70,72]. The microbial origin of these infections reflects that of the underlying infectious primary source. In reported series, the most common organism was *S aureus* followed by Enterobacteriaceae and streptococci [72]. As with other intravascular infections, blood cultures typically are positive and may be persistently so despite appropriate antimicrobial therapy. The traditional criterion diagnostic test is angiography, although both MRI and contrast-enhanced CT are useful and have the advantage of defining nonvascular sources of infection and complications.

Different management approaches for arterial infections of the head and neck have not been studied systematically, and therefore management must be individualized. Intravenous antimicrobial therapy guided by the specific infecting organism and underlying primary infection is essential. Because arterial infection shares many features in common and occurs frequently with endocarditis, antimicrobial selection and duration is reflective of that disease [74]. Neurologic and/or vascular surgical evaluation is required for all patients who have arterial infections. Medical treatment with prolonged antimicrobial therapy, serial imaging, and clinical reassessment may be chosen for small infected arterial aneurysms in noncritical sites. Those that are rapidly enlarging or in locations where rupture or thrombosis would be life-threatening or associated with major morbidity require surgical intervention that may include clipping, ligation, or resection with arterial reconstruction. Although endovascular approaches have emerged as a major modality for management of noninfective aneurysms, their role remains to be defined in infective aneurysms [75].

Subdural empyema and epidural abscess

Subdural empyemas and epidural abscesses are defined by pus collections between the dura mater and arachnoid and the dura mater and the skull, respectively [76,77]. These infections usually arise as complications of sinusitis, otogenic infections, and meningitis but also may follow trauma or surgery [1,3–8,34,78–81]. They may be diagnosed concurrently with and frequently are associated with dural sinus thrombosis [82]. Within the head and neck, almost all are intracranial in location [83–86].

Although the population incidence of these infections has not been well defined, they are observed infrequently, and rates vary dramatically worldwide. For example, approximately one to three cases per year of subdural empyema and/or epidural abscess typically have been reported from large tertiary care centers in the United States, Australia, Turkey, and Taiwan [1–4,77,79,80,87], whereas five cases per year were observed in a study from the Sultanate of Oman [88], and 50 cases per year were reported in a large series from South Africa [83,84,86]. Although rates vary among specific populations studied, subdural empyema and/or epidural abscesses probably complicate 1% or less of severe acute otogenic infections and paranasal sinusitis. These rates, however, may be substantially higher in chronic under- or untreated disease [1–3,5–7,34,79,87–89]. Subdural empyema and/or epidural abscess complicate 1% or less of cases of bacterial meningitis in adults, but this rate may be 10-fold higher in infants [78,90].

Subdural empyemas usually have an acute and severe onset and may be rapidly progressive because the infection may spread diffusely within the subdural space. The largest clinical experience reported with intracranial subdural empyema to date has been by Nathoo and colleagues [83] from South Africa, where 699 cases were managed during a 15-year period. In this series the underlying cause was paranasal sinusitis in 67% of cases, meningitis in 10%, otogenic sources in 9%, trauma in 8%, and dental infections in 1%. Common clinical signs were fever, neck stiffness, headache, and focal seizures. The overall mortality was 12%. They observed a higher proportion of sinusitis as the underlying cause than did other small series from other countries [1,3,77,79,87]. Pott's puffy tumor (subperiosteal abscess and osteomyelitis, usually in association with frontal sinusitis) was noted in a striking one third of the cases in this South African series but has been observed much less frequently elsewhere [1,3,77,79,87].

In contrast to subdural empyemas, where infection often is acute and rapidly progressive, epidural abscesses are limited anatomically by the tight adherence of the dura to bone. Presentation, therefore, often is less severe and of a more insidious onset [1,77]. Nathoo and colleagues [84] published a report from South Africa describing 82 cases of cranial epidural abscesses. Males and children and young adults predominated, and paranasal sinusitis was the most frequent underlying cause in 65%, followed by mastoiditis in 20%, trauma in 6%, and dental infections in 1%. Fever, neck stiffness, and periorbital edema were the most frequently observed clinical signs; seizures and focal neurologic deficit were relatively uncommon. As in their series with subdural empyemas, an unusually high proportion (one half) had Pott's puffy tumors. In contrast, the overall case-fatality rate of 1% was much lower for epidural abscesses [83,84]. It is noteworthy that Nathoo and colleagues [86] also reported 13 cases of infratentorial subdural empyema and nine cases of epidural abscess in South Africa. These cases were characterized by chronic otogenic origin of infection, and most were complicated by hydrocephalus. Five (23%) of the patients, all with subdural empyema, died [86].

The diagnosis of subdural empyema and epidural abscess usually is based on findings on contrast CT and/or MRI when a fluid collection is evident in association with an infective source (Fig. 3). Although enhanced CT identifies most intracranial collections, MRI is superior for identifying small and infratentorial collections and has the advantage of better distinction between infective and noninfective origin [91,92]. If CT is chosen as the initial imaging modality to assess for subdural empyema and/or epidural abscess, it is essential that it be contrast enhanced [3,91]. An MRI must be performed when clinical suspicion is high even in the setting of a negative enhanced CT.

Patients who have a subdural empyema and/or epidural abscess require appropriate intravenous antimicrobial therapy and urgent neurosurgical and otorhinolaryngologic surgical assessment to manage the infected collections and to treat the underlying causative infections. Empiric antimicrobial therapy should be selected to cover the most likely pathogens associated with the underlying infection source, but agents also should be chosen and dosed to achieve adequate central nervous system penetration. The empiric antimicrobial agents recommended and causative organisms are similar to those described for septic dural venous sinus thrombosis, although several studies have noted a particular importance of the *Streptococcus milleri* group species in subdural empyemas and epidural abscesses [1,4,79,83,84,93]. Usually a 4-week or longer duration of therapy is required, but duration depends on the clinical response, the adequacy of the surgical evacuation of the infected collection and underlying source of infection, and whether other complicating factors such as osteomyelitis are present.

Because infection may spread rapidly and be associated with severe intracranial complications, subdural empyema is a surgical emergency that requires urgent evacuation. Delayed and/or inadequate drainage is

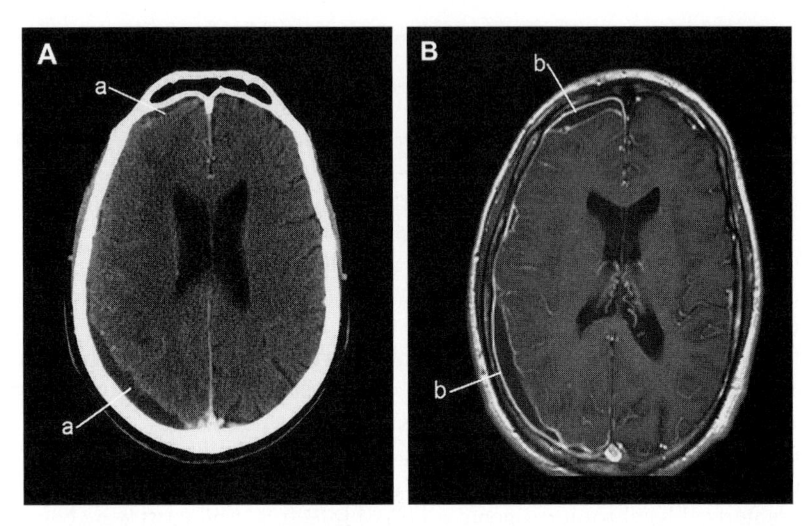

Fig. 3. Subdural empyema. (*A*) Contrast-enhanced CT image with right-sided crescentic hyperdense extracerebral fluid collection with faint rim enhancement (*a*). (*B*) Postgadolinium T1-weighted MR image with strong marginal enhancement (*b*) typical of subdural empyema. (*Courtesy of* James N. Scott, MD, FRCPC, Calgary, Alberta, Canada.)

associated with an adverse outcome. Surgical approaches may include craniectomy, craniotomy, and burr holes, with the main objectives being adequate drainage of the infected fluid and reduction of intracranial pressure [84,87]. Although epidural abscesses also require prompt surgical evaluation, some authors have reported that selected sinusitis-associated epidural abscesses in the absence of associated meningitis, intraparenchymal abscess, subdural empyema, raised intracranial pressure, or focal neurologic deficits in children may be managed successfully with sinus drainage procedures alone, without neurosurgical intervention [94]. When a more conservative neurosurgical approach is chosen, close clinical and radiologic assessment is required.

Acknowledgments

The author thanks James N. Scott, MD, FRCPC, Department of Diagnostic Imaging, Foothills Medical Centre, Calgary, Alberta, Canada for providing the figures and for expert review of the manuscript.

References

[1] Germiller JA, Monin DL, Sparano AM, et al. Intracranial complications of sinusitis in children and adolescents and their outcomes. Arch Otolaryngol Head Neck Surg 2006;132(9): 969–76.

[2] Glickstein JS, Chandra RK, Thompson JW. Intracranial complications of pediatric sinusitis. Otolaryngol Head Neck Surg 2006;134(5):733–6.

[3] Adame N, Hedlund G, Byington CL. Sinogenic intracranial empyema in children. Pediatrics 2005;116(3):e461–7.
[4] Leotta N, Chaseling R, Duncan G, et al. Intracranial suppuration. J Paediatr Child Health 2005;41(9–10):508–12.
[5] Seven H, Coskun BU, Calis AB, et al. Intracranial abscesses associated with chronic suppurative otitis media. Eur Arch Otorhinolaryngol 2005;262(10):847–51.
[6] Migirov L, Duvdevani S, Kronenberg J. Otogenic intracranial complications: a review of 28 cases. Acta Otolaryngol 2005;125(8):819–22.
[7] Luntz M, Brodsky A, Nusem S, et al. Acute mastoiditis—the antibiotic era: a multicenter study. Int J Pediatr Otorhinolaryngol 2001;57(1):1–9.
[8] Nathoo N, Nadvi SS, Van Dellen JR. Traumatic cranial empyemas: a review of 55 patients. Br J Neurosurg 2000;14(4):326–30.
[9] Hagelskjaer Kristensen L, Prag J. Human necrobacillosis, with emphasis on Lemierre's syndrome. Clin Infect Dis 2000;31(2):524–32.
[10] Brook I. Microbiology and management of deep facial infections and Lemierre syndrome. ORL J Otorhinolaryngol Relat Spec 2003;65(2):117–20.
[11] Ferro JM, Correia M, Pontes C, et al. Cerebral vein and dural sinus thrombosis in Portugal: 1980-1998. Cerebrovasc Dis 2001;11(3):177–82.
[12] Terazzi E, Mittino D, Ruda R, et al. Cerebral venous thrombosis: a retrospective multicentre study of 48 patients. Neurol Sci 2005;25(6):311–5.
[13] Ferro JM, Canhao P, Stam J, et al. Prognosis of cerebral vein and dural sinus thrombosis: results of the International Study on Cerebral Vein and Dural Sinus Thrombosis (ISCVT). Stroke 2004;35(3):664–70.
[14] Buonanno FS. Cerebral sinovenous thrombosis. Curr Treat Options Cardiovasc Med 2001; 3(5):417–27.
[15] McLean BN. Dural sinus thrombosis. Br J Hosp Med 1991;45(4):226–31.
[16] Southwick FS, Richardson EP Jr, Swartz MN. Septic thrombosis of the dural venous sinuses. Medicine (Baltimore) 1986;65(2):82–106.
[17] Kastenbauer S, Pfister HW. Pneumococcal meningitis in adults: spectrum of complications and prognostic factors in a series of 87 cases. Brain 2003;126(Pt 5):1015–25.
[18] Weisfelt M, van de Beek D, Spanjaard L, et al. Clinical features, complications, and outcome in adults with pneumococcal meningitis: a prospective case series. Lancet Neurol 2006;5(2): 123–9.
[19] DiNubile MJ, Boom WH, Southwick FS. Septic cortical thrombophlebitis. J Infect Dis 1990; 161(6):1216–20.
[20] Sagduyu A, Sirin H, Mulayim S, et al. Cerebral cortical and deep venous thrombosis without sinus thrombosis: clinical MRI correlates. Acta Neurol Scand 2006;114(4):254–60.
[21] Jacobs K, Moulin T, Bogousslavsky J, et al. The stroke syndrome of cortical vein thrombosis. Neurology 1996;47(2):376–82.
[22] Bousser MG. [Cerebral venous thrombosis. Report of 76 cases]. J Mal Vasc 1991;16(3): 249–54 [discussion: 254–5] [in French].
[23] Schmitt NJ, Beatty RL, Kennerdell JS. Superior ophthalmic vein thrombosis in a patient with dacryocystitis-induced orbital cellulitis. Ophthal Plast Reconstr Surg 2005;21(5):387–9.
[24] Sanchez TG, Cahali MB, Murakami MS, et al. Septic thrombosis of orbital vessels due to cutaneous nasal infection. Am J Rhinol 1997;11(6):429–33.
[25] Tveteras K, Kristensen S, Dommerby H. Septic cavernous and lateral sinus thrombosis: modern diagnostic and therapeutic principles. J Laryngol Otol 1988;102(10):877–82.
[26] Scott JN, Farb RI. Imaging and anatomy of the normal intracranial venous system. Neuroimaging Clin N Am 2003;13(1):1–12.
[27] Virapongse C, Cazenave C, Quisling R, et al. The empty delta sign: frequency and significance in 76 cases of dural sinus thrombosis. Radiology 1987;162(3):779–85.
[28] DiNubile MJ. Septic thrombosis of the cavernous sinuses. Arch Neurol 1988;45(5): 567–72.

[29] Zapanta PE, Chi DH, Faust RA. A unique case of Bezold's abscess associated with multiple dural sinus thromboses. Laryngoscope 2001;111(11 Pt 1):1944–8.
[30] Sneed WF. Lateral sinus thrombosis. Am J Otol 1983;4(3):258–62.
[31] Syms MJ, Tsai PD, Holtel MR. Management of lateral sinus thrombosis. Laryngoscope 1999;109(10):1616–20.
[32] Singh B. The management of lateral sinus thrombosis. J Laryngol Otol 1993;107(9):803–8.
[33] Migirov L. Computed tomographic versus surgical findings in complicated acute otomastoiditis. Ann Otol Rhinol Laryngol 2003;112(8):675–7.
[34] De Oliveira Penido N, Borin A, Iha LC, et al. Intracranial complications of otitis media: 15 years of experience in 33 patients. Otolaryngol Head Neck Surg 2005;132(1):37–42.
[35] Bhatia K, Jones NS. Septic cavernous sinus thrombosis secondary to sinusitis: are anticoagulants indicated? A review of the literature. J Laryngol Otol 2002;116(9):667–76.
[36] Ebright JR, Pace MT, Niazi AF. Septic thrombosis of the cavernous sinuses. Arch Intern Med 2001;161(22):2671–6.
[37] Chen JS, Mukherjee P, Dillon WP, et al. Restricted diffusion in bilateral optic nerves and retinas as an indicator of venous ischemia caused by cavernous sinus thrombophlebitis. AJNR Am J Neuroradiol 2006;27(9):1815–6.
[38] Rutar T, Zwick OM, Cockerham KP, et al. Bilateral blindness from orbital cellulitis caused by community-acquired methicillin-resistant Staphylococcus aureus. Am J Ophthalmol 2005;140(4):740–2.
[39] Friberg TR, Sogg RL. Ischemic optic neuropathy in cavernous sinus thrombosis. Arch Ophthalmol 1978;96(3):453–6.
[40] Pavlovich P, Looi A, Rootman J. Septic thrombosis of the cavernous sinus: two different mechanisms. Orbit 2006;25(1):39–43.
[41] Petty RK, Wardlaw J, Kennedy PG, et al. Panhypopituitarism after cavernous sinus thrombosis. J Neurol Neurosurg Psychiatry 1994;57(8):1010–1.
[42] Feinfeld DA, Al-Achkar G, Lipner HI, et al. Syndrome of inappropriate secretion of antidiuretic hormone: association with cavernous sinus thrombosis. JAMA 1978;240(9):856–7.
[43] Hoogendijk CF, Pretorius E. Cavernous sinus anatomy as a basis for interpretation of the clinical picture and radiological investigations in a case of Entomophthorales infection. Clin Anat 2006;19(6):535–9.
[44] Cannon ML, Antonio BL, McCloskey JJ, et al. Cavernous sinus thrombosis complicating sinusitis. Pediatr Crit Care Med 2004;5(1):86–8.
[45] Arat YO, Shetlar DJ, Rose JE. Blindness from septic thrombophlebitis of the orbit and cavernous sinus caused by Fusobacterium nucleatum. Arch Ophthalmol 2004;122(4):652–4.
[46] Quisling SV, Mawn LA, Larson TC 3rd. Blindness associated with enlarging mycotic aneurysm after cavernous sinus thrombosis. Ophthalmology 2003;110(10):2036–9.
[47] Ozsvath RR, Casey SO, Lustrin ES, et al. Cerebral venography: comparison of CT and MR projection venography. AJR Am J Roentgenol 1997;169(6):1699–707.
[48] Berge J, Louail C, Caille JM. Cavernous sinus thrombosis diagnostic approach. J Neuroradiol 1994;21(2):101–17.
[49] Ellie E, Houang B, Louail C, et al. CT and high-field MRI in septic thrombosis of the cavernous sinuses. Neuroradiology 1992;34(1):22–4.
[50] Gupta V, Keller A, Halliday W, et al. Cavernous sinus thrombosis presenting with diplopia in an allogeneic bone marrow transplant recipient. Am J Hematol 2004;77(1):77–81.
[51] Ferro JM, Correia M, Rosas MJ, et al. Seizures in cerebral vein and dural sinus thrombosis. Cerebrovasc Dis 2003;15(1–2):78–83.
[52] Levine SR, Twyman RE, Gilman S. The role of anticoagulation in cavernous sinus thrombosis. Neurology 1988;38(4):517–22.
[53] Harvey JE. Letter: streptokinase therapy and cavernous sinus thrombosis. Br Med J 1974; 4(5935):46.
[54] de Bruijn SF, Stam J. Randomized, placebo-controlled trial of anticoagulant treatment with low-molecular-weight heparin for cerebral sinus thrombosis. Stroke 1999;30(3):484–8.

[55] Einhaupl KM, Villringer A, Meister W, et al. Heparin treatment in sinus venous thrombosis. Lancet 1991;338(8767):597–600.
[56] Canhao P, Falcao F, Ferro JM. Thrombolytics for cerebral sinus thrombosis: a systematic review. Cerebrovasc Dis 2003;15(3):159–66.
[57] Lemierre A. On certain septicaemias due to anaerobic organisms. Lancet 1936;1:701–3.
[58] Hagelskjaer LH, Prag J, Malczynski J, et al. Incidence and clinical epidemiology of necrobacillosis, including Lemierre's syndrome, in Denmark 1990-1995. Eur J Clin Microbiol Infect Dis 1998;17(8):561–5.
[59] Chirinos JA, Lichtstein DM, Garcia J, et al. The evolution of Lemierre syndrome: report of 2 cases and review of the literature. Medicine (Baltimore) 2002;81(6):458–65.
[60] Wilson P, Tierney L. Lemierre syndrome caused by Streptococcus pyogenes. Clin Infect Dis 2005;41(8):1208–9.
[61] Hong P, MacCormick J, Lamothe A, et al. Lemierre syndrome: presentation of three cases. J Otolaryngol 2005;34(5):352–8.
[62] Cook RJ, Ashton RW, Aughenbaugh GL, et al. Septic pulmonary embolism: presenting features and clinical course of 14 patients. Chest 2005;128(1):162–6.
[63] Ramirez S, Hild TG, Rudolph CN, et al. Increased diagnosis of Lemierre syndrome and other Fusobacterium necrophorum infections at a Children's Hospital. Pediatrics 2003; 112(5):e380–5.
[64] Huang TT, Liu TC, Chen PR, et al. Deep neck infection: analysis of 185 cases. Head Neck 2004;26(10):854–60.
[65] Maalikjy Akkawi N, Borroni B, Magoni M, et al. Lemierre's syndrome complicated by carotid thrombosis. Neurol Sci 2001;22(5):403–4.
[66] Cloud GC, Rich PM, Markus HS. Serial MRI of a mycotic aneurysm of the cavernous carotid artery. Neuroradiology 2003;45(8):546–9.
[67] Takahashi K, Wakabayashi K, Watanabe Y, et al. [A case of cavernous sinus syndrome following a mycotic aneurysm of extracranial carotid artery]. Rinsho Shinkeigaku 2001;41(9): 606–11 [in Japanaese].
[68] Rout D, Sharma A, Mohan PK, et al. Bacterial aneurysms of the intracavernous carotid artery. J Neurosurg 1984;60(6):1236–42.
[69] Lansky LL, Maxwell JA. Mycotic aneurysm of the internal carotid artery in an unusual intra-cranial location. Dev Med Child Neurol 1975;17(1):79–83.
[70] Borazjani BH, Wilson SE, Fujitani RM, et al. Postoperative complications of carotid patching: pseudoaneurysm and infection. Ann Vasc Surg 2003;17(2):156–61.
[71] Bullock R, van Dellen JR, van den Heever CM. Intracranial mycotic aneurysms. A review of 9 cases. S Afr Med J 1981;60(25):970–3.
[72] Knouse MC, Madeira RG, Celani VJ. Pseudomonas aeruginosa causing a right carotid artery mycotic aneurysm after a dental extraction procedure. Mayo Clin Proc 2002;77(10): 1125–30.
[73] Blomquist IK, Bayer AS. Life-threatening deep fascial space infections of the head and neck. Infect Dis Clin North Am 1988;2(1):237–64.
[74] Baddour LM, Wilson WR, Bayer AS, et al. Infective endocarditis: diagnosis, antimicrobial therapy, and management of complications: a statement for healthcare professionals from the Committee on Rheumatic Fever, Endocarditis, and Kawasaki Disease, Council on Cardiovascular Disease in the Young, and the Councils on Clinical Cardiology, Stroke, and Cardiovascular Surgery and Anesthesia, American Heart Association: endorsed by the Infectious Diseases Society of America. Circulation 2005;111(23): e394–434.
[75] Johnston SC, Higashida RT, Barrow DL, et al. Recommendations for the endovascular treatment of intracranial aneurysms: a statement for healthcare professionals from the Committee on Cerebrovascular Imaging of the American Heart Association Council on Cardiovascular Radiology. Stroke 2002;33(10):2536–44.
[76] Greenlee JE. Subdural empyema. Curr Treat Options Neurol 2003;5(1):13–22.

[77] Tsai YD, Chang WN, Shen CC, et al. Intracranial suppuration: a clinical comparison of subdural empyemas and epidural abscesses. Surg Neurol 2003;59(3):191–6 [discussion: 196].
[78] van de Beek D, de Gans J, Tunkel AR, et al. Community-acquired bacterial meningitis in adults. N Engl J Med 2006;354(1):44–53.
[79] Oxford LE, McClay J. Complications of acute sinusitis in children. Otolaryngol Head Neck Surg 2005;133(1):32–7.
[80] Dill SR, Cobbs CG, McDonald CK. Subdural empyema: analysis of 32 cases and review. Clin Infect Dis 1995;20(2):372–86.
[81] Laupland KB, Bosch JD. Acute group A streptococcal mastoiditis complicated by pneumocephaly in a previously healthy adult. Scand J Infect Dis 2006;38(8):719–21.
[82] Kamouchi M, Wakugawa Y, Okada Y, et al. Venous infarction secondary to septic cavernous sinus thrombosis. Intern Med 2006;45(1):25–7.
[83] Nathoo N, Nadvi SS, van Dellen JR, et al. Intracranial subdural empyemas in the era of computed tomography: a review of 699 cases. Neurosurgery 1999;44(3):529–35 [discussion: 535–6].
[84] Nathoo N, Nadvi SS, van Dellen JR. Cranial extradural empyema in the era of computed tomography: a review of 82 cases. Neurosurgery 1999;44(4):748–53 [discussion: 753–4].
[85] Chen MH, Huang JS. Cervical subdural empyema following acupuncture. J Clin Neurosci 2004;11(8):909–11.
[86] Nathoo N, Nadvi SS, van Dellen JR. Infratentorial empyema: analysis of 22 cases. Neurosurgery 1997;41(6):1263–8 [discussion: 1268–9].
[87] Yilmaz N, Kiymaz N, Yilmaz C, et al. Surgical treatment outcome of subdural empyema: a clinical study. Pediatr Neurosurg 2006;42(5):293–8.
[88] Tewari MK, Sharma RR, Shiv VK, et al. Spectrum of intracranial subdural empyemas in a series of 45 patients: current surgical options and outcome. Neurol India 2004;52(3):346–9.
[89] Quraishi H, Zevallos JP. Subdural empyema as a complication of sinusitis in the pediatric population. Int J Pediatr Otorhinolaryngol 2006;70(9):1581–6.
[90] van de Beek D, de Gans J, Spanjaard L, et al. Clinical features and prognostic factors in adults with bacterial meningitis. N Engl J Med 2004;351(18):1849–59.
[91] Kastrup O, Wanke I, Maschke M. Neuroimaging of infections. NeuroRx 2005;2(2):324–32.
[92] Tsuchiya K, Osawa A, Katase S, et al. Diffusion-weighted MRI of subdural and epidural empyemas. Neuroradiology 2003;45(4):220–3.
[93] Laupland KB, Ross T, Church DL, et al. Population-based surveillance of invasive pyogenic streptococcal infection in a large Canadian region. Clin Microbiol Infect 2006;12(3):224–30.
[94] Heran NS, Steinbok P, Cochrane DD. Conservative neurosurgical management of intracranial epidural abscesses in children. Neurosurgery 2003;53(4):893–7 [discussion 897–8].

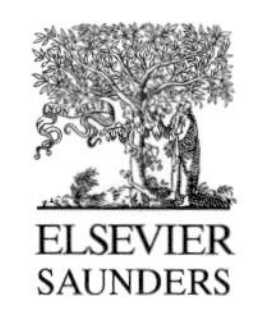

ELSEVIER
SAUNDERS

INFECTIOUS
DISEASE CLINICS
OF NORTH AMERICA

Infect Dis Clin N Am 21 (2007) 591–599

Index

Note: Page numbers of article titles are in **boldface** type.

doi:10.1016/S0891-5520(07)00050-5

D

E

W